Concise **Medical Immunology**

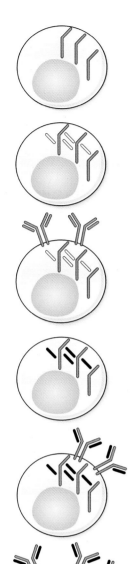

Concise
Medical Immunology

Thao T. Doan, MD
Medical Director
Abbott Laboratories
Waukegan, Illinois

Roger Melvold, PhD
Professor and Chair, Department of Microbiology and Immunology
University of North Dakota School of Medicine and Health Sciences
Grand Forks, North Dakota

Carl Waltenbaugh, PhD
Professor, Department of Microbiology-Immunology
Feinberg School of Medicine, Northwestern University
Chicago, Illinois

LIPPINCOTT WILLIAMS & WILKINS
A **Wolters Kluwer** Company
Philadelphia • Baltimore • New York • London
Buenos Aires • Hong Kong • Sydney • Tokyo

Editor: Betty Sun
Developmental Editor: Kathleen H. Scogna
Marketing Manager: Joe Schott
Production Editor: Kevin Johnson
Designer: Holly McLaughlin
Compositor: Maryland Composition
Printer: Quebecor Versailles

Printed in the United States of America

First Edition, 2005

Library of Congress Cataloging-in-Publication Data

Doan, Thao.
  Concise medical immunology / Thao Doan, Roger Melvold, Carl Waltenbaugh.—1st ed.
    p. ; cm.
  Includes bibliographical references and index.
  ISBN 0-7817-5741-X
 1. Clinical immunology.
  [DNLM: 1. Immune System. 2. Immunity. 3. Immunologic Factors. 4. Immunotherapy.]
I. Melvold, Roger. II. Waltenbaugh, Carl. III. Title.
  RC582.D63 2005
  616.07′9—dc22

                                                              2004027771

The publishers have made every effort to trace the copyright holders for borrowed material. If they have inadvertently overlooked any, they will be pleased to make the necessary arrangements at the first opportunity.

To purchase additional copies of this book, call our customer service department at (800) 638-3030 or fax orders to (301) 824-7390. International customers should call (301) 714-2324.

Visit Lippincott Williams & Wilkins on the Internet: http://www.LWW.com. Lippincott Williams & Wilkins customer service representatives are available from 8:30 am to 6:00 pm, EST.

 01 02 03 04 05
1 2 3 4 5 6 7 8 9 10

Dedicated to our medical students who were instrumental in making us simplify immunological concepts and to the late Dr. Roy Patterson who was the creative spark for this book.

Preface

Concise Medical Immunology is aimed primarily at readers in areas of human health, and at medical students in particular. It focuses on human immunology, with only minimal reference to non-human organisms where necessary to illustrate a particular point or process. In this text, the authors have attempted to distill the information necessary for understanding the basic role of the immune system in human health and disease during the early years of medical training. The text is not designed to be comprehensive and provide the molecular, evolutionary, and genetic detail that several excellent texts already provide. Rather it attempts to introduce the subject in a more general and perhaps less intimidating way. This approach will lay the groundwork for a more focused and detailed study of immunology during subsequent training.

This approach should also make *Concise Medical Immunology* an appropriate selection for those learning human immunology in other health science contexts–including nursing, clinical laboratory science, pre-medical undergraduates, or practitioners wishing to refresh their knowledge.

HOW THE TEXT IS ORGANIZED

The text follows a logical sequence. We begin with a discussion of some of the most immediate and basic immunological responses—those of the so-called "innate" immune system—in which cells and molecules of the innate immune system respond to molecules widely expressed on or by invasive organisms. We then transition from innate to "adaptive" immune responses or those that require recognition by highly specialized lymphocyte receptors that recognize molecules expressed on or by a very limited number of invasive organisms. Lymphocytes view microbes and other potential threats in very narrow terms and permit the development of immunological memory—the ability to remember previously encountered threats and respond more

rapidly and vigorously against them in subsequent encounters. In these defensive actions, the adaptive system often recruits elements of the innate system for assistance.

We begin by describing the function of the individual immune system components, then how these components interact to form a system that protects the body. Immune responses can be viewed as part of a long and continuing form of warfare between the body and the world of infectious agents—an ever spiraling arms race in which each side has developed new weapons and counter-measures against the other. In the development of a body system capable of attack, the risk of failure or misuse exists, and we include consideration of the consequences that occur when the immune system is incomplete or too vigorous or becomes inappropriately directed against the body it is meant to protect.

Unique features

A number of unique features distinguish this book:

- Clinical Application boxes highlight the clinical aspects of immunology and help readers make the connection between basic science and real-life clinical application.
- Patient Vignettes introduce a patient with a set of signs and symptoms and then pose a question to the reader regarding diagnosis, treatment, or etiology. Patients are distinguished as male, female, or child by special icons. "Answers" to the questions posed are also included in the vignettes.
- Side bars present interesting facts and current research findings about immunology and help keep the reading experience lively and informative.
- Review questions, included in every chapter, allow readers to test themselves on the information presented. Answers with explanations are included in Appendix D.
- A glossary of immunologic terms provides a

resource for the health science student. The glossary is extensive, listing much of the terminology that is used in immunology and its related clinical fields.

We have enjoyed writing this text and we hope that our interest and excitement in the subject matter is conveyed to the reader. We hope that readers will find the book sufficient in detail and coverage without becoming so overwhelming that the view of the "immunological forest" is obscured by all of the "immunological trees," and that the text will prepare the reader to go on to greater depth in the area should their future interests and training lead them to do so.

ACKNOWLEDGMENTS

We would like to thank Kathleen Scogna, Senior Developmental Editor, for her efficient guidance in this project. In addition, we thank Betty Sun, Executive Editor, for her encouragement. Thanks also to Kevin Johnson, Production Editor, Matt Chansky, the Illustrator Coordinator, Heidi Pongratz, Project Manager, and the staff at Lippincott Williams & Wilkins for their expertise and assistance. Finally, we thank Dr. Robert F. O'Dea, Dr. Roger H. Kobayashi, and Jan Lips for their advice on some sections, particularly the Patient Vignettes.

Abbreviations List

A

Ab	Antibody
ABO	Major blood group system in humans
ADA	Adenosine deaminase
ADCC	Antibody-dependent cell-mediated cytotoxicity
Ag	Antigen
AIDS	Acquired immune deficiency syndrome
ALL	Acute lymphoblastic leukemia
AML	Acute myelocytic leukemia
ANA	Anti-nuclear antibody
AP-1	Activation protein-1
APC	Antigen-presenting cell

B

B	A component of the alternative complement pathway (see Bf)
B cell	Bone-marrow derived lymphocyte
B-1 cell	Self-renewing B cell population
B-2 cell	Conventional B cell
BA	*Brucella abortus*
β_2m	Beta 2 microglobulin
BALT	Bronchial-associated lymphoid tissue
BCG	Bacille Calmette-Guerin
BCGF	B cell growth factor, *also called* IL-4
BCR	Antigen-specific B cell receptor
Bf	Factor B of the alternative complement pathway
BM	Bone marrow
BSE	Bovine spongiform encephalitis
btk	B-cell tyrosine kinase gene

C

C	Complement
C region	Constant region of a molecule or gene
C2, C3, C4, *etc*	Components of classical or lectin-binding pathways of complement
C3R	Receptor for the third component of complement
CAM	Cell adhesion molecule
CD	Cluster of differentiation *also* Contact dermatitis
CDR	Complementarity-determining (hyper-variable) region
CEA	Carcinoembryonic antigen

CF	Complement fixation *or* cystic fibrosis
CFM	Chemotactic factor for macrophages
CFU	Colony-forming unit
CGD	Chronic granulomatous disease
C_H	Heavy chain constant region(s) of immunoglobulin
CJD	Creutzfeld-Jacob disease
C_L	Constant region of immunoglobulin light chain
CLIP	Class II-associated invariant chain peptide
CLL	Chronic lymphoblastic leukemia
CMI	Cell-mediated immunity
CML	Cell-mediated lysis *also* Chronic myelocytic leukemia
Con A	Concanavalin A, a mitogen
COOH	Carboxyl terminus of an amino acid or protein
CS	Contact sensitivity *also* Contact dermatitis
CR	Complement receptor
CRP	C-reactive protein
CSF	Colony-stimulating factor
CTL	Cytotoxic T lymphocyte *also called* Tc

D

D	Component of the alternative complement pathway
DAF	Decay accelerating factor
DH	Delayed (-type) hypersensitivity, *see also* DTH
DIC	Disseminated intravascular coagulation
DMARD	Disease-modifying antirheumatic drug
DN	Double negative cell
DNA	Deoxyribonucleic acid
DP	A human MHC class II region *also* double positive cell
DPT	Diptheria-tetanus-pertussis vaccine
DR	A human MHC class II region
DTH	Delayed (-type) hypersensitivity
DQ	A human MHC class II region

E

E	Effector cell in MLR or CTL assay, *also* Symbol for erythrocyte
EBV	Epstein-Barr virus
ECF-A	Eosinophil chemotactic factor of anaphylaxis

ECP	Eosinophil cationic protein
EDN	Eosinophil-derived neurotoxin
EIA	Enzyme immunosorbent assay *also called* ELISA
ELISA	Enzyme-linked immunosorbent assay *also called* EIA
EPO	Eosinophil peroxidase

F

Fab	Univalent antigen-binding fragment of immunoglobulin
F(ab')$_2$	Divalent antigen-binding fragment of immunoglobulin
FACS	Fluorescence-activated cell sorter, a flow cytometer
Fas	Fas protein
FasL	Fas ligand
Fc	Constant or crystallizable fragment of immunoglobulin
FcR	Receptor for Fc region of immunoglobulin
Fd	Heavy chain portion of Fab fragment of immunoglobulin
FDA	Food and Drug Administration
FDC	Follicular dendritic cell
FIA	Fluorescence immunoassay
FITC	Fluorescein isothiocyanate, a green fluorescent dye
FR	Framework region of antibody molecule

G

GALT	Gut-associated lymphoid tissue
GAS	Group A streptococci
GEF	Guanine-nucleotide exchange factor
GM-CSF	Granulocyte-monocyte colony stimulating factor
GVH	Graft *versus* host
GVHD	Graft-versus-host disease

H

H2 *or* H-2	Major histocompatibility complex of the mouse
H	Component of the alternative complement pathway
HA	Hemagglutinin
HAT	Hypoxanthine aminopterin thymidine selective culture medium
H chain	Heavy chain of antibody molecule
HCV	Hepatitis C virus
HDN	Hemolytic disease of the newborn

HEV	High endothelial venule
HGPT	Hypoxanthine-guanine phosphoribosil transferase
HIV	Human immunodeficiency virus
HLA	Human leukocyte antigen, human MHC
HRF	Homologous restriction factor
HSP	Heat shock protein
HTLV	Human T cell leukemia virus
HVG	Host *versus* graft

I

I	Component of the alternative complement pathway
ICAM	Intercellular adhesion molecule
iC3b	Incomplete C3b
Id	Idiotype
IDDM	Insulin-dependent diabetes mellitus
IEL	Intestinal epithelial lymphocyte
IEP	Immunoelectrophoresis
IFN	Interferon, often followed by α, β or γ
Ig	Immunoglobulin
Ii	Invariant chain associated with MHC class II
IκB	Inhibitor of NF-κB
IL	Interleukin
IP$_3$	Inositol triphosphate
ITAM	Immunoreceptor tyrosine activation motif
ITIM	Immunoreceptor tyrosine inhibition motif
IVIG	Intravenous immunoglobulin

J

J chain	Joining chain of some antibody molecules
J region	Joining region of Ig and TCR genes

K

kappa (κ)	Kappa (κ) light chain of immunoglobulin
KAR	Killer activation receptor
kDa	kiloDalton
KIR	Killer inhibition receptor

L

LAD	Leukocyte adhesion deficiency syndrome
LAK	Lymphokine-activated killer cell
Lambda (λ)	Lambda (λ) light chain of immunoglobulin
L chain	Light chain of antibody molecule *also* κ *or* λ
LAD	Lymphocyte activating determinant
LAF	Lymphocyte activation factor

LAK	Lymphokine-activated killer cell
LAT	Linker of activation for T cells
LCMV	Lymphocytic choriomeningitis virus
LD	Lymphocyte defined determinant
LFA	Leukocyte functional antigen
LGL	Large granular lymphocyte
LMP	Low molecular weight proteins
LN	Lymph node
LPS	Lipopolysaccharide (endotoxin)

M

M cells	Microfold cells
mAb	Monoclonal antibody
MAC	Membrane attack complex of complement
MAF	Macrophage-activating factor
MAGE	Melanoma-associated antigen (tumor antigen)
MALT	Mucosal-associated lymphoid tissue
MAP	Mitogen-activate protein
MBL	Mannan-binding lectin *also* mannose-binding lectin
MBP	Major basic protein of eosinophils *or* myelin basic protein
MCF	Macrophage chemotactic factor
MCP	Macrophage chemotactic protein *or* membrane cofactor protein
MHC	Major histocompatibility complex
MIP	Macrophage inhibitory protein
MLC	Mixed lymphocyte culture
Mls	Minor lymphocyte-stimulating locus

N

NADH	Nicotinamide adenine dinucleotide phosphate
NBT	Nitroblue tetrazolium
NF-κB	Nuclear factor kappa B
NK	Natural killer (cell)
NKT	T cell with NK properties
NSAID	Nonsteroidal anti-inflammatory drug

P

P	Properdin of the alternative complement pathway
PAF	Platelet-activating factor
PALS	Periarteriolar lymphoid sheath
PAMP	Pathogen-associated molecular patterns
PBL	Peripheral blood leukocyte (or lymphocyte)
pCTL	Pre-cytotoxic T lymphocyte
PE	Phycoerythrin, a red fluorescent dye

PEG	Polyethylene glycol
PHA	Phytohemagglutinin, a mitogen
PIP$_2$	Phosphatidylinositol 4,5-biphosphate
P-K	Prausnitz-Kustner reaction
PKC	Protein kinase C
PLC-γ	Phospholipase C-gamma
PMA	Phorbol myristate acetate
pMHC	Peptide bound by major histocompatibility complex molecule
PMN	Polymorphonuclear leukocyte or neutrophil
PMT	Photomultiplier tube
PNP	Purine nucloside phosphorylase
PRR	Pattern recognition receptor
PWM	Pokeweed mitogen

R

RA	Rheumatoid arthritis
RAG	Recombination-activating gene
Ras	Rat sarcoma
RAST	Radioallergosorbent test, IgE-specific ELISA
RBC	Red blood cell
RES	Reticuloendothelial system
RF	Rheumatoid factor
Rh	Rhesus, a human blood group antigen system
RIA	Radioimmunoassay
RID	Radial immunodiffusion, *also called* Mancini technique
RNA	Ribonucleic acid
ROI	Reactive-oxygen intermediates

S

S	Stimulator cell in the MLR or CTL assay
SAP	Stress-activate protein
SC	Secretory component of IgA
SCID	Severe combined immune deficiency
SD	Serologically defined determinant
SLE	Systemic lupus erythematosis
Src	Sarcoma kinase(s)
SRS	Slow reacting substance

T

T cell	Thymus-derived lymphocyte
TAA	Tumor associated antigen(s)
TAP-1, TAP-2	Transporter associated with antigen-presentation
TB	Tuberculosis
Tc	Cytotoxic T cell *also called* CTL

TCGF	T lymphocyte growth factor, *also called* IL-2
TCR	Antigen-specific T cell receptor
TGF	Tumor growth factor
TdT	Terminal deoxynucleotidyl transferase
Th	Helper T cell
TIL	Tumor infiltrating lymphocytes
TK	Thymidine kinase *or* tyrosine kinase
TLR	Toll-like receptor
TNF	Tumor necrosis factor
Treg	Regulatory T cell
Ts	Suppressor T cell
TSA	Tumor-specific antigen(s)
TSTA	Tumor-specific transplantation antigen(s)

U

UNOS	United network for organ sharing

V

V$_H$	Variable region of immunoglobulin heavy chain
V$_L$	Variable region of immunoglobulin light chain
VLA	Very late antigen
V region	Variable region of a molecule or gene

W

WBC	White blood cell, leukocyte

X

X-SCID	X-linked severe combined immune deficiency
XLA	X-linked agammaglobulinemia

Z

ZAP-70	70-kDa cytoplasmic tyrosine kinase

Contents

Introduction to the Immune System: Antigens and the Concept of Self versus Nonself

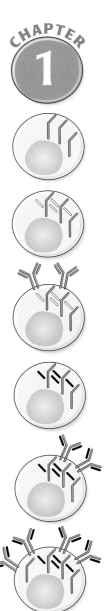

Chapter Outline

Introduction *Who am I? Who are you?* These simple questions are critical for survival. The body must be able to distinguish between self (or that which is identical to self) and nonself (or foreign). And, in identifying nonself, there is also an urgent need to be able to distinguish that which is threatening from that which is not threatening. Organisms must interact with the environment, recognizing and responding to external and internal threats to increase the opportunity for survival and reproduction (Fig. 1-1). The immune system is charged with the defense of the individual and is the subject of this book.

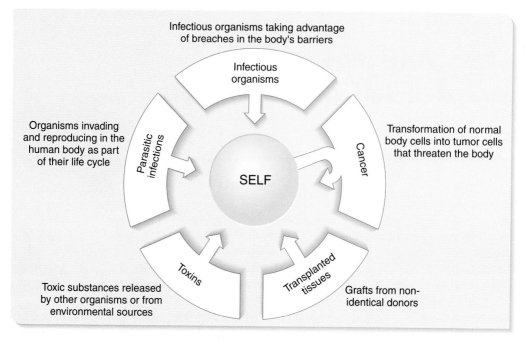

FIGURE 1-1. Threats encountered by the immune system. Infectious and parasitic organisms are present in the surrounding environment, as are biological (e.g., bee venom) and chemical (e.g., chemicals encountered in industrial work sites) toxins. Transformed cells arise within the body itself. Transplanted tissues, although not intended as a threat, are perceived as "foreign" by the immune system.

The immune system constantly guards against microbial invasion. Basically, a constant state of war exists between would-be pathogens and the host, and the immune system is responsible for defending the body against the threat of pathogenic attack. The immune system may be viewed both as an armory—where tools and weapons are constructed for use in defense of the host—and as an army capable of wielding them. Both cellular and molecular weapons are wielded with extreme ferocity, often resulting in the death and degradation of invasive organisms. Each cellular or molecular weapon has at least one deadly use; many have multiple uses. And, like any tool, it can harm its user if not properly operated. The analogy of weaponry is a useful one to keep in mind as we explore the various ways that the immune system defends the host.

Almost every form of life has some type of defense system. Even unicellular organisms such as bacteria have evolved mechanisms to protect against invasion by other infectious agents. With the appearance of structures enabling multicellular forms of life, cells needed to know whether adjoining cells belonged within the structure or were invaders—"self" or "nonself." And if the intruding cells represented a threat, some means had to be devised to remove or deflect the threat.

The mammalian immune system is a complex collection of defensive mechanisms acting in concert, functioning at different levels, and employing a wide variety of defensive mechanisms. These include both ancient forms of defense, shared with most other life forms, and more recently evolved mechanisms that provide greater degrees of discrimination and a more intense focus in the targeting of immune responses.

CLINICAL APPLICATION
CONSEQUENCES OF LOSS OF IMMUNE FUNCTION

Human Immunodeficiency Virus (HIV), the virus that causes AIDS (acquired immune deficiency syndrome), disables the immune system by targeting a specific group of immune cells responsible for coordinating immune responses. People infected with HIV often develop numerous opportunistic infections such as *Mycobacterium avium* complex infection, *Candida albicans* esophagitis, and *Pneumocystis carinii* pneumonia. These infections often involve agents that rarely cause infections in normal healthy individuals.

The immunological concept of self

The idea of individuality (the concept of *self*) seems a rather simple one. A quick glance in the mirror each morning gives us visual cues assuring us that, indeed, it is our "self" staring back at us. Strangers may require the presentation of some type of document, often with a photograph, to ensure that we are who we say we are and that we belong where we are. Individuals can be distinguished visually by gender, facial shape, eye and (sometimes) hair color, skin tone, and other physical attributes. Evaluation of these same characteristics often allows us to distinguish related from nonrelated individuals—family group from nonfamily group.

When the immune system encounters cells or molecules, it must determine whether they belong to the body—whether they are self or nonself. This decision is made without the benefit of such visual clues. Instead, the immune system uses a variety of soluble molecules and cell-bound surface receptors to determine whether the molecules that it encounters are self or nonself. Those molecules may be simple independent structures; they may be part of a larger molecular complex; or they may constitute part of a virus or cell.

The need to distinguish "self" and "nonself" and to counter threats from nonself has been met in many different ways. These include development of physical or chemical barriers to prevent the entry of external agents into the body, special molecules designed to detect and distinguish "self" and "nonself," and special cells and molecules that destroy and remove material identified as "nonself." Some immune systems, as in humans, have also developed the ability to identify and recall threats previously encountered. This **immunological memory** provides the body with an enhanced ability to deal with threats encountered on more than one occasion and to deal with them differently upon subsequent occasions (Fig. 1-2). And, like many biological systems, the immune system employs redundancy—multiple mechanisms with overlapping functions—to ensure that if one mechanism is not effective, another may be.

Biological defense mechanisms are diverse. Unicellular and simple multicellular organisms can detect the entry of infectious microbes (even of cells from adjacent members of their same species), and are able to attack and destroy those that actually make contact. Even plants have evolved mechanisms for detecting the presence of infectious organisms and respond by producing proteins (toxins) that kill would-be pathogens. As more complex animal forms developed—from worms and clams to amphibians, reptiles and mammals—more and more types of defensive "weaponry" appeared. In response, infectious agents developed ways to counter or circumvent those weapons, and these, in turn, stimulated development of even newer defensive mechanisms. The hostile interactions between hosts and infectious organisms represent a spiraling arms race as each side continuously responds to new developments by the other.

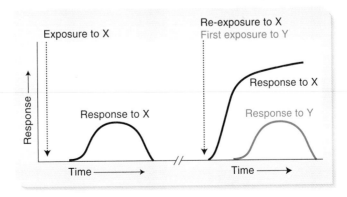

FIGURE 1-2. **Immunological memory.** If a substance X is encountered on more than one occasion, the response on the second occasion may be faster, more vigorous, and longer-lasting than that generated by the first exposure. These changes are specific for each stimulus. If a different stimulus (substance Y) is administered for the first time at the same time that substance X is administered for a second time, the heightened response to X is not reflected in the response to Y. If Y were to be administered again in the future, a heightened response to Y could then be seen.

The human immune system is complex, composed of multiple organs, cell types, and molecules that must work together. At times, the immune system appears to be a collection of paradoxes. It is diffusely distributed throughout the body, yet many of its cells are concentrated within specific lymphoid organs. It can be very general and yet highly specific in detecting and responding to potential threats. Many cells and molecules of the immune system act unilaterally, but almost all of its actions are determined *"by committee."* The immune system is highly regulated to ensure that it functions properly, but it can sometimes become confused or so intense that it begins to harm the body that it is trying to protect.

CLINICAL APPLICATION
RHEUMATIC HEART DISEASE

Rheumatic heart disease is an inflammation of the heart resulting in heart valve deformities. The disease can occur following a group A *Streptococcus* pharyngeal or skin infection, and is due to the similarity between certain molecules on the streptococcal bacteria and those on human heart tissue (*"molecular mimicry"*). As a result, immune responses generated against the bacteria also attack and damage the heart tissue of the infected individual.

The immune system, along with the endocrine and nervous systems, is one of the great communication systems of the body. The immune system approaches threats in three fundamental ways: killing them, consuming them, and overgrowing them. Some of the cells and molecules of the immune system destroy and ingest microbial cells. Infected or altered host cells are destroyed by disrupting their membranes or inducing them to undergo **apoptosis**, a form of "programmed suicide" in which they destroy their own nucleic acids. The very act of capturing and ingesting microbes—live or dead—and cellular debris provokes many **phagocytic** or **pinocytotic** cells to increase their activity. The ingestion and subsequent degradation of microbes or cellular debris also triggers some phagocytic cells to secrete molecules that selectively activate other elements of the immune system. Finally, many cells of the immune system proliferate rapidly upon perceiving the presence of a threat in order to generate sufficient numbers of themselves to deal with the hostile stimuli.

Communication among the elements of the immune system relies on activities that are ubiquitous among biological systems. Receptors on cell surfaces are used to detect the presence of invasive cells or molecules, as well as to receive signals transmitted by other cells. Cells exchange "messages," either by cell-to-cell interaction of cell surface molecules or by soluble molecules secreted by one cell that bind to surface receptors on another cell. Communication can even occur between soluble molecules. Mechanistically, these basic biological functions are quite similar to those used by the endocrine system to regulate other body structures through hormones, by cells of the nervous system to transmit signals, and by migrating cells to examine the nature of other cells and tissues with which they come into contact.

The innate and adaptive immune systems

Initial protection against infection is provided by mechanical (e.g., skin and membranes) and chemical (e.g., microcidal molecules secreted by some skin cells) barriers that are usually effective in barring the entry of microbes into the body. These barriers constitute an important part of the innate immune system. However, these barriers can be breached, and when microbes succeed in entering the body, the immune system must become involved in a more active way to resist and eliminate the infection.

Humans use two immune systems to combat invasion by infectious organisms (Fig. 1-3). One is an ancient system of self-defense, the **innate immune system** (sometimes called the "nonspecific immune system"). The other is the **adaptive immune system** (sometimes called the "specific immune system"). The innate and adaptive systems work together in the development of protective immunity. The innate system uses **pattern-recognition receptors** (PRRs) that are genetically encoded and are expressed by a variety of **leukocytes** (or "white blood cells"). These include phagocytic cells such as **dendritic cells** and **macrophages**, granulocytic cells such as **eosinophils** or **neutrophils** that can destroy or engulf microbes, and **natural killer** (NK) cells that can identify stressed or infected host cells and destroy them. These receptors recognize and bind to molecules found on a wide variety of microbial cells, and on damaged or infected host cells, and thus recognize in a broad and general way the presence of infectious agents. Upon

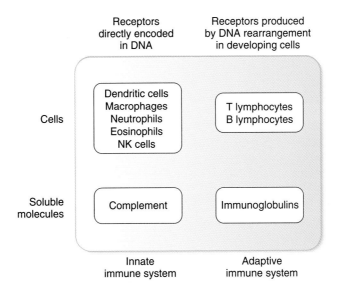

FIGURE 1-3. **The innate and adaptive immune systems.** The innate and adaptive immune systems include both cellular and soluble components. The receptors of the innate immune system are directly encoded by specific genes within the DNA. The receptors of the adaptive immune system are generated in developing lymphocytes by rearranging and splicing of DNA segments and the elimination of the intervening DNA.

encountering microbes, these cells are activated and can quickly differentiate into short-lived effector cells that can attack and usually clear the infection. In addition, the innate immune system includes **complement**, a set of soluble molecules that can bind to certain molecules common to microbial cells. This binding can lead to the direct destruction of the microbe and can also trigger increased activity by phagocytic cells.

Sometimes, however, the innate immune system cannot quickly eliminate the infectious agents. In such instances, cells of the innate system interact with **T lymphocytes** (T cells) and **B lymphocytes** (B cells) to initiate adaptive immune responses against those microbes that pose the immediate threat. The adaptive immune system is based on lymphocytes that bear receptors that are not directly encoded within the germline DNA. Instead, the receptors of lymphocytes are generated by rearrangement of DNA segments, a process that is described in detail in Chapter 4. Such receptors are able to identify and bind a far greater range of substances than can be detected by the PRRs of the innate system. Lymphocytes can detect, with extraordinary specificity, very narrowly defined threats and proliferate rapidly to act against them in a highly targeted manner. The structures recognized and bound by these receptors are termed **antigens**.

The interaction between the innate and adaptive immune responses begins when certain phagocytic cells break down microbial molecules and display them in a way that leads to activation of the T lymphocytes. The activated T cells can then interact with a variety of other cells, including B lymphocytes and other T lymphocytes. Some T lymphocytes become directly involved in attacks against the infection, while others regulate or orchestrate the immune response. B lymphocytes produce **immunoglobulins**. Unlike the innate system that operates at a relatively constant level, adaptive immune responses generate memory B and T lymphocytes that produce more rapid and vigorous responses upon subsequent encounters with the same antigen. Once initiated by cells of the innate system, adaptive responses lead to a clonal expansion in the numbers of lymphocytes able to recognize and bind the antigen in question, and culminate with active responses by those lymphocytes targeted very specifically against that antigen. In responding to an antigen, the lymphocytes not only act directly upon the antigen providing the threatening stimulus, but may also recruit cells (e.g., phagocytic cells) and molecules from the innate system and focus their destructive capabilities upon the threat. Figure 1-4 provides a "map" of the immune system, illustrating the interactions between and within the innate and adaptive immune responses, which may be helpful in remembering these relationships as they are discussed in future chapters.

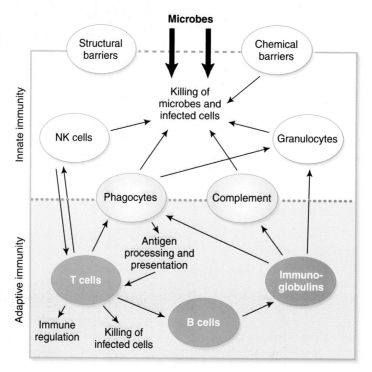

FIGURE 1-4. Interactions between the innate and adaptive immune systems. Extensive communication and interaction exists between the elements of the innate and adaptive immune systems. Some elements of the innate system, such as the phagocytic cells and complement, participate in both innate and adaptive responses. Lymphocytes and immunoglobulins can recruit phagocytic cells and complement and focus their activities upon specific targets identified by the adaptive immune system.

Patient Vignette 1.1

The patient vignettes introduce a set of patient cases that we will return to throughout the text at appropriate points as new information is presented that bear upon the patients' conditions.

 Leona T. is a 24-year old medical technician who has sustained a needle stick injury. One hour ago, she tried to draw blood from a patient with a known history of viral hepatitis B infection. On her third attempt, she inadvertently stuck her right thumb with the needle.

How will her body combat the possible invasion of the viral hepatitis B infection?

Both the innate and adaptive immune systems will be used. The innate system will provide immediate protection. This system includes the phagocytic cells, granulocytic cells, and natural killer cells that express pattern recognition receptors capable of recognizing

(continued)

Patient Vignette 1.1 (Continued)

pathogen-associated molecular patterns on viruses. Since the technician received a viral Hepatitis B vaccination many months prior to starting her job, the adaptive responses such as antibodies and lymphocytes capable of destroying infected cells are also activated and should provide rapid protection.

ANTIGENS

What is an antigen?

Soluble or cell-bound molecules recognized and bound by the specific membrane-bound receptors of T and B lymphocytes are known as **antigens**. Antigens can also be bound by soluble immunoglobulins. Depending upon circumstances, the recognition and binding may involve the entire antigen or only a portion of the antigen. The smallest identifiable part of an antigenic molecule that can be recognized by a given T or B cell receptor is called a **determinant** or **epitope** (Fig. 1-5). Some antigens are very simple, bearing only one or very few epitopes. Others may be complex, containing numerous different epitopes (Fig. 1-6). In general, the more complex the antigen, the more stimulatory or **immunogenic** it will be in eliciting an immune response. Very small, simple antigens are less immunogenic. The physical state of an antigen may also affect its **immunogenicity**.

In the innate immune system, glycoproteins and glycolipids are more stimulatory than are proteins. The immunoglobulins produced by B lymphocytes can readily bind protein and carbohydrate antigens. The antigen-specific receptors of T lymphocytes, on the other hand, are primarily attuned to protein antigens.

Immunogens, haptens, and tolerogens

There are three types of antigens: immunogens, haptens, and tolerogens.

Immunogens are molecules that can, by themselves, both stimulate an immune response and, in turn, be a target of an immune response (Fig. 1-7). Subsequent exposures to the same immunogen generally lead to heightened secondary responses by the adaptive immune system.

Haptens are small molecules that, by themselves, cannot stimulate an immune response. However, when coupled to an immunogenic molecule (a "**carrier**"), they can become stimulatory and prompt the immune system to generate responses against the hapten and against the carrier (Fig. 1-7). This phenomenon involves interactions between different lymphocytes and is discussed in greater detail in Chapter 5. As with immunogens, responses to haptens can be elevated upon subsequent re-exposure to the same hapten-carrier conjugate.

Tolerogens are molecules that, like immuno-

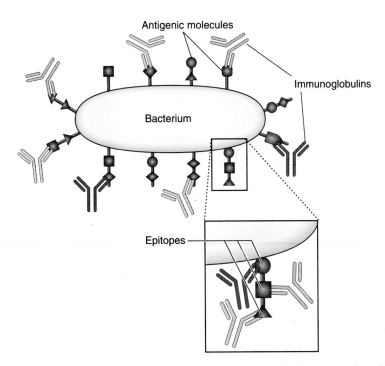

FIGURE 1-5. **Antigenic molecules.** Invasive microbes express many antigenic molecules that can be individually identified by different antigen receptors (e.g., immunoglobulins). Therefore, the antibody response against a microbe can consist of many different immunoglobulins recognizing different specific sites on the microbe. An individual molecule can even consist of smaller parts that are specifically recognized by different immunoglobulins. The smallest individual entity that can be detected by a receptor is termed an epitope.

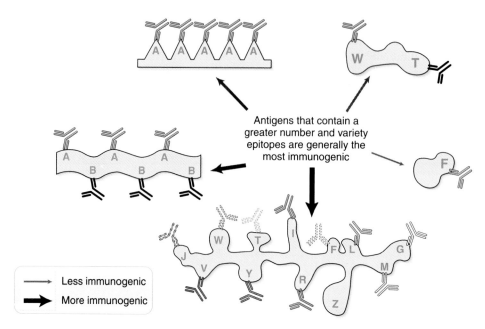

FIGURE 1-6. Immunogenicity. Antigens that are more complex in structure tend to have more binding sites and express a greater variety of different epitopes. Antigens that can be recognized by the greatest range of available T and B cell receptors, and antibodies will generally stimulate the strongest overall immune responses (i.e., they have greater immunogenicity).

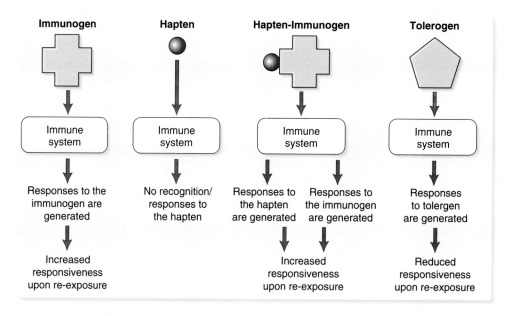

FIGURE 1-7. Immunogens, haptens and tolerogens. Immunogens and tolerogens, by themselves, can both stimulate and serve as targets of immune responses. Haptens cannot stimulate responses on their own, but can serve as targets of responses generated if the hapten is attached to an immunogen. Reexposure to immunogens and haptens (attached to the same immunogens) usually generate heightened responses. Reexposures to tolerogens usually result in diminished responses.

gens, can both stimulate immune responses and serve as targets of those responses (Fig. 1-7). Unlike immunogens, subsequent exposure of the immune system to the same tolerogen leads to diminished responsiveness against it.

Variability of immune responses

If a sample of several individuals (excluding identical twins) were tested for their ability to respond to the same set of antigens, two results would be evident. First, no one would be able to respond to every antigen. Second, the pattern of responsiveness would vary among the individuals —different individuals would respond to different subsets of those antigens.

A given antigen may provoke different responses in different individuals. A molecule that is immunogenic for one person may be tolerogenic for another and perhaps unrecognized by a third person (Fig. 1-8). Four major factors account for this variability. The first is the genetic constitution of each individual. Several genes influence how our immune system responds to a given antigen, and these can differ considerably among individuals. The second factor is the physical state of the antigen. For example, antigens denatured by heat or chemical treatment may be seen differently from their native form by the immune system and the responses against them may be different, as well. The third factor is often re-

lated to therapeutic treatment where application of chemical or physical agents (e.g., drugs or irradiation) can alter an individual's immune response. As a result, an antigen that was previously tolerogenic to that individual may subsequently be seen as immunogenic or vice versa. Finally, all individuals have "holes" in their immunologic repertoires. While the lymphocytes of an individual can, in theory, initially generate antigen-specific receptors against all antigens, the intervening steps involved in the "education" of the immune system, together with the random element of chance, results in the loss or inactivation of many lymphocytes and the receptors they bear. The lymphocytes and receptors that are lost vary among individuals, so that one person may respond well against a particular antigen or infectious agent while another may not because he or she lacks a lymphocyte subpopulation bearing the necessary receptors.

The diversity of the immune response is protective. While it may be improbable for an individual to generate an immune response to every antigenic epitope on a particular microbe, many (if not most) individuals can generate an immune response to at least one of the many epitopes displayed by that microbe. Thus, for almost any infectious agent that might move through the population, there are likely to be at least some individuals able to resist the infection and survive. The consequences of an absence of such diversity are seen in genetically homogenous populations, such as inbred strains of experimental animals, where a single type of infectious agent can sometimes kill every individual.

SELF AND NONSELF

All cells, including those of the immune system, use a variety of surface receptors to recognize the general characteristics of their environment, as well as the nature of the cells and molecules they encounter (Fig. 1-9). Many cell receptors detect signals transmitted between the various cells of the body, but some receptors are dedicated to monitoring for potential threats. These receptors vary in their discrimination. Some receptors bind structures that have a very limited distribution (e.g., they are found only on particular substrains of particular species of microbes). Others bind a variety of molecular structures sharing some basic characteristic but distributed widely among many

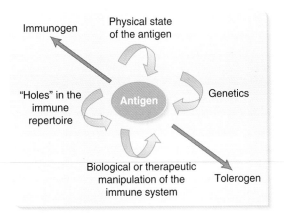

FIGURE 1-8. Variability of the antigenic response. A given antigen may provoke different types of responses in different individuals. The type of response generated can be affected by the genetic makeup of the individual; the collective influences that determine the spectrum of receptors ("immunologic repertoire") generated by an individual's immune system; the influence of therapy on the individual's immune system; and the physical form of the antigen.

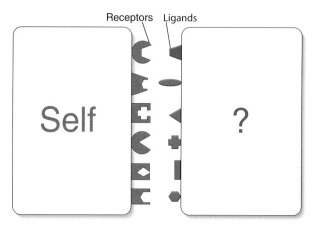

FIGURE 1-9. Cell surface receptors. Receptors on cells allow them to "inspect" other cells to determine the nature of those cells and to influence if and how they might interact with those cells.

molecules or organisms.

The detection of different molecules (including antigens) by these receptors influences the subsequent actions of the cells bearing those receptors. For example, a cell may have to determine whether a molecule that it has bound arose from within the body or entered from the environment. Self molecules presumably present no threat, but alien or nonself molecules have the potential to forewarn of an impending microbial invasion. Based on the information gathered by their receptors, cells go on to make decisions about what must be done to protect the body.

> **CLINICAL APPLICATION**
> **GRAVE'S DISEASE**
>
> Grave's disease is an autoimmune disease characterized by the presence of antibodies directed against thyroid stimulating hormone (TSH) receptors of the thyroid gland. The condition is caused by failure of the immune regulatory system to prevent activation of self reactive lymphocytes.

Recognition

The statement is often made that the antigen-specific receptors of the immune system recognize "foreign" antigens. This is only partially correct. Some T and B lymphocytes receptors do recognize foreign or nonself antigens, but others recognize self antigens. In fact, the body's immune system learns what is nonself by first learning what is self—a process we refer to as "education." The ability to respond to nonself is the basis for protection against environmental threats and is generally, but not always, beneficial. The ability to recognize self, while critical to immunologic education, is potentially dangerous. When self-reactive lymphocytes become inappropriately activated, they can attack the body's own cells and tissues and lead to autoimmune responses (see Chapter 9). Several mechanisms exist to eliminate or control potentially autoreactive lymphocytes, providing protection against autoimmunity that is successful for most individuals.

Surface receptors often have cytoplasmic tails that span the cell membrane and extend into the cytoplasm. In some cases, surface receptors that lack cytoplasmic tails are associated with accessory molecules that do possess cytoplasmic tails. When such a surface receptor is bound by an antigen or other molecule, that information is relayed into the cytoplasm and often to the nucleus. This process, known as **signal transduction**, involves a series of steps that activate sequential sets of enzymes leading to the activation of their substrate molecules. The "knowledge" gained by the cell when a particular receptor is engaged can be used to alter its metabolism, movement, and even the pattern of genes that are transcribed and translated into proteins. As a result, cells can be induced to proliferate and differentiate, becoming more specialized with capabilities for new activities. We discuss the signal transduction pathways that are most relevant to immune function in Chapter 5.

Distinguishing self from nonself

In a world shared with an almost unlimited number of other organisms, individuals need to be able to detect the inappropriate presence of such organisms. This recognition involves two considerations: self versus nonself and threat versus nonthreat. Cells of the immune system distinguish self from nonself through cell-surface receptors. The immune system faces a formidable task in generating these receptors. On one hand, immune cells must produce receptors that recognize self molecules and respond accordingly to them. On the other hand, immune cells must also generate receptors for an enormous number of nonself molecules months, years or decades *prior to* encountering those molecules. Many receptors are generated that probably never encounter the molecules that they are designed to recognize and bind.

Recognition of common self epitopes

Different sets of receptors may be used by cells to ask different types of questions in making the distinction between self and nonself (Fig. 1-10). Some receptors are designed to recognize and bind self. They are used by cells to determine if an encountered molecule or cell has the appropriate structures to show that it is a part of the body. In essence, the immune system is asking "*Do you have what I expect you to have?*" These self structures are normally absent from invasive microbial cells, and may also be absent from some abnormal cells of the body (e.g., some cancer cells), and from cells of other individuals of the same species (e.g., a transplanted graft). The absence of such self indicators can trigger an attack upon the invader. For example, natural killer (NK) cells bear **killer inhibition receptors** (KIRs) that recognize MHC I molecules. MHC I molecules should be present on every nucleated cell of the body, but are highly variable from one individual to another, even within the same species, and their structure and functions are discussed in further detail in Chapters 4 and 5. When NK cells make contact with another cell, they assess whether that "target" cell carries appropriate MHC I molecules and in normal quantities. If the cell under assessment does not carry the same array of MHC I molecules as does the NK cell itself, or if those molecules are present but in abnormally low quantities, the NK cell will kill the target cell. The actions of NK cells will also be discussed in greater detail in Chapter 3.

The other form of self recognition asks "*Do you and I have anything in common?*" In this case, the recognition is not as strict. Instead, the "sharing" of at least one copy of some critical structure

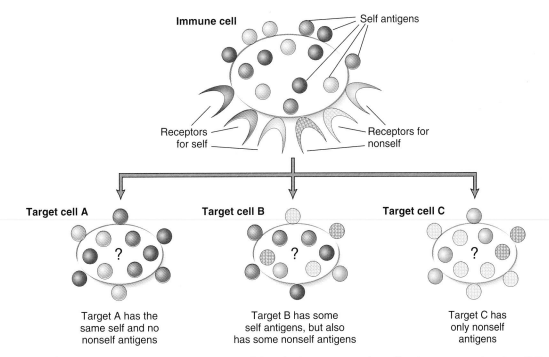

FIGURE 1-10. Self and nonself receptors. Immune cells have both receptors against self and receptors against nonself. By examining other cells for the presence of both self and nonself molecules, immune cells can determine the relationship of those cells to the body and, ultimately, what kind of threat they might pose.

identifies the intruding cell as similar enough to be considered self, even though the intruder may also express some nonself structures, as well (Fig. 1-8). While human immune systems rely primarily on a strict definition of self, recognition via "sharing" may occur in a very few special situations. This form of self recognition is widely used throughout the biological world and may represent the most ancient means for distinguishing self from nonself.

Recognition of widely expressed foreign epitopes

Some receptors are designed to recognize and bind structures that are not normally present within the body. They ask the question, "*Do you have something that I don't have?*" This form of recognition enforces "identity"—the absence of structures alien to the body—and is triggered by the presence of nonself (Fig. 1-8). For example, the pattern recognition receptors (PRRs) identify structures that are typically associated with microbes but not with human cells. Thus, they identify the presence of something that is foreign to the body (nonself).

Recognition of foreign epitopes by somatically generated receptors

In many instances, T cell receptors (TCRs) and B cell receptors (BCRs) generated by DNA rearrangement recognize unfamiliar or foreign epitopes. Once activated, T cells and B cells launch a powerful and lethal response that ultimately leads to the destruction of the cells or molecules bearing a foreign determinant. Before such a powerful response is unleashed, it is vital that these cells do not respond to cells or molecules of the body itself. You will see in Chapter 5 that T and B cells must meet several requirements before they become activated.

Avoidance of adverse responses

The identification of an intrusive cell or molecule as nonself does not necessarily require the generation of an active immune response against it. A second level of assessment occurs, whereby the immune system decides whether or not the structure identified as "nonself" represents a sufficient threat to trigger a defensive action. The decision as to whether and how to respond to a particular stimulus is generally determined by interactions between several types of cells within the immune

system. Examples of situations where the immune system may perceive nonself to be nonthreatening include the movement of food that passes through the gastrointestinal system, and the presence of commensal microbes on the skin and in the intestine. Immune responses constantly mounted against harmless nonself molecules can be undesirable, as seen in individuals with food allergies.

Patient Vignette 1.2

 Peter H. is a 3-year-old boy with a family history of allergy. He has developed generalized pruritus (itching) and hives (swollen, reddish bumps or patches on the skin) after eating a peanut.

His symptoms became increasingly severe with each subsequent exposure to peanuts.

What immunologic factors might be involved in his problems?

This child's clinical symptoms are consistent with peanut allergy. Peanut protein is a common food allergen (antigen) in both adults and children. Clinical symptoms associated with peanut allergy can be localized (hives), or severe and systemic (anaphylactic shock), a life-threatening condition causing the circulatory collapse and respiratory failure. For this child, a peanut (or some component), is presumably an immunogen, as it provokes a positive immune response that increases upon subsequent exposures.

However, it should be noted that the surface of the skin, the lining of the respiratory tract, and the lumen of the gastrointestinal tract are topographically outside of the body proper. Nonself encountered within the tissues of the body proper, on the other hand, is less likely to be viewed as nonthreatening. In addition, the decision to mount an immune response against a particular form of nonself is sometimes influenced by genetics and may therefore differ from one individual to another.

"Self-education"

In many cases, the structures of cellular receptors are fixed and uniform because they are directly encoded in the DNA and have been shaped by evolutionary selection. This is the case for the pattern recognition receptors (PRRs) expressed by leukocytes. In contrast, the antigen-specific receptors of T and B lymphocytes that are the basis for the adaptive immune response are generated anew within the lymphocytes as they undergo development within each individual. This process is initially random and results in the generation of receptors that may fall into one of three general categories: (1) those that will appropriately identify nonself; (2) those that are potentially reactive against self; and (3) those (for T lymphocytes) that will be unable to function in the body within which they are generated. As will be discussed further in Chapter 5, the body must develop a system by which the body attunes its immune system by amplification of lymphocytes in the first category and elimination of those lymphocytes in the second and third categories. Education involves a series of selective events in which the ability to develop lymphocytes to engage their receptors may be either a fatal event (negative selection) or a necessary event (positive selection). By these and other means, each individual adjusts their adaptive response to their own genetic and environmental circumstances.

Summary

- The immune system must be able to distinguish self—that which belongs within the body—from nonself. Nonself may enter the body from the outside or represent an unacceptable change within the body (e.g., a normal cell becoming cancerous).
- The human immune system is complex, composed of multiple organs, cell types, and molecules that must work together.
- Initial protection against infection is provided by mechanical barriers (such as the skin and mucous membranes) and by chemical barriers (such as microcidal molecules secreted by some skin cells) that can quite effectively bar the entry of microbes in the body.
- We use two immune systems to combat invasion by infectious organisms. One is an ancient system of self-defense—the innate immune system (sometimes called the "nonspecific" immune system). The other is the antigen-specific adaptive immune system (sometimes called the "specific" immune system).
- Using a variety of surface receptors, cells can sample not only the general characteristics of their environment, but also the nature of the cells and molecules with which they come into contact.

- An antigen is a structure that can be recognized and bound by the specific receptors of T and B lymphocytes. Antigens may be proteins, carbohydrates, lipids, or combinations such as glycoproteins or glycolipids. A given antigen may provoke different responses in different individuals.
- The smallest identifiable part of an antigenic molecule that can be recognized by a T or B cell receptor is called an epitope or determinant.
- Immunogens are antigenic molecules that can, by themselves, both stimulate an immune response and, in turn, be a target of an immune response. Subsequent exposures usually elicit heightened responses against that specific immunogen.
- Haptens are small molecules that, by themselves, cannot stimulate an immune response, but can be recognized by the immune system if bound to an immunogenic molecule.
- Tolerogens are molecules that, like immunogens, can both stimulate immune responses and serve as targets of those responses, but subsequent exposures result in diminished response to that specific tolerogen.
- The process in which a surface receptor transfers information into the cytoplasm and often to the nucleus is known as signal transduction. This process involves a series of steps that activate sequential sets of enzymes that can modify their substrate molecules to become biologically active.
- The adaptive immune response is initially random and results in T and B cell receptors that (1) appropriately identify nonself, (2) are potentially reactive against self, or (3) that will (in the case of T lymphocytes) be unable to function in the body.

Suggested readings

Abbas AK, Lichtman AH. General properties of immune responses. In *Cellular and molecular immunology*, 5th ed. Philadephia: WB Saunders Co., 2003.

Berzofsky JA, Berkower IJ. Immunogenicity and antigen structure. In Paul WE, ed. *Fundamental immunology*, 5th ed. Philadephia: Lippincott Williams & Wilkins, 2003.

Chaplin DD. Overview of the immune response. *J Allergy Clin Immunol* 2003;111:S442.

Janeway CA, Jr. Evolution of the immune system. In Janeway CA Jr, Travers P, Walport M, Shlomchik P, eds. *Immunobiology: The immune system in health and disease*, 6th ed. Philadephia: Garland Publishing, 2004:665–682.

Paul WE. The immune system: An introduction. In Paul WE, ed. *Fundamental immunology*, 5th ed. Philadephia: Lippincott Williams & Wilkins, 2003.

Review questions

DIRECTIONS: Each of the numbered items or incomplete statements in this section is followed by answers or by completions of the statement. Select ONE lettered answer or completion that is BEST in each case.

1. Which one of the following statements accurately describes the human immune system?
   (A) The primary function of the immune system is the prevention of inbreeding
   (B) The human immune system includes only mechanisms that are unique to mammals
   (C) The human immune system has evolved to include a complex collection of defensive mechanisms, acting in concert with one another
   (D) The immune system is designed to recognize only "nonself"

2. Humans use two immune systems to combat invasions by infectious organisms. They are:
   (A) innate and adaptive immune systems
   (B) adaptive and specific immune systems
   (C) innate and pathogenic immune systems
   (D) adaptive and cellular immune systems

3. A 30-year-old man has a *Mycobacterium avium* complex infection, *Candida albicans* esophagitis, and *Pneumocystis carinii* pneumonia, all of which are opportunistic infections. He has a history of an excessive number of repeated infections that do not respond well to standard treatments. His infections often involve agents (e.g., *Candida* and Pneumocystis) that rarely cause infections in normal healthy individuals. What type of underlying disease might you most suspect that this man has?
   (A) A disease in which his immune system is attacking his own body (autoimmune disease)
   (B) A disease in which his body lacks the ability to generate a normal immune response (immune deficiency)
   (C) An occupationally related disease, in which he is repeatedly exposed to infectious agents
   (D) A disease in which he cannot tolerate the antibiotic drugs usually given to fight infections

4. A 67- year-old woman with a family history of a disease developed Graves' disease, an autoimmune disease characterized by the presence of antibodies directed against TSH receptors in the thyroid gland. Her condition is due to:
   (A) the failure of her immune system to generate an innate immune response
   (B) an implanted "foreign" thyroid gland from an unrelated donor
   (C) the failure of her immune system to prevent activation of self-reactive lymphocytes
   (D) a shortage of B lymphocytes

5. Properties of haptens include:
   (A) immunogenicity (the ability to initiate an immune response) and reactivity (ability to be recognized by an immune response)
   (B) reactivity but not immunogenicity
   (C) immunogenicity but not reactivity
   (D) neither immunogenicity nor reactivity
   (E) chemical complexity and macromolecular nature

6. Pattern recognition receptors (PRRs) are able to identify structures that are typically associated with:
   (A) macrophages
   (B) red blood cells
   (C) platelets
   (D) microbes

7. Natural killer (NK) cells have killer inhibitor receptors (KIRs) that recognize:
   (A) major histocompatibility complex (MHC) II molecules
   (B) MHC I molecules
   (C) complement
   (D) red blood cells

8. The adaptive immune response process results in the generation of numerous receptors that:
   (A) are capable of detecting self only
   (B) are expressed by phagocytic cells
   (C) are capable of detecting nonself only
   (D) detect self in some cases and nonself in others

9. The smallest identifiable part of an antigenic molecule that can be recognized by a T or B cell receptor is called:
   - (A) an epitope
   - (B) a signal
   - (C) an immunoglobulin
   - (D) a receptor

10. Properties of immunogens include:
    - (A) immunogenicity (the ability to initiate an immune response) and reactivity (ability to be recognized by an immune response)
    - (B) reactivity but not immunogenicity
    - (C) immunogenicity but not reactivity
    - (D) neither immunogenicity nor reactivity
    - (E) a small, simple molecular structure

11. Tolerogens are molecules that:
    - (A) are not recognized at all by the immune system
    - (B) can generate elevated secondary responses upon reexposure to the immune system
    - (C) can lead to diminished responses upon subsequent reexposure to the immune system
    - (D) eliminate responses to immunogens

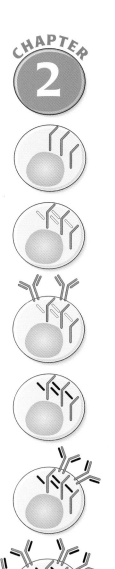

Cells, Cell-surface Molecules, and Organs

Chapter Outline

Introduction White blood cells or **leukocytes** may be likened to the soldiers of the immune system. They police the tissues and organs of the body, using both the lymphatic and blood circulatory systems, and serve as sentinels and defenders against infection. Like soldiers, leukocytes often have specialized roles to play in combating infection; some cells are involved in "hand-to-hand" combat, others wield the "slings and arrows," and yet others serve as field marshals by regulating the assault. Leukocytes bivouac as individuals or as accumulations with varying degrees of organization that constitute the organs and tissues of the immune system, namely, the spleen, thymus, lymph nodes, tonsils, Peyer's patches, and appendix. Understanding the roles of each leukocyte type, how it traverses the body, and how leukocyte accumulations are organized is important to the understanding of immune function.

CELL-SURFACE MOLECULES

Leukocytes, like soldiers, often display badges of rank. Although leukocytes display a number of molecules on their cell surfaces, several are useful for distinguishing their function and role in immune defense. Cell surface molecules that are useful in distinguishing leukocytes include immunoglobulin (Ig), cluster of differentiation (CD), receptors, and major histocompatibility complex (MHC) molecules.

Immunoglobulin molecules

Immunoglobulin molecules play a pivotal role in a number of immune functions. Not only do immunoglobulins show exquisite specificity, but some also serve as signals for increased phagocytosis, as cell surface receptors, and as activators of lytic molecules. We discuss the structure of immunoglobulins in greater detail in Chapter 4. However, an understanding of the landmarks of immunoglobulin molecules helps in understanding leukocyte classification. Immunoglobulin

molecules have a basic paired structure containing two identical light chains and two identical heavy chains, and the structure is linked by disulfide bonds (Fig. 2-1). The amino (NH_2) terminus of each heavy-light chain pair contains the sites that specifically recognize antigens.

> **SIDEBAR 2.1 DISTINCTION BETWEEN IMMUNOGLOBULIN AND ANTIBODY**
>
> The term "immunoglobulin" is generic; any globular molecule that migrates in an electrical field is a globulin. Not all immunoglobulins are antibodies, however. Remember the old adage that a cat is a quadruped, but not all quadrupeds are cats? We will (properly) use the term "antibody" when the antigen-binding specificity of an immunoglobulin molecule is known.

> **SIDEBAR 2.2 ANTIBODIES AS DIAGNOSTIC REAGENTS**
>
> A readily detectable molecule (e.g., a fluorochrome, radioactive molecule, or enzyme) bound covalently to an antibody provides the basis for a number of clinical diagnostic and immune function tests. Several commonly used assays are described in Appendix A.

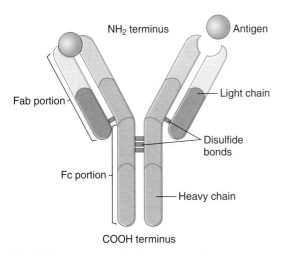

FIGURE 2-1. Immunoglobulin molecule. The basic immunoglobulin structural unit contains four polypeptides, two identical heavy chains, and two identical light chains. Heavy and light chains are linked by disulfide bonds (in red). The amino (NH_2) terminus of each polypeptide contains a variable amino acid sequence. The combination of heavy and light chain variable regions forms an antigen-binding pocket and every immunoglobulin has at least two. This is the so-called antigen-binding portion of the molecule or Fab (for antigen-binding fragment). The constant portion of the heavy chain or Fc (for crystalizable or constant fragment) undergoes a conformational change when antigen is bound. Complement receptors and Fc receptors recognize and bind Fc immunoglobulin regions that have been altered in this way.

Cluster of differentiation molecules

Blood cells originate from stem cell precursors. As they mature and differentiate into specialized leukocytes, these cells begin to express different cell-surface molecules that are indicative of both their cell type and their stage in development. In addition, leukocyte subpopulations sometimes express cell-surface molecules that are unique to their functional or maturation stage of the cell. A series of over 250 distinguishing molecules have been identified so far. They are called **cluster of differentiation** (CD) molecules and are identified by number (e.g., CD1, CD2, etc.). We will introduce CD molecules on a "need to know basis" as we discuss immune function. A partial listing of the currently identified CD molecules is given in Appendix B.

Cell-surface receptors

Cells sense their environment through a variety of **cell-surface receptors**. As major defenders of the body, cells of the immune system may kill or severely impair cells that they perceive as foreign. Therefore, it is extremely important that leukocytes do not mistakenly react against cells of the body (Chapter 9) or do not fail to recognize foreign cells (Chapter 7). The receptors expressed may be used to identify a particular class or population of leukocytes. Some leukocytes express receptors for the Fc portion of the immunoglobulin molecule (FcR) or for an activated component of complement (complement receptor or CR), enabling these leukocytes to phagocytize and kill cells that are coated with antibody and/or complement.

Major histocompatibility complex molecules

All nucleated cells of the body express molecules that are markers of self. These are the **major histocompatibility complex (MHC) class I molecules**. Dendritic cells, monocytes, and certain lymphocyte populations constitutively express **MHC class II molecules**. Some T lymphocytes express MHC class II upon activation. The presence or absence of MHC class II on the cell surface is an important distinguishing characteristic for several leukocyte subsets. MHC class I and II molecules are critical to the activation of T lymphocytes and the initiation of adaptive immune responses. Their functions are discussed in greater detail in Chapter 5.

CLINICAL APPLICATION
HISTOCOMPATIBILITY

Histocompatibility is the ability to transplant tissues between individuals without triggering tissue rejection. One of the preoperative immunological evaluations for organ transplantation includes matching of the donor's and recipient's MHC proteins of the human leukocyte antigen (HLA) system.

LEUKOCYTES

Five morphologically distinct types of leukocytes are commonly found in the circulation and may be classified as **granular** (containing cytoplasmic granules—polymorphonuclear cells, basophils and eosinophils) or as **agranular cells** (lymphocytes and monocytes). Although it is difficult to distinguish between cells within a particular class by light microscopy, cell-surface molecules are very often helpful in understanding the function of leukocytes.

Leukocytes or their products are responsible for most immune functions. Each of the five different types of leukocytes performs a specific task in defending the host from invasive organisms. Leukocyte types can often be readily distinguished morphologically. However, those within a particular type may be more difficult to distinguish from one another.

CLINICAL APPLICATION
NEUTROPENIA

A neutrophil count of less than 1,000 cells/μl is called **neutropenia** and indicates an increased risk of infection. Gram-negative bacteria and fungi are common types of organisms infecting patients with neutropenia. The most common causes of neutropenia are drugs or bone marrow toxicity due to a viral infection.

Lymphocytes

Although **lymphocytes** look alike by both light and electron microscopy, they are sometimes categorized according to size as small (4 to 7 μm), medium (7 to 11 μm), or large (11 to 15 μm). Stimulated lymphocytes often transform into large **blast** cells (up to 30 μm). Morphologically similar, lymphocytes may differ widely in function (Fig. 2-2A). Lymphocytes are broadly categorized by the organs in which they undergo the major part of their development—**B lymphocytes** in the bone marrow and **T lymphocytes** in the thymus. The terms "B cell" and "T cell" are used interchangeably with "B lymphocyte" and "T lymphocyte."

T lymphocytes or T cells

Arising from stem cells resident in the bone marrow, immature lymphocytes known as **prothymocytes** migrate to a lymphoid organ known as the **thymus**. The thymus serves as an indoctrination center where the lymphocytes, now known as **thymocytes**, must learn to distinguish self from nonself. Thymocytes that cannot make this distinction are eliminated. Those that can may further differentiate, mature, and "graduate" as thymus-derived lymphocytes or T cells and enter the circulation. Collectively, T cells display a number of diverse functions. Although T cells cannot synthesize antibody, they often function to initiate, regulate, and fine-tune antibody or humoral immune responses. T cells are often are key players in the immunological battle. In this role, T cells are called *effector cells* and are responsible

for the various types of *cell-mediated immune responses*, i.e., lacking antibody involvement. Types of cell-mediated responses are:

- *Delayed (-type) hypersensitivity (DTH) responses.* An example of a DTH response would be the cellular infiltration causing swelling following a tuberculin skin test.

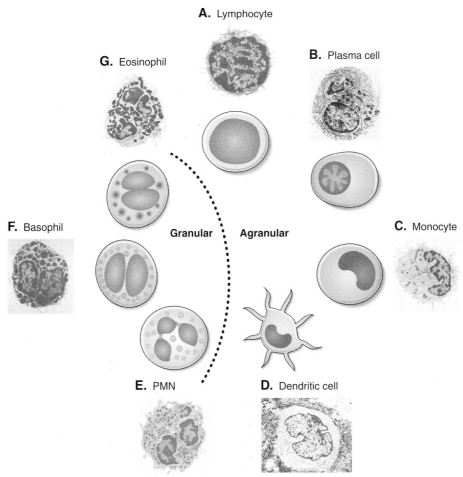

FIGURE 2-2. Leukocytes. Five morphologically distinct leukocytes are normally found in the circulation. Leukocytes may be broadly divided into agranular and granular forms, based upon the absence or presence of cytoplasmic inclusions. **(A)** Lymphocytes are the workhorses of the adaptive immune system. Although they look similar by light microscopy, they have quite different functions. Lymphocytes that mature within the thymus are known as T cells and those that differentiate within bone marrow are known as B cells. **(B)** Upon further maturation, B cells may further differentiate into immunoglobulin-secreting cells known as plasma cells. Plasma cells are rarely found in the circulation. **(C)** Monocytes are phagocytic cells found in the circulation; when they cross the endothelium into the tissues, they are known as macrophages. **(D)** Dendritic cells are phagocytes that are important for the clearance of cellular debris, invading microorganisms, and for the initiation of adaptive immune responses. These cells, named for their tree branch-like projections, are rarely identified in the circulation. **(E)** Neutrophils or polymorphonuclear (PMN) cells are the most prominent leukocyte found in the circulation. Their nuclei may be in two to five lobes, depending upon their maturation stage, and give rise to the name *polymorphonuclear*. Their other name, *neutrophils*, reflects the presence of neutral staining cytoplasmic granules that contain antimicrobial enzymes. **(F)** Basophils have a bilobed nucleus and cytoplasmic granules that contain vasoactive amines. So named because they stain with basic dyes, basophils are important mediators of allergic reactions. Functionally related cells in the tissues are known as mast cells. **(G)** Eosinophils have bilobed nuclei and cytoplasmic granules that stain with acid dyes. Eosinophils are important in defending against parasitic infection. (All photos reprinted from Rubin E, Gorstein F, Rubin R, et al. *Rubin's pathology: Clinicopathologic foundations of medicine*, 4th ed. Baltimore: Lippincott Williams & Wilkins, 2005.)

- *Contact sensitivity (CS) responses.* These responses cause cellular infiltration leading to swelling and itching, e.g., following exposure to poison ivy. Contact sensitivity is a form of DTH directed against chemicals applied to the skin or mucous membranes that react with and bind to cells.
- *Transplantation immunity.* Graft rejection is usually initiated by T cells.
- *Cytotoxic T lymphocyte or (T_c or CTL) responses.* When activated, these T cells make direct contact with other cells to cause their destruction by lysis.

CLINICAL APPLICATION
TUBERCULOSIS

Nearly a third of the world's population is infected with *Mycobacterium tuberculosis*. Approximately 5–10% of those infected with *M. tuberculosis* become sick or infectious some time in their lifetimes, developing a disease known as tuberculosis (TB). Approximately 8 million people worldwide develop TB annually resulting in nearly two million deaths each year. The Mantoux skin test is a useful screening test to identify people who have been infected with TB. It involves injection of 5 TU (tuberculin units) of purified protein derivative (PPD, tuberculin), usually 0.1 mL, intradermally. Induration (swelling) is assessed at 48 to 72 hours. A positive response is an example of DTH.

T cells have a variety of characteristic cell-surface molecules that include (but are not limited to) the following:

SIDEBAR 2.3 THE ANTIGENIC UNIVERSE

Scientists estimate that the antigenic universe contains between 10^6 and 10^7 epitopes. This means that there are at least 10^6 and 10^7 epitope-specific T cells and B cells. When the term *antigen-specific* is used, it means that there is a cell (B and/or T cell) resident in the immune system for each of the 10^6 to 10^7 epitopes!

- *T-cell receptor.* The T-cell receptor (TCR) is a heterodimeric cell-surface molecule composed of either an α–β or a γ–δ polypeptide-chain pair. The amino acid sequence of the antigen-recognition portion of each chain is determined by genetic recombination, meaning that each T cell or its progeny expresses multiple copies of this unique TCR that recognize a narrowly defined epitope (Fig. 2-3). It has been estimated that human T cells can recognize at least 10^6 to 10^7 different epitopes. Since each T cell expresses a different TCR, this means that there are *at least* 10^6 to 10^7 epitope-distinct T cells in the immune system! The TCR lacks a

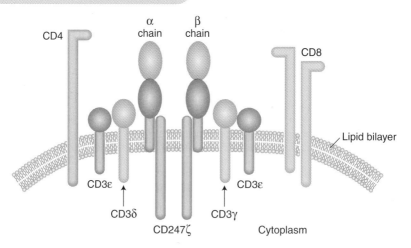

FIGURE 2-3. T cell receptor (TCR) complex. Thymus-derived lymphocytes or T cells display an antigen-specific cell surface receptor (TCR). The TCR is a heterodimer containing α–β or γ–δ polypeptide chains. The combination of the variable portions of the two polypeptides forms an peptide-binding pocket in the amino terminus of the molecules. The TCR lacks a cytoplasmic tail that would allow direct cytoplasmic signaling of peptide engagement by the TCR. Signals are conveyed through a group of six invariant accessory molecules collectively known as the CD3 complex (2 CD3ε + 1 CD3γ +1 CD3δ + 2 ζ or CD247 chains). In addition, mature T cells express CD4 or CD8 molecules in association with the TCR complex.

cytoplasmic tail that would allow direct cyto-plasmic signaling once the TCR binds an epi-tope. Cytoplasmic signal transduction occurs through invariant accessory chains, known collectively as CD3, that noncovalently associ-ate with the TCR.

- *CD3 complex.* The CD3 complex is composed of a group of six invariant accessory molecules: one CD3γ, one CD3δ, two CD3ε, and an in-tracytoplasmic homodimer of ζ (or CD247) chains. The CD3 complex is essential for both the cell-surface expression of the TCR and for signal transduction once the TCR recognizes an antigen.
- *CD4 or CD8.* Most mature T cells express CD4 or CD8 molecules. CD4 and CD8 molecules function as important coreceptors in associa-tion with the TCR. By binding to invariant por-tions of the MHC I (CD8) or MHC II (CD4), they serve to increase the interaction of the MHC-bound antigenic fragment and the TCR. A useful mnemonic is **the rule of eight**: CD4 recognizes MHC class II ($4 \times 2 = 8$), and CD8 recognizes MHC class I ($8 \times 1 = 8$).

CLINICAL APPLICATION
HUMAN IMMUNODEFICIENCY VIRUS

The first case of AIDS (acquired immune defi-ciency syndrome), which is caused by the hu-man immunodeficiency virus infection (HIV), was reported in 1981. Since then, the disease has become a worldwide problem. HIV at-taches to the CD4[+] T cell-surface molecule. The CD4[+] T cell is the main target of HIV be-cause CD4[+] T cells express high levels of this surface receptor. After infection, the virus then causes progressive dysfunction and de-struction of the infected cell and the immune system. The disease is devastating because of the elimination of the major cell coordinat-ing immune responses. Monitoring CD4[+] T cell counts is important in the management of HIV infection and AIDS.

B lymphocytes or B cells

B lymphocytes or **B cells** are responsible for the production of immunoglobulins and antibodies. In birds, the **Bursa of Fabricius** serves as the site for development and maturation of these cells. In mammals, the **bone marrow** serves as the equiva-lent site. The term "B cell" is a mnemonic for the

bursal or bone marrow origin of these cells. Dis-tinguishing surface characteristics of B cells are:

- *Surface immunoglobulin.* By definition, B cells synthesize and express both surface and cyto-plasmic immunoglobulin. Immature or pre-B cells express cytoplasmic but not surface im-munoglobulin. Cells that secrete immunoglob-ulin are termed **plasma cells** (Fig. 2-2B). More-over, B cells are specific, i.e., a single B cell produces immunoglobulin of *only one* antibody specificity that recognizes *only one* epitope!
- *Fc receptor (FcR).* The FcR recognizes the Fc portion of the immunoglobulin molecule. It is thought that the FcR binds serum immuno-globulin and serves to concentrate antigen bound by that antibody at the B cell surface.
- *Complement receptors (CR1 and CR2).* These receptors bind activated fragments of comple-ment. **Complement** is a collective term for 20+ serum proteins that act in concert to lyse cells. Complement is discussed in greater de-tail in Chapter 3. CR1 binds fragments of the third (C3) and fourth (C4) components of complement, C3b and C4b, respectively. CR2 binds fragments of C3. At least one pathogen, Epstein-Barr virus (EBV), the cause of infec-tious mononucleosis, specifically binds to CR2.
- *MHC class II molecules.* Like dendritic cells and macrophages, B cells are able to degrade in-gested antigen and "present" fragments on MHC II molecules that can be recognized by the TCR of CD4[+] T cells.

CLINICAL APPLICATION
MONONUCLEOSIS

Infectious *mononucleosis* is caused by the Epstein-Barr virus (EBV) and occurs frequently in young adults. Symptoms of mononucleosis may include fever, sore throat, enlarged lymph nodes, enlarged spleen, and increased lymphocytes. The lymphocytes affected are atypical and primarily activated CD8[+] cyto-toxic T cells. EBV attaches to the CR2 (C3d complement receptor, also known as CD21) cell-surface receptor of the B lymphocyte.

Natural killer cells

T cells (60% to 70%) and B cells (5% to 20%) do not account for all peripheral blood lymphocytes. Large granular non-T, non-B lymphocytes are known as **natural killer** (NK) cells. Because NK cells do not require prior exposure to antigen for their activity, they play an important role in innate immunity. NK cells are thought to be responsible for immunity against virally infected cells and spontaneously arising tumors, thus acting in immune surveillance. They do not express immunoglobulin or T cell receptors, but instead use other means of recognition, including the ability to recognize and kill cells with reduced levels of surface MHC I molecules. Reduced MHC I expression is often caused by some viruses or alterations in control of cell growth. NK cells also express Fc receptors that enable them to recognize and kill foreign cells that have antibody bound to them. This process is called **antibody-dependent cell-mediated cytotoxicity** (ADCC). NK cells are the major cell type mediating this reaction, although other leukocytes, such as eosinophils, macrophages, and neutrophils, can also do so.

Phagocytic mononuclear cells

Phagocytes are found in all multicellular invertebrate animals as they are in all vertebrates. They are the scavengers or garbage collectors of the body, serving a vital housekeeping role and acting as a basic defense against microbial infection. Phagocytic cells internalize cellular debris, foreign cells, and particles and degrade them enzymatically. Although a number of phagocytes perform this vital function, we will be concerned here with only two, macrophages and dendritic cells.

Monocytes/macrophages

Circulating mononuclear phagocytes known as monocytes eventually migrate into the tissues where they are called macrophages (Fig. 2-2C). These phagocytic cells are found in large numbers in the connective tissue, the lung, spleen, liver (where they are also known as Kupffer cells), peritoneal cavity, and gastrointestinal tract. Monocytes/macrophages are morphologically and functionally distinct from lymphocytes. They have the following cell-surface characteristics:

- *FcγR and FcαR*. These surface receptors bind the Fcγ portion of IgG (IgG$_1$ and IgG$_3$ isotypes) and the Fcα portion of IgA molecules that are bound to a microbe or other antigen. Note that monocytes/macrophages do not synthesize immunoglobulin.
- *CR1, CR3, CR4*. These cell-surface receptors bind activated fragments of complement. CR1

binds fragments of the third (C3) and fourth (C4) components of complement; CR3 and CR4 bind incomplete C3b (iC3b).
- *MHC class II*. These molecules "present" peptide fragments to the TCRs of CD4$^+$ T cells.

Macrophages and monocytes engulf molecules by phagocytosis, enzymatically degrade the molecules, and display the degraded material on their cell membranes; this process is called **antigen presentation**. T cells must recognize both processed antigen and an MHC molecule as a necessary initiation step in an adaptive immune response. Cells that display peptide fragments bound by MHC class II molecules (pMHC class II) are called **antigen-presenting cells** (APCs).

Dendritic Cells

Dendritic cells are named for their tree branch-like projections (Fig. 2-2D). Like macrophages, dendritic cells sample their environment for foreign cells by phagocytosis. Unlike macrophages, dendritic cells constitutively sample the extracellular fluid by **macropinocytosis**. Unlike macrophages and B cells, dendritic cells are the only APCs known to induce the activation of resting (naïve) T cells and, thus, they are important in the activation of an adaptive immune response.

Granulocytes

Granular leukocytes contain cytoplasmic granules that are readily discernable by light microscopy. Granulocytes have multilobed nuclei and cytoplasmic granules that contain amines (stained by basic dyes), basic proteins (stained by acidophilic or eosinophilic dyes), or both (neutral staining). As a group, granulocytes include both the most numerous (neutrophils) and least numerous (basophils and eosinophils) of the leukocytes found in the blood.

Polymorphonuclear cells

Polymorphonuclear (PMN) cells, also known as **neutrophils**, comprise approximately 60% of blood leukocytes (3,000 to 6,000 per μl) in peripheral blood. They are 10 to 12 μm in diameter. Approximately 100 billion PMNs enter the circulation daily in normal adults. Characteristically, PMNs have cytoplasmic granules and multisegmented nuclei. The number of nuclear lobes reflects the maturational state of the cell (Fig. 2-2E). PMNs arise in the bone marrow and early stages have an elongated nucleus, often referred to as a "band form." Constrictions occur in the nucleus as the cell matures, resulting first in bilobed nuclei and, eventually, nuclei of up to five lobes or segments. PMNs contain smaller, so-called specific granules and larger, reddish purple staining azurophil cytoplasmic granules. The specific granules have little affinity for either basic or acidic dyes and stain a neutral color. They contain lysozyme, collagenase, and lactoferrin. The less numerous azurophilic granules contain anti-microbial enzymes such as myeloperoxidase, lysozyme, and defensins as well as acid hydro-lases. PMNs serve as the first line of defense in microbial infection and their numbers increase rapidly in response to infection. Accumulation of living and dead PMNs at the site of infection is known as *pus*.

Basophils and mast cells

Basophils account for less than 0.5% of blood-borne leukocytes. **Mast cells** are similar to basophils in many aspects but are morphologically distinct. Both cell types are thought to derive from a common hematopoietic bone marrow precursor. Basophils are 10 to 12 μm in diameter and have a characteristic bilobed nucleus that is nearly obscured by purple-staining or basophilic cytoplasmic granules (Fig. 2-2F). Mast cells are 10 to 15 μm and are generally round, oval, or spindle-shaped with numerous surface projections. First, free IgE molecules (not bound to antigen) must bind by the Fc region to high affinity receptors (Fc$_\varepsilon$RI) expressed exclusively on basophils and mast cells. Then, the crosslinking of receptor-bound IgE antibody by antigen, i.e., an allergen, causes receptor aggregation that leads to degranulation and release of the vasoactive amines. Mast cell or basophil degranulation is involved in the development of allergic reactions to common substances such as pollen and pet dander.

Eosinophils

Mature **eosinophils** are slightly larger than PMNs, with a diameter of 12 to 17 μm. The nucleus is bilobed and the cytoplasmic granules readily stain with acidic dyes such as eosin, giving the cell its name (Fig 2-2G). Basic proteins within the granules, such as major basic protein (MBP), eosinophil cationic protein (ECP), eosinophil-derived neurotoxin (EDN), and eosinophil peroxidase (EPO), serve as potent agents in resistance to

infection by parasitic worms. It is not surprising that eosinophils are commonly found at the sites of parasitic infection.

> **CLINICAL APPLICATION**
> **EOSINOPHILIA**
>
> *Eosinophilia* occurs when the eosinophil count is greater than 700 cells/μl. Some common causes of eosinophilia include neoplasms, Addison's disease, allergy, asthma, drug allergy, collagen vascular diseases, and parasites.

> **Patient Vignette 2.1**
>
> Seepa M., a 43-year old female immigrant from Southeast Asia, worries that she may have tapeworms.
>
> *Elevated levels of which type of white blood cell may help to diagnose tapeworm infection?*
>
> *Taenia solium*, the pork tapeworm, is prevalent in many areas including Southeast Asia, Mexico, and Africa. Patients with intestinal infection of this tapeworm may be asymptomatic or complain of nonspecific epigastric discomfort. The diagnosis is made by detecting the presence of eggs or proglottids in the stool. Also, eosinophils often increase in number and are found in association with tissues containing parasites. Eosinophils and IgE are the main components of the immune defense in response to parasitic infection.

IMMUNE ORGANS

Lymphoid tissues can be classified as organs (thymus, spleen, and lymph nodes) and lymphoid accumulations (Peyer's patches and lymphocytes within the lamina propria, etc.). Lymphoid organs are classified as **primary lymphoid organs and secondary lymphoid organs**. Differentiation occurs within a primary organ. Mature T and B cells are generated and develop within primary organs, the thymus and bone marrow, respectively. The secondary lymphoid organs, lymph nodes, and lymphoid accumulations trap and concentrate immunogens and provide a site where large numbers of immune cells can make contact with each another. Specific immune reactions are actually initiated in secondary lymphoid organs.

Thymus

The bilobed **thymus** is the first lymphoid organ to develop during ontogeny. It increases in size during fetal and neonatal life and progressively involutes following puberty. The organization and trafficking of cells through the thymus is shown in Fig. 2-4A. Stem cells called prothymocytes, derived from the bone marrow and committed to the T cell lineage, migrate via the circulation to the thymic cortex. In this new environment, they are called **cortical thymocytes**. Subsequently, they migrate through the cortico-medullary border into the medulla where they mature. Mature thymocytes enter the circulation and are known as T cells. It

takes about 3 days for a prothymocyte to mature into a T cell and in the process they learn to distinguish nonself from self. Tremendous numbers of cells go through this process in the thymus, but less than 5% of the thymocytes successfully complete this process. This process of "thymic education" is more fully described in Chapter 5. The thymus is highly active at birth and continues to grow until puberty. After puberty, the thymus begins to involute and becomes progressively inactive.

Spleen

The *spleen*, the largest lymphoid organ, clears particulate matter from the blood and concentrates

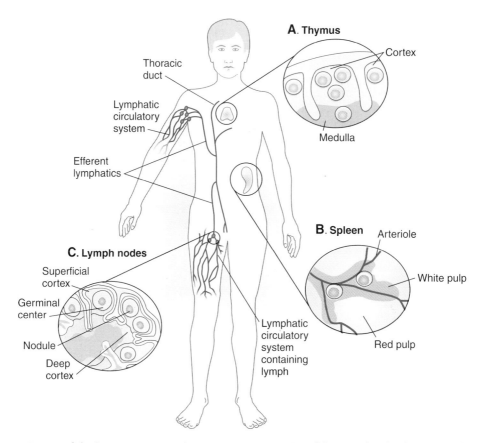

FIGURE 2-4. Organs of the immune system. Diagrammatic representation of the major lymphoid organs in relationship to the body. **(A)** The *thymus*. Prothymocytes originating in the bone marrow migrate via the circulation to the cortex of the thymus, where they encounter specialized dendritic cells. It is here that these cortical thymocytes acquire the ability to distinguish self from nonself. The entire maturational process takes 3 to 5 days, and less than 5% successfully "learn" in this process of thymic education (Chapter 5). **(B)** The *spleen*. Lymphocytes are located around small arteries and arterioles and, because this area is relatively erythrocyte-free, it is called the white pulp. **(C)** *Lymph node*. Lymph nodes are leukocyte accumulations surrounding lymphatic vessels. They function to filter the lymph and both clear the lymph (the fluid contained within the lymphatic vessel) of debris and sample it for the presence of nonself substances. Lymph enters via afferent lymphatics, percolates through the B cell-rich cortex, then the T cell-rich deep cortex, and finally through the medulla prior to exiting the node via the efferent lymphatic circulation. The efferent lymphatics join with the thoracic duct, and the contents of the thoracic duct empty into the subclavian vein, where the lymph enters the circulation.

blood-borne antigens and microbes. It is histologically divided into the lymphocyte-rich **white pulp** and erythrocyte-rich **red pulp** (Fig. 2-4B). Lymphocytes are concentrated around small arteries and arterioles. Immediately surrounding the arteriole is a thymic-dependent area of diffuse B cell-rich lymphoid tissue. The thymic-independent area surrounds the thymic-dependent area and is T cell-rich.

Lymph nodes

Lymph nodes, small round or oval-shaped peripheral or secondary lymphoid organs, are leukocyte accumulations occurring periodically throughout the lymphatic circulatory system (Fig. 2-4C). They function as filters to purify **lymph**, the fluid and cellular content of the lymphatic circulatory system, and as sites for initiation of the immune response. Anatomically, the node is divided into the cortex and medulla. The **reticulum** or framework of the organ is composed of phagocytes and specialized kinds of reticular or dendritic cells. Lymphocytes are distributed mainly in two areas of the cortex. The **superficial cortex** is closely packed with clusters of lymphocytes forming **nodules** or **follicles**. It is sometimes called the thymus-independent area and contains mostly B cells. When an immune response takes place, the follicles develop a central area with large proliferating cells, termed a **germinal center**. The **deep cortex** is the T cell-rich area.

> ### CLINICAL APPLICATION
> ### ENLARGED LYMPH NODES
>
> Common causes of enlarged lymph nodes include infections and cancer. The enlargement is due to the high rate of cell proliferation within the nodes.

Other lymphoid accumulations

Lymphocytes, plasma cells, dendritic cells, and macrophages are often found at potential portals of microbial entry. Included are the **tonsils** that form a ring around the nasopharynx, the **appendix** at the ilio-cecal junction, and **Peyer's patches** found in the submucosa of the small intestine. Additional diffuse accumulations are found in the lamina propria of the small intestine. Also, leukocytes transiently accumulate at the sites of microbial invasion as part of the process of inflammation (Chapter 3).

LEUKOCYTE TRAFFICKING AND ANTIGEN TRAPPING

Lymphocyte trafficking

Lymphatics comprise a network of vessels and nodes that parallels the blood circulation and contains lymph. The lymph enters nodes via the **afferent lymphatic vessels**, and exits via the **efferent lymphatic vessels**. The lymph eventually drains into the major lymphatic vessels, such as the thoracic duct and the right lymphatic duct, which, in turn, empty into the venous circulation. The node is the major area where blood-borne lymphocytes cross into the lymphatic circulation. T cells enter primarily through the arterial circulation and adhere to the **postcapillary venules** in the deep cortex of the node. The postcapillary endothelial cells are tall and bear special surface proteins that facilitates the passage of lymphocytes through the blood vessel wall and into the lymph node. A typical lymphocyte recirculates through the deep cortex for about one day and exits through the efferent lymphatic vessel. About 95% of the lymphocytes in an unstimulated node are derived from the blood circulation and are not formed in situ.

Dendritic cell trafficking

Immature dendritic cells serve as sentinels of the immune system and express a number of pattern-recognition receptors (Chapter 1). Immature dendritic cells are located in the skin, where they efficiently sample their environment by both macropinocytosis and phagocytosis. Those located in the stratum spinosum of the skin are known as Langerhans cells. Unlike other APCs, immature dendritic cells display only small amounts of MHC class II on molecules on their cell surface. The binding of an antigen to an immature dendritic cell provides a maturation signal that causes the cell to decrease or cease its phagocytic activity and increase surface MHC class II. The now mature dendritic cell migrates through the tissue and/or lymphatic circulation to the closest (downstream) lymph node, where it takes up residence and displays its antigenic fragments, together with MHC class II, to both resident and transient T cells.

Antigen trapping

Antigens are trapped in either the sinuses or deep cortex by the lymph node reticular cells or by cells that migrate to the lymph node. This is an important step in the induction of immune responses. Most of the antigen taken up by dendritic cells or macrophages is enzymatically digested, but some molecules escape total breakdown and are used to interact with lymphocytes.

As soon as antigen is taken up by dendritic cells within a lymph node, inductive events occur whereby lymphocytes recognize and interact with some of the trapped antigen molecules. Within 24 hours of this interaction, the number of lymphocytes leaving the node markedly decreases. Presumably, lymphocytes keep entering the node from the postcapillary venules.

Two to 5 days later, lymphocytes leaving the node *increasing* in number, and more lymphocytes enter the node from the postcapillary venules. Lymphocytes that are specifically reactive with the antigen *remain* in the node. The cellularity of the node increases, which often results in swelling (a sign that the physician looks for during physical diagnosis). Lymphocyte proliferation becomes abundant in the deep cortex and the first antibody-containing cells appear in the deep and superficial cortex. Development of the superficial cortex proceeds and germinal centers become evident. The germinal centers and interfollicular areas are abundant with plasma cells.

After another 5 days (8 to 11 days total elapsed time), total numbers of cells leaving the node are reduced. However, lymphocytes that have reacted with the antigen (called **primed** or **activated** cells) now leave the node and are disseminated throughout the tissues.

Summary

- Five morphologically distinct **leukocytes** are commonly found in the circulation and may be classified as **granular** (containing cytoplasmic granules—polymorphonuclear cells, basophils, and eosinophils) or **agranular** cells (lymphocytes and monocytes).
- Cell surface molecules that are useful in distinguishing leukocytes include immunoglobulin, cluster of differentiation molecules, receptors, and major histocompatibility complex (MHC) molecules.
- **Immunoglobulin** molecules have a basic paired structure containing two identical light chains and two identical heavy chains, linked by disulfide bonds.
- Leukocyte subpopulations express a wide variety of cell-surface proteins depending upon their functional or developmental stage, referred to as **cluster of differentiation** (CD).
- All nucleated cells of the body express **MHC class I molecules** that are markers of self.
- Dendritic cells, monocytes, and certain lymphocyte populations constitutively express **MHC class II molecules**.
- **T lymphocytes** regulate and mediate immune responses. T cells express antigen-specific T cell receptors. Mature T cells express CD4 or CD8 molecules and immature thymocytes simultaneously express both CD4 and CD8 molecules.
- **B lymphocytes** are responsible for the production of immunoglobulins. Distinguishing surface characteristics of B cells are surface immunoglobulin, Fc receptors, cell surface receptors, and MHC class II molecules.
- **Natural killer cells** are large, granular non-T, non-B lymphocytes and are thought to be responsible for immunity against virally-infected cells and spontaneously arising tumors.
- **Antibody-dependent cell-mediated cytotoxicity** is a process where cells have receptors that recognize and kill foreign cells that have antibody bound to them.
- Phagocytic cells (macrophages/monocytes) internalize cellular debris, foreign cells, and particles and degrade them enzymatically.
- Granulocytes include **neutrophils, basophils**, and **eosinophils**. Neutrophils (or polymorphonuclear cells) have cytoplasmic granules and multisegmented nuclei. Eosinophils have cytoplasmic granules that readily stain with acidic dyes such as eosin and bilobed nuclei. Basophils have a bilobed nucleus with basophilic cytoplasmic granules.
- Lymphoid tissues can be classified as organs (thymus, spleen, and lymph nodes) and lymphoid accumulations (Peyer's patches and lymphocytes within the lamina propria). The thymus is the first lymphoid organ to develop during development.
- The **spleen**, the largest lymphoid organ, clears particulate matter from the blood and concentrates blood-borne antigens and microbes. It is histologically divided into the lymphocyte-rich white pulp and erythrocyte-rich red pulp.

- The **lymph nodes** (secondary lymphoid organs) function as filters to purify lymph, the fluid and cellular content of the lymphatic circulatory system, and as sites for initiation of the immune response.
- Immature **dendritic cells** are located within the dermis, where they efficiently sample their environment by both macropincytosis and phagocytosis.

Suggested readings

Crivellato E, Vacca A, Ribatti D. Setting the stage: An anatomist's view of the immune system. *Trends Immunol* 2004;25:210.

Ross MH, Kaye GI, Pawlina W. Blood. In *Histology, a text and atlas*, 4th ed. Philadelphia: Lippincott Williams & Wilkins, 2003.

Ross MH, Kaye GI, Pawlina W. Lymphatic system. In *Histology, a text and atlas*, 4th ed. Philadelphia: Lippincott Williams & Wilkins, 2003.

Théry C, Amigorena S. The cell biology of antigen presentation in dendritic cells. *Curr Opin Immunol* 2001;1313:45.

Review questions

DIRECTIONS: Each of the numbered items or incomplete statements in this section is followed by answers or by completions of the statement. Select the ONE lettered answer or completion that is BEST in each case.

1. Mast cells are similar to:
   (A) eosinophils
   (B) basophils
   (C) neutrophils
   (D) lymphocytes

2. The largest lymphoid organ is the:
   (A) thymus
   (B) spleen
   (C) lymph node
   (D) Peyer's patch

3. The precursors of active immunoglobulin-secreting cells are the:
   (A) B cells
   (B) T cells
   (C) plasma cells
   (D) mast cells

4. Natural killer (NK) cells identify target cells for destruction by assessing:
   (A) whether they express sufficient amounts of self MHC I molecules
   (B) whether they express foreign antigens
   (C) the presence of CD4 or CD8 on their surface
   (D) whether or not they are secreting histamine

5. T and B lymphocytes can be distinguished from one another
   (A) visually by size, B lymphocytes being larger

   (B) by the type of nucleus, T lymphocytes having multilobed nuclei
   (C) by the presence or absence of cell surface molecules such as immunoglobulin or CD3
   (D) by granularity of the cytoplasm, B lymphocytes being granular

6. Antibody-dependent cellular cytotoxicity (ADCC) results in the death of invasive organisms coated by antibodies. This function is performed by:
   (A) T lymphocytes
   (B) natural killer cells
   (C) neutrophils
   (D) mast cells

7. Wendy C., a 12-year-old girl, develops symptoms of sneezing, runny nose, and itchy eyes when she is near cats. This patient has symptoms consistent with allergic rhinitis due to cat dander. Which of the following is true?
   (A) Crosslinking of receptor-bound IgE antibody by the allergen (cat dander) activates neutrophils.
   (B) Crosslinking of receptor-bound IgE antibody by the allergen (cat dander) activates mast cells
   (C) Crosslinking of receptor-bound IgG antibody by the allergen (cat dander) activates neutrophils.
   (D) Crosslinking of receptor-bound IgG antibody by the allergen (cat dander) activates mast cells.

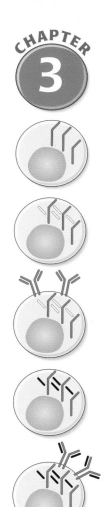

The Innate Immune Response

Introduction We live in a microbe-filled world. Bacteria, viruses, fungi, and protozoa live in close proximity to our skin and mucous membranes, in varying degrees. For the most part, these microorganisms are innocuous and, in some cases, beneficial in providing an essential symbiotic relationship with our bodies. However, a microbe that crosses the skin or mucus membranes and "sets up housekeeping" within the body is another matter entirely, causing a pathological condition—an infection. Most microbes reproduce rapidly and would quickly overwhelm the body in the time that it takes to develop an antigen-specific adaptive immune response. Fortunately, we have an initial immune barrier called the **innate immune system** that responds rapidly to infection and can provide protection while antigen-specific lymphocytes prepare to act. Among our defense forces, the elements of the innate system are the rapidly mobilized forces that rush to meet the enemy at the gates. This system utilizes a limited number of germline-encoded receptors that recognize **conserved molecules** (molecules commonly expressed by a large number of species) produced by microbes, but not by host cells. **Pattern recognition receptors** (PRRs) on host cells and certain soluble molecules can recognize **pathogen-**

associated molecular patterns (PAMPs), with profound consequences. The first is the activation of phagocytic cells and soluble molecules leading to **inflammation** that serves to contain and destroy the
infectious agents. The second is participation in the induction of adaptive immune responses. Innate (sometimes called nonspecific) immune responses are generally initiated without the engagement of the
antigen-specific lymphocytes. Innate responses differ from the lym-
phocyte-based **adaptive** (or **specific**) **immune responses** in several important ways. In normal individuals, cells and molecules of the innate
system are constitutively activated or can be rapidly induced or activated upon encounter with a microbe. In addition, innate immune responses are an important step leading to the induction of adaptive immunity. Thus, innate responses begin almost immediately (within
minutes to hours) after infection, unlike adaptive responses that require days to weeks to develop.

PRRs are expressed by more than one cell
type. In contrast, antigen-specific receptors of
the adaptive immune system are generated by
DNA rearrangement so that each T or B lymphocyte (and its descendants) expresses multiple
copies of a unique T cell receptor (TCR) or B
cell receptors (BCR). Unlike adaptive immune
responses, innate responses do not increase
upon repeated microbial exposure, nor does the
innate system display recall or memory responses. Recall or memory immune responses
are solely a property of B and T lymphocytes in
adaptive responses.

PHYSICAL, CHEMICAL, AND MECHANICAL BARRIERS OF THE INNATE IMMUNE SYSTEM

The initial protective and nonspecific devices of
the body are the barriers that guard its interface
with the environment (Fig. 3-1). These include
the skin; the mucous membranes of the gastrointestinal, respiratory, and urogenital tracts; and
other membranous surfaces (e.g., the eye). The
skin and mucous membranes of the body actually
comprise a vast surface area that is potentially
available for pathogenic invasion, but they also
contain a variety of protective mechanisms to
minimize or prevent entry of potential pathogenic organisms into the body. In our military
analogy, these are the moats, walls, and mine
fields of the immune system.

The skin is nearly waterproof, enabling the
relatively fluid human body to exist in dry air
without dehydration, and to be immersed in
fresh water without swelling and in salt water
without shrinking. The skin also provides a
highly resistant barrier to invasive microbes.
The outer layer of the **epidermis** continuously
sloughs dead cells and microbes associated with
them. The **keratinocytes** of the epidermis provide a waterproof barrier that effectively inhibits entry of microbes except when breached
by damage that might expose underlying cells
and tissues. The **sebaceous glands** of the dermal layer of the skin secrete **sebum** that contains **lactic acid**, and a variety of fatty acids
whose low pH gives them a microcidal activity.
In addition, skin secretions and mucosal
surfaces contain microcidal molecules such as
β-defensins, small proteins that kill microbes
by disrupting their membranes. So effective are
these molecules are that laboratory personnel
wear protective gloves to prevent direct skin
contact from affecting biochemical or molecular
procedures. Finally, the skin is populated by an
extensive colony of harmless microbes whose

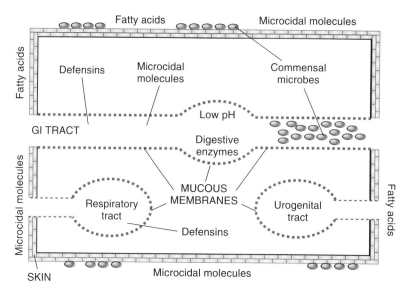

FIGURE 3-1. Mechanical, chemical, and biological barriers of the innate immune system. Mechanical barriers include the skin and mucous membranes. Chemical barriers include microcidal molecules, fatty acids, and the low pH of the stomach. Commensal microbes on the skin and in the gut act as biological barriers to colonization by new and potentially harmful microbial populations.

presence deters colonization by more pathogenic microbes.

Mucosal surfaces consist of moist epithelium and present a formidable challenge for the body. They must allow the secretion and absorption of molecules but at the same time resist microbial invasion. The gastrointestinal tract defends against infection in a variety of ways. The oral cavity and stomach contain digestive enzymes that can destroy many potential pathogens, as can the low pH of the stomach. Some epithelial cells of the intestine secrete microcidal molecules such as **α-defensins** and **cryptidins**. Like the skin, the gastrointestinal tract is also normally colonized by a variety of commensal microbes. This microbial population assists in the digestive process, but also discourages the establishment of more harmful microbes.

> **CLINICAL APPLICATION**
> **PSEUDOMEMBRANOUS COLITIS**
>
> *Pseudomembranous colitis* is a condition caused by *Clostridium difficile*, a bacterium that colonizes in the gastrointestinal tract. Patients with this disease have symptoms of watery diarrhea, abdominal cramps, and fever. The disease may occur during or following a course of broad-spectrum antibi-

> **CLINICAL APPLICATION (Continued)**
> otics. The underlying cause of this disease is complex. However, one explanation is that the antibiotics suppress the normal bacteria of the gastrointestinal tract. This permits the overgrowth by the *Clostridium difficile*, which produces a toxin that causes damage to the gastrointestinal tract.

The respiratory tract is protected by mucous secretions in the nasal and bronchial passages that entrap inhaled particles and microbes. The ciliary action of the epithelia lining these passages moves the secretions outward for expulsion by coughing and sneezing. Some cells of the respiratory epithelium also secrete microcidal molecules (β-defensins) and a variety of other molecules in the mucous that can attach to microbes and render them more susceptible to ingestion and destruction by phagocytic cells.

> **CLINICAL APPLICATION**
> **CYSTIC FIBROSIS**
>
> **Cystic fibrosis** (CF) is a common, fatal genetic disorder attributed to a defective gene product that interferes with the normal chloride ion permeability. This defect leads to thickened and viscous secretions in the respiratory tract. The secretions obstruct

(continued)   *(continued)*

The eyes and urogenital tract are protected by mechanical and chemical barriers. The eyes are protected, in part, through constant washing by **lysozyme**-containing secretions of the lacrymal glands. Lysozyme is an enzyme that hydrolyzes peptidoglycan molecules found in the cell walls of most bacteria. Urination helps inhibit movement of microbes from the environment up the urinary tract and into the bladder and kidneys. The acidic fluids of the vaginal tract also inhibit microbial growth.

Phagocytic cells also participate in innate immunity. Phagocytic cells that detect invasive microbes and act against these infectious organisms, both directly and indirectly, protect the skin, mucosal surfaces, and their underlying tissues. These include **dendritic cells**, **macrophages**, **mast cells**, and **neutrophils**. The broad antimicrobial activity of these cells is augmented by a group of highly specialized defense molecules that comprise the **complement system**. Certain complement components recognize and bind microbial-associated molecules and initiate a sequence of enzymatic steps that lead to the destruction of the microbes. We will return to the complement system later in this chapter.

INNATE RECOGNITION BY MEMBRANE-BOUND RECEPTORS

A wide range of organisms, including plants, use PRRs to recognize and counter infectious agents. Among the PRRs are a set of receptors known as the **toll-like receptors** (TLRs). Their name is derived from their structural relationship to a protein named "toll" (from the German for *great!* or *super!*) that was originally discovered in the fruit fly *Drosophila melanogaster*. At least ten different TLRs have been identified in humans, and their cellular distribution and binding specificities are given in Table 3-1. TLRs contain structural motifs that bind a diverse range of viral, bacterial, and fungal components. Which TLRs are bound is determined by the type of microbe encountered. Some TLRs also recognize molecules produced by host cells in response to stress or damage by, for example, infection.

Binding of a TLR triggers cells that participate in some aspect of inflammation. TLRs are found on phagocytic cells such as macrophages and dendritic cells that ingest and degrade microbes; on mast cells that produce many soluble molecules that promote inflammation; and on some types of epithelial cells. Some are even found on B lymphocytes that can bind and ingest microbes and cellular debris prior to becoming involved in adaptive immune responses and the secretion of immunoglobulins. TLR binding activates several pathways of cytoplasmic signaling that lead to changes in nuclear gene transcription and a subsequent alteration in cell activity called **activation**.

Activated phagocytes: macrophages and dendritic cells

Activated macrophages and dendritic cells are characterized by increases in size and in the rate of production of degradative enzymes and microcidal molecules. The rate at which they seek and destroy microbes is also increased (Fig. 3-2). In addition, they begin to secrete a range of soluble molecules called cytokines and chemokines that attract and activate other cells involved in innate immune responses (Table 3-2). Some cytokines [e.g., interleukin-1 (IL-1) and interleukin-6 (IL-6)], induce production of protective proteins by the liver and cause metabolic changes leading to elevated body temperature. Others such as Tumor necrosis factor-α (TNF-α) and interleukin-1 (IL-1) affect the local vascular epithelium to increase its permeability, permitting cells and soluble molecules to move from the vasculature into the tissues. Still others such as interleukin-8 (IL-8) and interleukin-12 (IL-12) attract and activate cells such as neutrophils and natural killer cells.

In addition to TLRs, most phagocytic cells also bear receptors that recognize molecules that bind to the microbial cell surface, thus "tagging" them for destruction. When such receptors are used to increase the phagocytic destruction of microbes or other material, the process is known as **opsonization**. The presence of an opsonin on a microbe makes it more "attractive" to phagocytic cells, and the ensuing ingestion of microbes

TABLE 3-1. HUMAN TOLL-LIKE RECEPTORS (TLRS)

	Expressed on	Recognizes and binds	Found on
TLR1	Monocytes/macrophages Dendritic cell subset B lymphocytes	Multiple tri-acyl lipopeptides	Bacteria
TLR2	Monocytes/macrophages Subset of dendritic cells Mast cells	Multiple glycolipids Multiple lipopeptides Multiple lipoproteins Lipotechonic acid Peptidoglycan HSP70 Zymosan Numerous other molecules	Bacteria Bacteria Bacteria Bacteria Gram$^+$ bacteria Host cells Fungi
TLR3	Dendritic cells B lymphocytes	Viral DNA (double-stranded)	Viruses
TLR4	Monocytes/macrophages Dendritic cell subset Mast cells Intestinal epithelium	Lipopolysacharide Several heat shock proteins Fibrinogen (host cell product) Heparan sulfate fragments Hyaluronic acid fragments Numerous other molecules	Gram$^-$ bacteria Bacterial/host cells Host cells Host cells Host cells
TLR5	Monocytes/macrophages Dendritic cell subset Intestinal epithelium	Flagellin	Bacteria
TLR6	Monocytes/macrophages Mast cells B lymphocytes	Multiple lipopeptides (di-acyl)	Mycoplasma
TLR7	Monocytes/macrophages Dendritic cell subset B lymphocytes	Imidezoquinoline Loxoribine Bropirimine	Synthetic compound Synthetic compound Synthetic compound
TLR8	Monocytes/macrophages Dendritic cell subset Mast cells	Unknown	Unknown
TLR9	Monocytes/macrophages Dendritic cell subset B lymphocytes	CgG motif of bacterial DNA	Bacteria
TLR10	Monocytes/macrophages B lymphocytes	Unknown	Unknown

through opsoniztion can activate the phagocytic cells and increase their activity.

Natural killer (NK) cells

Most cells of the innate system use receptors that detect pathogen-encoded molecules. NK cells, on the other hand, use a recognition mechanism that detects alterations in host cells that are induced by infection or transformation. Although NK cells do not have receptors generated by genetic recombination like B and T lymphocytes, they are able to determine whether cells are of self or foreign origin. The exact nature of NK receptors is not fully understood; however, several types of NK recognition are known that allow them to use several mechanisms for recognizing target cells to be killed (Fig. 3-3A). First, NK cells recognize antibody-coated cells through a low-affinity receptor (CD16, App. B). NK cells lyse antibody-coated targets by **antibody-dependent cell-mediated cytotoxicity** (ADCC), a process that is addressed in Chapter 5. Second, NK cells express type 3 and type 4 complement receptors (CR3 and CR4, respectively) that recognize and bind to membrane-bound C3b (see "Complement," below). Third, certain NK receptors recognize "stress-induced" proteins [e.g., heat shock proteins (HSPs), adhesion molecules, etc.] that are found on normal cells but are rapidly increased in cells subjected to a pathologic insult or transformation.

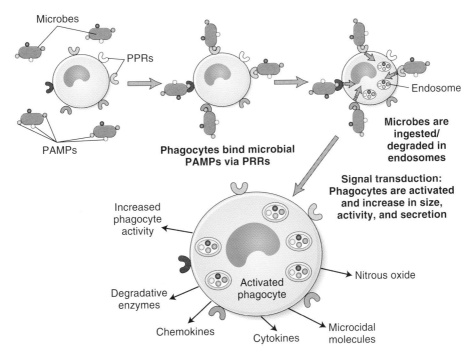

FIGURE 3-2. Activation of phagocytic cells through binding of PRRs. Binding of PRRs to PAMPs on microbial cells stimulate phagocytes to become activated, increasing their size, phagocytic activity, production of antimicrobial substances, and production of cytokines and chemokines to attract and activate other components of the immune system.

A fourth way by which NK cells distinguish normal cells from infected or transformed cells is by monitoring the amount of surface MHC class I molecules (Fig. 3-3B). In an apparent attempt at stealth and infiltration, some infectious organisms, upon entry into host cells, decrease MHC class I expression by those cells, trying to evade immune recognition by the adaptive immune response. Likewise, in some malignant transformations, cancer cells also decrease their MHC class I expression. NK cells bear a **killer activation receptor** (KAR), called *NKG2D* in humans, that recognizes and binds certain molecules (called *MICAs* and *MICBs* in humans) that appear on cells that are undergoing stress such as infection, malignant transformation, etc. This binding provides a "kill signal" that will induce the NK cell to kill the target cell. However, once contact is made with the stressed target cells, NK cells use a second set of receptors, the **killer inhibitory receptors** (KIRs), to examine the target cell surface for the expression and levels of self MHC class I molecules. If the KIRs locate and bind sufficient MHC class I molecules on the target cell surface, the "kill

TABLE 3-2. CYTOKINES AND CHEMOKINES OF THE INNATE IMMUNE RESPONSE PRODUCED BY ACTIVATED PHAGOCYTES

Cytokine/Chemokine	Acts on	Causes
Interleukin-1 (IL-1)	Vascular endothelium	Increased permeability of vascular endothelium Stimulates production of IL-6
Interleukin-6 (IL-6)	Liver	Production of acute phase proteins (e.g., C-reactive protein); elevated temperature (fever)
Interleukin-8 (IL-8)	Vascular endothelium	Activation of vascular endothelium Attraction/activation of neutrophils
Interleukin-12 (IL-12)	NK cells	Activates NK cells Influences lymphocyte differentiation
Tumor necrosis factor-α (TNF-α)	Vascular endothelium	Increased permeability of vascular endothelium Activation of vascular endothelium

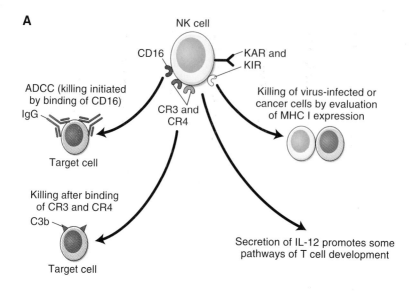

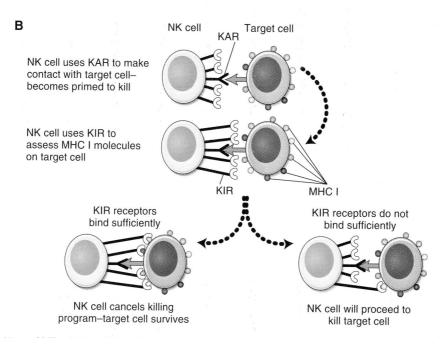

FIGURE 3-3. Natural killer (NK) cells. (A) NK cells use a variety of receptors to identify target cells to be killed. These include Fc receptors, complement receptors, and receptors that assess the MHC I molecules present on target cells. In addition, NK cells can influence the development of T cells in the initiation of adaptive immune responses. **(B)** NK cells utilize killer activation receptors (KARs) to recognize cells undergoing stress. Once engaged, KARs activate the NK cell to kill the target. Killer inhibitory receptors (KIRs) "examine" the target for sufficient levels of "self" MHC I molecules. If KIRs are sufficiently engaged, the killing program is terminated. If not, killing of the target cell proceeds.

signal" is overridden to prevent the killing of the target cells. NK cytotoxic activity is augmented in the presence of type I interferons, interferon-α (IFN-α), and interferon-β (IFN-β) produced by virally infected cells and by cytokines such as IL-12 produced by phagocytic cells activated by the presence of infectious agents (Table 3-2).

Type I interferons produced by infected cells

Some virally infected cells detect the presence of the foreign viral nucleic acids and respond by increasing secretion of type I interferons, IFN-α and IFN-β. Type I IFNs also stimulate synthesis of host cell proteins that can inhibit viral replication. In addition, IFN-α and IFN-β are secreted by infected cells and bound by receptors of neighboring uninfected cells. In doing so, the uninfected cells respond by increasing their production of host cell products that help resist infection. They spread the alarm that hostile invaders have struck. Lysis of infected cells by NK cells is also amplified in the presence of IFN-α and IFN-β.

Patient Vignette 3.1

Robert M. has come down with the latest strain of influenza to sweep through the nation. He became infected two days ago, and his innate immune system is providing him some level of protection until his adaptive response rises to protective levels. Some of his infected cells have begun to produce IFN-α and IFN-β.

What do these molecules induce the uninfected neighboring cells to produce?

Interferon-α and IFN-β stimulate the production of molecules that inhibit viral replication both within themselves and in neighboring uninfected cells, as well as stimulating NK cells to seek and kill virally infected cells.

COMPLEMENT: INNATE RECOGNITION BY SOLUBLE MOLECULES

Rapid responses by cellular components of the innate immune system can occur only after those cells encounter a pathogen. What happens if a pathogen evades contact with cells of the innate system? **Complement** provides a soluble means of defense. The complement system is a complex set of enzymes and nonenzymatic proteins that provide essential functions for both innate and adaptive immunity. Once activated, components of the classical, alternative, or MBL pathways interact serially to destroy microbes by damaging their membranes, increase phagocytosis of microbes, and attract and activate other cells and molecules of the immune system to the site of infection. Complement can be activated in three different ways:

- Antigen-antibody complexes and certain negatively charged structures initiate the **classical pathway.**

- Several molecules commonly found on microbial surfaces activate the **alternative pathway.**
- Particular carbohydrate structures on microbes initiate the **mannan-binding lectin (MBL) pathway.**

The classical pathway, because of its activation by antigen-antibody complexes, is an adjunct to the adaptive immune response and is covered in detail in Chapter 4. The alternative and MBL pathways are integral to the innate immune response.

Mannan-binding lectin (MBL) pathway

Recognition

As a member of the collectin family of proteins, MBL recognizes carbohydrate structures through its carbohydrate-recognition domain (CRD). MBL binds to a variety of microbial carbohydrate structures, including glucans, lipophosphoglycans, and glycoinositol-phospholipids with terminal mannose, glucose, fucose, or N-acetyl-glucosamine hexoses. When MBL binds to one of these carbohydrates, it can then interact with an enzyme called MBL-activated serine protease (MASP).

Enzymatic activation

Activation of MASP: This leads to enzymatic activation of sequential complement components that constitute the MBL pathway of complement activation (Fig. 3-4).

Activation of C4: The MBL/MASP complex cleaves C4 into a small fragment (C4a) and a larger fragment (C4b). It is important to realize that C4b binds to the microbial membrane.

Activation of C2: The MBL/MASP complex cleaves C2 into a small fragment (C2a) and a larger fragment (C2b) and C2b binds to C4b.

Activation of C3: C4b2b, a C3 convertase, is formed by the activation of C4 and C2 and readily cleaves C3 into C3a and C3b. Although some C3b binds to the C4b2b complex, most of the C3b binds directly to the microbial cell surface. C3 convertase acts as an amplification loop, generating chemoattractant fragments (C3a) and membrane adherent (C3b) fragments. C3a acts as a soluble signal, drawing neutrophils and other leukocytes to the site of infection. C3b acts as an opsonin, tagging the microbial cell for ingestion by phagocytic cells bearing receptors for membrane-bound C3b.

Activation of C5: The combination of C4b2b and C3b forms C4b2b3b, a C5 convertase that cleaves C5 into C5a and C5b.

Terminal or lytic pathway

The fixation or attachment of C5b to biological membranes initiates a rapid sequence of events leading to formation of the **membrane attack complex** (MAC) and lysis of the cell. This **terminal or lytic sequence** can be entered from the MBL, classical (Chapter 4), or alternative pathways.

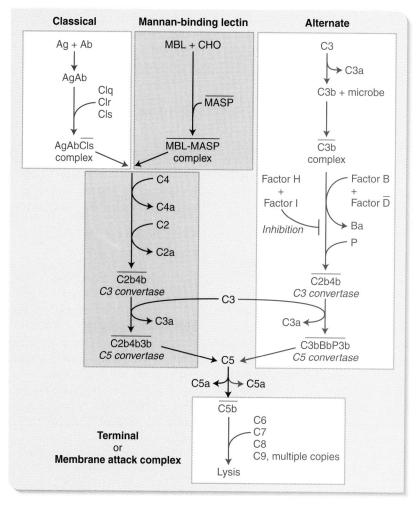

FIGURE 3-4. The mannan-binding lectin (MBL) pathway of complement activation. Binding of mannan on microbial membranes by MBL triggers the serial activation of complement components C4, C2, and C3 to produce a C3 convertase, a C5 convertase, and C3b.

Assembly of the membrane attack complex

C5b, whether produced as a result of the MBL, alternative, or classical pathway, forms a stable macromolecular complex serving as the building block for the remaining complement components (Fig. 3-5). It interacts with C6, C7, and C8 on the microbial surface to set the stage for multiple C9 molecules to form a pore in the microbial membrane.

Lysis

C8 inserts itself into the microbial surface and facilitates the subsequent insertion of numerous C9 molecules into the surface (Fig. 3-6). The C9 molecules form a pore in the microbial membrane

surface, damaging its integrity and permitting bidirectional flow of ions and macromolecules. As a result, the osmotic balance of the microbe is disrupted. This disruption ultimately causes the death of the microbe.

CLINICAL APPLICATION
COMPLEMENT DEFICIENCY

Individuals who lack some of the complement components, particularly the terminal components C5 through C9, are susceptible to meningococcal infections. The components C5 through C9 are responsible for destroying the organism.

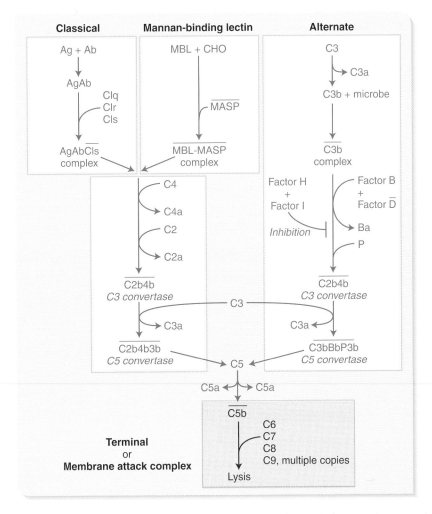

FIGURE 3-5. The terminal or lytic pathway of complement activation. The terminal, or membrane attack complex, pathway is initiated by C5b, which (together with C6) inserts into the cell membrane, to be followed by C7 and C8. After membrane insertion of C8, multiple C9 molecules are inserted to form a pore in the membrane, leading to cell lysis.

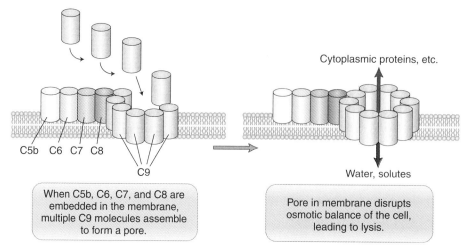

Cytoplasmic proteins, etc.

C5b C6 C7 C8

C9

When C5b, C6, C7, and C8 are embedded in the membrane, multiple C9 molecules assemble to form a pore.

Pore in membrane disrupts osmotic balance of the cell, leading to lysis.

Water, solutes

FIGURE 3-6. The membrane attack complex (MAC). The assembly of multiple C9 molecules completes the MAC by forming a pore in the membrane that leads to cell lysis.

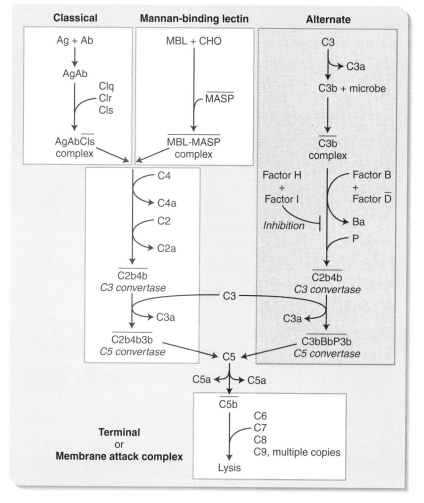

FIGURE 3-7. The alternative pathway of complement activation. Binding of C3b to microbial surfaces triggers the serial activation of complement components B and C3, a C3 convertase, and a C5 convertase and amplifies the amount of C3b. Regulatory factors D and P contribute to the activation, while factors H and I act as inhibitory regulatory elements.

Alternative pathway

The alternative pathway is activated on the surfaces of microbes in the absence of antibody. Spontaneous breakdown of serum C3 creates a short-lived C3b fragment. Binding of C3b to a microbial surface can initiate a second means of complement activation, the alternative pathway (Fig. 3-7). The alternative pathway does not involve MBL, C2, or C4, but another major component—factor B (Bf)—and several other elements (factors D, H, I, and P) that promote the stability or dissolution of some of the molecular complexes to which factor B contributes.

Recognition

The alternative pathway can be activated by a number of substances, including:

- Complex polysaccharides (e.g., peptidoglycan) on bacterial cell walls
- Lipopolysaccharides (endotoxin) on bacterial cell walls
- Yeast cell walls (zymosan)
- Immune complexes (aggregates of antibodies and antigens), especially those involving IgG, IgA, and IgE, although less efficiently than the classical pathway
- Constituents of leukocyte granules
- Cellophane (the membrane used in kidney dialysis)

The precise mechanism that activates the alternative pathway is unknown. The most likely possibility is that C3b plays this recognition role when it binds to one of the surfaces or substances listed above.

Regulation of C3b

As we have seen, C3b is important for the creation of a C5 convertase that leads to the formation of the MAC. The large number of C3b molecules produced upon entering the circulation could trigger the lytic sequence and wreak havoc on the tissues of the body. **Factor H** has evolved to limit this possibility by inhibiting the binding of C3b to Bb (formed by the cleavage of **Factor B** into fragments Ba and Bb by C3b). Factor H is the necessary cofactor for the inactivation of C3b by **Factor I**. An orderly sequence of events leading to lysis, either by the classical or alternative pathway, requires that some C3b molecules must remain active. Therefore, **Factor B** acts to stabilize C3b and

prevents inhibition by Factor H. In fact, both Factor B and Factor H compete for the same site on the C3b molecule.

ENZYMATIC ACTIVATION.

- *Formation of the alternative pathway C3 convertase:* C3b bound to the microbial cell surface, in the presence of Factor D, cleaves factor B to yield small (Ba) and large (Bb) fragments. The C3bBb complex is the alternative pathway C3 convertase.
- *Stabilization of alternative pathway C3 convertase:* A molecule known as **properdin** or **Factor P** (Latin "perdere," to destroy) stabilizes the alternative pathway C3 convertase by binding to C3bBb and extending its half-life.
- *Activation of C3 and C5:* C3bBbP, the stabilized C3 convertase, cleaves native C3 to produce C3bBbP3b. The stabilized C3 convertase serves the same function as in the MBL pathway—it generates chemoattractant C3a and opsonic C3b fragments and produces C3b that complexes with C3bBbP. The C5 convertase of the alternative pathway, C3bBbP3b, cleaves C5 into C5a and C5b. The formation of C5b allows the formation of a stable membrane-bound complex that initiates the MAC.

Cell-surface complement receptors

Complement fragments, such as C3b, are effective opsonins because phagocytic cells have receptors for membrane-bound C3b. There are several such complement receptors (CRs) that can mediate these activities (Table 3-3). CR1, CR2, CR3, and CR4 can all recognize and bind C3b or smaller fragments of C3b, and CR1 can also bind C4b.

Macrophages, monocytes, neutrophils, and some dendritic cells bear CR1, CR3, and CR4. These cells are active in binding to and ingesting of microbes. B lymphocytes, which are able to ingest and degrade some materials, bear CR1 and CR2.

Anaphylatoxins: C3a, C4a, C5a

In many cases, the smaller "a" fragments of complement also have biological activity. Called **anaphylatoxins**, they function as short-range hormone-like molecules that serve as chemoattractants and activators of other cells involved in local

TABLE 3-3. COMPLEMENT RECEPTORS (CRS)

Receptor	Found on	Binds	Leads to
CR1	Macrophages Monocytes Neutrophils Eosinophils Erythrocytes B lymphocytes Dendritic cell subset	C3b, iC3b*, C4b	Increased phagocytosis (opsonization) Transport of Ag-Ab complexes by erythrocytes to sites for disposal Accelerated destruction of C3b and C4b
CR2	B lymphocytes Dendritic cell subset	C3b, iC3b	B cell activation Increased phagocytosis Receptor for Epstein-Barr Virus
CR3	Macrophages Monocytes Neutrophils NK cells Dendritic cell subset	iC3b	Increased phagocytosis
CR4	Macrophages Monocytes Neutrophils NK cells	iC3b	Increased phagocytosis

* iC3b (incomplete C3b) designates breakdown products of C3b.

inflammatory responses (Table 3-4). Those with significant activity are C5a, C3a, and C4a (in decreasing order of their potency). All have the potential to stimulate release of histamine by mast cells, and C5a and C3a are also effective in attracting neutrophils to the site of inflammation and activating them upon their arrival. C5a and C3a fragments can activate local vascular endothelium to increase its expression of adhesion molecules that will enhance the recruitment of cells from the vasculature into the tissue site of inflammation. In addition, C5a and C3a induce macrophages and neutrophils drawn to the site of infection to increase the expression of adhesion molecules on their surfaces. Expression of these molecules helps these cells bind to vascular endothelium and the movement of cells from the vasculature into the tissues.

> **Patient Vignette 3.2**
>
>
> After ignoring a small cut on her ankle the previous day, Lois D. has developed an active bacterial infection at the site. Since her adaptive immune response has not yet responded to the situation, she must rely on her innate immune system for the time being.
>
> *(continued)*

> **Patient Vignette 3.2 (Continued)**
>
> *What signals are being recognized by her innate immune system that indicate the presence of infectious agents?*
>
> Pathogen-associated molecular patterns (PAMPs) are the initial signal for activation of the innate immune response here. The production of cytokines by phagocytes and the activation of complement components occur in response to recognition and binding of PAMPs. Antibodies are generally considered to be part of the adaptive response rather than the innate response.

Regulators of the complement system

The ability of enzymatic complexes such as C4b2b, C4b2b3b, C3bBb, and C3bBb3b to attach to membranes raises the question of whether they can also attach to host cell surfaces, and, if so, whether they can lead to damage or destruction of host cells. The answer is that they can, but, fortunately, host cells carry additional enzymes on their surfaces that disrupt and destroy the enzymatic complexes before they can damage the host cell. Microbial cells lack these protective enzymes and are unable to prevent attachment of complement

TABLE 3-4. FUNCTIONS OF C5a, C3a, C4a—LISTED DECREASING IN ORDER OF POTENCY

Anaphylotoxin	Acts on	Actions
C5a	Phagocytic cells	Increased phagocytosis
	Endothelial cells	Activation of phagocytes
	Neutrophils	Activation of vascular endothelium
	Mast cells	Attraction and activation of neutrophils
		Mast cell degranulation
C3a	Phagocytic cells	Increased phagocytosis
	Endothelial cells	Activation of phagocytes
	Mast cells	Activation of vascular endothelium
C4a	Phagocytic cells	Increased phagocytosis

components and complexes on their surfaces, and are thus damaged while host cells are not. A number of human diseases result from defects or deficiencies in these protective enzymes. These diseases are discussed in detail in Chapter 7.

Several mechanisms exist to prevent unnecessary activation (Table 3-5). Some of these act by disrupting the enzymatic complexes that are formed during complement activation. Others act to prevent deposition of complement fragments on the surfaces of host cells. Factor H, Factor I, and **decay accelerating factor** (DAF) can bind to C3b in order to inactivate and disperse the enzymatic complexes in which the C3b is participating. C4-binding protein (C4BP) does the same for C4b. A molecule called **membrane cofactor protein** (MCP) inactivates C3b and C4b fragments attaching to host cell membranes. Likewise, CD59 prevents the formation of the MAC on host cell surfaces. The presence of these protective molecules on host cells, but not on microbial cells, allows the activation of complement in order to destroy invasive microbes while sparing host cells. However, as will be discussed in Chapter 7, some individuals lack these protective molecules and suffer disease as a result of unregulated episodes of complement activation.

INFLAMMATION

Inflammation is a condition in which multiple innate and adaptive immune responses are targeted at particular antigenic stimuli (Fig. 3-8). In a sense, the immune system is throwing every bit of weaponry at its disposal at the perceived threat, in the expectation that some will be successful in destroying the invader. All of these responses can occur simultaneously. Contributions of the innate immune response to an inflammatory response include:

- Activation of complement (via the lectin-binding and alternative pathways)
- Heightened activity of activated macrophages and other phagocytic cells
- NK cell activity
- Secretion of Type I interferons by infected cells
- Secretion of cytokines and chemokines by activated macrophages
- Alterations in vascular permeability to facilitate entry of cells and molecules into tissues
- Attraction and activation of neutrophils
- Release of inflammatory mediators by mast cells, basophils, and eosinophils
- Increased body temperature

TABLE 3-5. REGULATORY MOLECULES OF THE LECTIN-BINDING AND ALTERNATIVE COMPLEMENT PATHWAYS

Regulatory molecule	Action
C4-Binding Protein (C4BP)	Facilitates breakdown of C4b
Factor H	Acts with Factor I to facilitate breakdown of C3b
Factor I	Acts with Factor I to facilitate breakdown of C3b
Factor P (properdin)	Stabilizes interaction of C3b and Bb
Membrane Cofactor Protein (MCP)	Inactivates C3b and C4b fragments binding to host cell membranes
Decay Accelerating Factor (DAF)	Breaks down C3 convertases (C3bBb and C4bC2b)
CD59	Prevents formation of MAC on host cell membranes

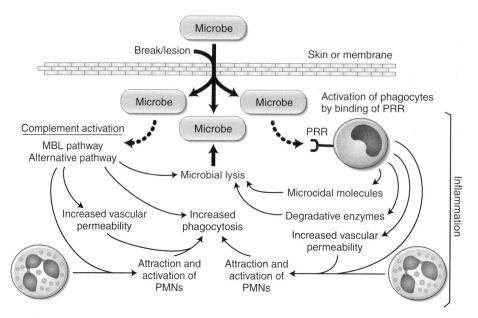

FIGURE 3-8. Inflammation. Inflammation is the summation of multiple processes generated in response to stimuli such as infection. The activation of serum complement leads to the direct killing of infectious microbes and to the attraction and activation of neutrophils. The activation of phagocytic cells leads to elaboration of a number of secreted molecules that attack microbes directly and that attract and activate other elements of the immune system. Increased vascular permeability facilitates their passage from the vasculature into the infected tissues.

Inflammation has four primary characteristics or "cardinal signs"—swelling, redness, warmth, and pain. Each of these signs is derived from the activities cited above. Inflammation is the battlefield where total war is being waged; where the host forces are throwing all of their weaponry at the invader. Changes in local vasculature permit cells and fluid to enter the tissues from the vasculature, which produces swelling. In addition, blood flow to the area is increased, resulting in heightened red color and heat. Finally, several of the chemical mediators released by granulocytic cells such as mast cells, basophils, and eosinophils stimulate nerves and cause pain (the actions of these various inflammatory mediators will be discussed in Chapter 8). Neutrophils are drawn to the site of inflammation in large numbers as well, in response to the cytokines and chemokines secreted by activated phagocytes and by anaphylatoxins. They contribute greatly to the clearance of infectious organisms and cellular debris. Their numbers increase significantly during infection; in fact, an elevated neutrophil level in the blood is evidence of an infection active somewhere in the body. The inflammatory response continues until the threat or stimulus is removed, at which point the healing process begins. In cases where inflammation becomes chronic, the damage it inflicts may become the ba-

sis for immune-mediated diseases (e.g., rheumatoid arthritis and systemic lupus erythematosus).

Patient Vignette 3.3

 Sara N. is tending her rose garden when she pricks her thumb on a particularly nasty thorn. She momentarily ignores the injury while she finishes her work, but notices a few hours later that the area around the wound has become red and swollen. When she presses it, it feels warm and the pressure of her touch is quite painful.

What is the source of the redness?

The source of redness of an inflamed area is increased blood flow at the injury site.

What is the primary source of the swelling?

The primary source of swelling in an inflamed area is primarily caused by the entry of fluid from the vasculature into the tissues as a result of the "loosening" of the vascular endothelium in response to signals from activation of phagocytes and complement. In

(continued)

Patient Vignette 3.3 (Continued)

some cases, cells entering the tissues from the vasculature may contribute to the swelling as well.

What is the source of the warmth?

As with the redness, the warmth in an inflamed area results from the increased blood flow that brings with it body core warmth.

The presence of microbial products such as lipopolysaccharide (LPS) leads to a marked rise in certain serum proteins known as **acute phase proteins** that serve to curtail the spread of infectious organisms. Included among this group are complement (alternative and lectin pathways), type I interferons, coagulation proteins (fibronectin), protease inhibitors, TNF, and IL-1. IL-1 secreted by activated monocytes stimulates local blood flow to the affected area and the synthesis of **C-reactive protein** (CRP) by the liver. Within 24 to 48 hours of an infection, serum CRP levels increase by a thousand-fold. CRP readily binds to phosphocholine molecules expressed on certain microorganisms and acts as an opsonin binding to receptors on monocytic cells, thus targeting the microbe for phagocytosis. IL-1 and TNF increase vascular permeability to facilitate the movement of inflammatory cells and molecules from the vasculature into the infected or damaged tissues.

In addition, some activities that fall within the realm of the adaptive immune response (e.g., immunoglobulins, T lymphocytes) contribute to inflammation. Their contributions are discussed in greater depth in Chapter 8.

Summary

- Innate immune responses occur without the participation of the antigen-specific receptors of T or B lymphocytes.
- These responses begin almost immediately after infection and do not display memory.
- Recognition of microbial-associated molecules is achieved in innate responses through membrane-bound receptors (PRRs) and by particular sets of soluble molecules (complement). Infectious organisms display a wide range of molecules that express pathogen-associated molecular patterns that are not typically found on cells of the infected hosts. Toll-like

receptors (TLRs) are pattern recognition receptors that are found on phagocytic cells such as macrophages and dendritic cells, mast cells, some types of epithelial cells, and even on B lymphocytes. Toll-like receptors contain structural motifs capable of binding a diverse range of viral, bacterial and fungal products.
- The initial protective defenses of the body include the skin and the mucous membranes of the gastrointestinal and respiratory tract, and other membranous surfaces (e.g., the eye and the urogenital tract).
- Opsonization is an increased ingestion of microbes or other material by phagocytic cells.
- NK cells distinguish normal from infected cells, in part by detecting the level of MHC class I molecules on their surfaces.
- Many virally infected cells detect the presence of the viral nucleic acid sequences and respond by secreting type I interferons (α- and β-interferon).
- Two innate complement cascades are known: the mannan-binding lectin (MBL) and the alternative pathways. The MBL pathway involves the sequential activation of five components—MBL, C4, C2, C3, and C5. The alternative pathway sequentially activates components C3, B, P, C3, and C5.
- The membrane attack complex (MAC) is initiated by the binding of C5b to the cell surface and is followed by the rapid sequential binding of C6, C7, C8 and multiple copies of C9.
- Some complement fragments, such as C3b, also function as efficient opsonins in stimulating phagocytosis.
- Anaphylatoxins are the smaller fragments released during the cleavage of C5, C3, or C4. They serve as chemoattractants and activators of other cells involved in local inflammatory responses.
- Activation of the complement system can induce inflammation, a condition in which multiple innate and adaptive immune responses are targeted simultaneously at particular antigenic stimuli. The four primary characteristics or "cardinal signs" of inflammation are swelling, redness, warmth, and pain.

Suggested readings

Abbas AK, Lichtman AH. Innate immunity. In *Cellular and molecular immunology*, 5th ed. Philadephia: WB Saunders Co., 2003.

Feizi T. Carbohydrate-mediated recognition systems in innate immunity. *Immunol Rev* 2000;173:79.

Gadjeva M, Theil S, Jensenius JC. The Mannan-binding-lectin pathway of the innate immune response. *Curr Opin Immunol* 2001;13:74.

Greenberg S, Grinstein S. Phagocytosis and innate immunity. *Curr Opin Immunol* 2003;15:396.

Janeway CA Jr. How the immune system works to protect the host from infection: A personal view. *Proc Natl Acad Sci USA* 2002;98:7461.

Janeway CA Jr, Medzhitov R. Innate immune recognition. *Annu Rev Immunol* 2002;20:197.

Janeway CA Jr, Travers P, Walport M, Shlomchik P. Innate immunity. In *Immunobiology: The immune system in health and disease*, 6th ed. Philadephia: Garland Publishing, 2004.

Janssens S, Beyaert R. Role of toll-like receptors in pathogen recognition. *Clin Microbiol Rev* 2003;16:637.

Natarajan K, Dimasi N, Wang J, et al. Structure and function of natural killer cell receptors: Multiple solutions to self, non-self discrimination. *Annu Rev Immunol* 2002;20:853.

Prodinger WM, Wurzner R, Stoiber H, Dierich MP. Complement. In Paul WE, ed. *Fundamental immunology*, 5th ed. Philadelphia: Lippincott Williams & Wilkins, 2003:1077–1103.

Review questions

DIRECTIONS: Each of the numbered items or incomplete statements in this section is followed by answers or by completions of the statement. Select the ONE lettered answer or completion that is BEST in each case.

1. The lectin-binding pathway of complement activation can be initiated by the binding of mannan-binding lection (MBL) to _____ on microbial cells.
   (A) lipopolysaccharide (LPS)
   (B) mannan
   (C) penicillin
   (D) C3

2. The critical products produced at the completion of the lectin-binding pathway and the alternative pathway of complement activation are:
   (A) the components comprising the membrane attack complex.
   (B) factors H and I.
   (C) C5 convertases and C3b fragments.
   (D) C3 convertases and C4b fragments.

3. C3b is an effective
   (A) C5 convertase.
   (B) opsonin.
   (C) anaphylatoxin.
   (D) inhibitor of the MAC.

4. Successful formation of the MAC on a microbial membrane leads to:
   (A) opsonization of the microbe.
   (B) cleavage of C3 to C3a and C3b.
   (C) lysis of the microbe.
   (D) induction of fever.

5. Virally infected cells can be recognized as such and killed by:
   (A) components of the lectin-binding complement pathway.
   (B) mast cells.
   (C) natural killer (NK) cells.
   (D) basophils.

6. Virally infected cells can alert their unaffected neighboring cells and natural killer cells to the viral presence by the production and release of:
   (A) immunoglobulins.
   (B) Interleukin-12 (IL-12).
   (C) Interferon-α and interferon-β.
   (D) Interferon-γ.
   (E) Interleukin-2 (IL-2).

7. Human natural killer (NK) cells become activated to kill infected or otherwise stressed cells through the binding of _____ on the NK cells to _____ on the target cells.
   (A) T cell receptor/pMHC I
   (B) Interleukin-2 (IL-2)/IL-2 receptor
   (C) CD40/CD40 ligand
   (D) NKG2D/MICA and MICB
   (E) KIR/self MHC I

8. Human natural killer (NK) cells are inhibited from killing infected or otherwise stressed cells through the binding of _____ on the NK cells to _____ on the target cells.
   (A) T cell receptor/pMHC I
   (B) Interleukin-2 (IL-2)/IL-2 receptor
   (C) CD40/CD40 ligand
   (D) NKG2D/MICA and MICB
   (E) killer inhibitory receptors (KIR)/self MHC I

9. Binding of microbial molecules by toll-like receptors (TLRs) on a phagocytic cell should lead to:
   (A) activation of the phagocyte.
   (B) death of the phagocyte by apoptosis.
   (C) production of Interleukin-2 (IL-2) and IL-2 receptors by the phagocyte.
   (D) induction of CD3 expression on the phagocyte membrane.
   (E) formation of the membrane attack complex (MAC).

10. C-reactive protein (CRP) acts as a(n):
    (A) integrin.
    (B) signaling receptor.
    (C) cytokine.
    (D) opsonin.
    (E) addressin.

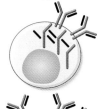

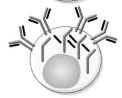

CHAPTER 4

Molecules of the Adaptive Immune System

Chapter Outline

INTRODUCTION

IMMUNOGLOBULINS
- Basic structure
- Landmarks
- Variable region
- Constant region
- Additional degrees of immunoglobulin variation
- Allelic exclusion
- Antibody-antigen reactions
- Direct effects of antibody
    Agglutination
    Neutralization
- Indirect effects of antibody
    Complement activation
    Opsonization

T CELL RECEPTORS
- Basic structure
- Variable region

MAJOR HISTOCOMPATIBILITY COMPLEX MOLECULES
- Class I molecules
- Class II molecules
- Class III molecules

CLUSTER OF DIFFERENTIATION MOLECULES
- CD3
- CD4
- CD8

CYTOKINES AND CHEMOKINES

ADHESION MOLECULES

CHAPTER SUMMARY

SUGGESTED READINGS

REVIEW QUESTIONS

Introduction Humans use two immune systems, the innate and the adaptive, to combat invasion by infectious organisms. Upon microbial encounter, cells of the innate immune system rapidly differentiate into short-lived functionally active immune cells, often called **effector cells** or **effectors**, that usually clear the infection. Although the innate system contains a large number of leukocytes, they are genetically "hardwired" to produce a relatively limited variety of **pattern-recognition receptors** (PRRs) that recognize genetically conserved **pathogen-associated molecular patterns** (PAMPs) expressed by microbes. Genetically selected over evolutionary time, PRRs do not recognize self molecules, allowing the cells of the innate system to act rapidly and autonomously in response to potential pathogens. The innate immune response does not increase in intensity upon repeated antigenic encounters (i.e., it does not develop immunologic memory).

In contrast, lymphocytes of the **adaptive immune system** generate antigen-specific, B cell- and T cell-surface receptors (BCRs and TCRs) by gene rearrangement for a wide variety of antigens that an individual may potentially encounter during her or his lifetime. Even the most basic appreciation of adaptive immunity depends upon understanding the role that these molecules play in the function of the immune system. These molecules include immunoglobulins, T cell receptors, cell determinant or **cluster of differentiation** (CD) molecules, **human leukocyte antigen** (HLA) molecules, cytokines, and complement. **Immunoglobulins**, a major component of the humoral immune response, are synthesized by B cells, some of which further differentiate into immunoglobulin-secreting *plasma cells*. Immunoglobulins also serve as antigen-specific B cell receptors (BCR) on the surfaces of B cells. **T cell receptors** (TCRs) are cell-surface molecules on the T lymphocyte that recognize and bind antigens. They are associated with other molecules such as CD3, CD4, or CD8 that assist the TCR. *CD molecules* are cell-surface molecules that are often useful indicators of the functional capacities of lymphocytes and other cells. **HLA molecules** are the products of distinct genetic loci in the MHC that encode proteins of three different types called class I, II, or III MHC molecules. **Cytokines** are protein molecules that act as messengers between cells and affect cell behavior. **Complement** is a set of serum proteins involved in many biological defense mechanisms such as destruction and ingestion of cells and molecules, and the attraction and activation of cells involved in inflammation (Chapter 3).

IMMUNOGLOBULINS

Immunoglobulin is a generic term that refers to a diverse group of molecules found in the blood and tissue fluids. As the name implies, they are globulin molecules, soluble in mild (e.g., 0.15M) salt solutions, and they generally migrate in an electrophoretic field at or near the gamma (γ) globulin fraction of serum proteins. An **antibody** is an immunoglobulin molecule capable of combining specifically with a known substance (**antigen**). Throughout this text we will refer to immunoglobulins of known antigen specificity as **antibodies**. If antigen specificity is not known, we will use the term **immunoglobulin**. **Humoral immune responses** involve the actions of immunoglobulins or antibodies. Immunoglobulins

are synthesized by **B lymphocytes** (B cells) and by terminally differentiated B cells or **plasma cells**. Antibodies are soluble proteins that are capable of binding to both intact antigens and to fragments of antigens. They can act directly upon the antigen to which they bind to render it harmless or, often, they "tag" the antigen for destruction and removal by some other component of the immune system. In doing so, antibodies facilitate the ability of numerous other cells and molecules in the immune system to identify and interact with antigens.

Basic structure

The basic **immunoglobulin monomer** is defined as containing four polypeptides, two light (L) and two heavy (H) glycoprotein chains linked by disulfide bonds (Fig. 4-1). The **immunoglobulin heavy chain** is larger than the light chain. There are five different types of heavy chains, termed α, δ, ε, γ, and μ. The **immunoglobulin light chain** is present in all immunoglobulin monomers. There are two types of light chains, κ (kappa) and λ (lambda). An individual B cell or immunoglobulin monomer expresses either κ or λ, but not both. Within any single immunoglobulin molecule, both of the light chains (either κ–κ or λ–λ) and both of the heavy chains (α–α, δ–δ, ε–ε, γ–γ or μ–μ) are identical. Some immunoglobulin molecules are basic monomers and others are composed of multiple copies (dimers or pentamers) of identical immunoglobulin monomers (Table 4-1).

CLINICAL APPLICATION

All immunoglobulins are found in human breast milk, but sIgA (secretory IgA) is the most abundant during the weeks before the infant can produce its own sIgA to protect the oropharynx and gastrointestinal tracts. The sIgA from the mother's milk provides immunity for the infant before the endogenous production of sIgA occurs.

Both heavy and light chains can be divided into **regions** or **domains**, homologous portions of an immunoglobulin chain, each composed of approximately 110 amino acids and containing an intra-domain disulfide bridge (Fig. 4-1 inset). Light chains contain two regions, a **variable** (V_L) and a **constant** (C_L) domain. Heavy chains contain a single variable (V_H) and multiple constant

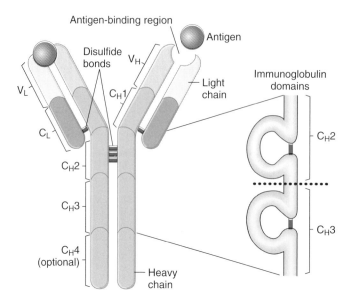

FIGURE 4-1. **Basic immunoglobulin structure.** The basic monomeric structures of immunoglobulin molecules contain two identical heavy and light polypeptide chains. Both heavy and light chains contain variable (V_H and V_L, respectively) and constant (e.g., C_H1, C_H2 or C_L, respectively) region domains of approximately 110 amino acids each that contain an intradomain disulfide bond (see insert). Together, the variable portions of a single heavy and single light chain form an antigen-binding region. Light chains contain a single C region (C_L) and heavy chains contain three or four C regions (C_H1, C_H2, C_H3, and, in some cases, C_H4). Some immunoglobulins are composed of dimers or pentamers of identical monomers (Table 4-1).

domains (C_H1, C_H2, C_H3, and sometimes C_H4). Variable regions in both heavy and light chains are so-named because of the extensive variation in the amino acid sequences found in Ig molecules made by different B cells. The amino acid sequence determines the conformational structure of V_H and V_L. The combination of a light variable and a heavy variable region forms a pocket that constitutes the **antigen-binding region** of the Ig molecule.

Landmarks

The V and C regions of immunoglobulin are located at the amino and carboxyl ends of the molecule, respectively. Other portions of the molecule are also functionally important. Immunoglobulin molecules can be enzymatically cleaved into discrete fragments by either pepsin or papain [Fig. 4-2]. *Disulfide bonds* hold the heavy and light chains together. Disulfide bonds join the heavy chains at or near a flexible, proline-rich *hinge region*, which confers flexibility on the Ig molecule.

The fragments of immunoglobulin are:

- *Fab* or antigen-binding fragment is produced by *papain* cleavage of the immunoglobulin molecule. It is monovalent with regard to antigen-binding sites, and consists of V_H, C_H1, V_L, and C_L.
- *Fc* or constant (crystallizable) fragment is produced by cleavage of the immunoglobulin molecule with papain. The Fc portion contains the C_H2, C_H3, and (sometimes) C_H4 regions of the antibody molecule. It is responsible for biologic activities that occur following engagement of antigen by antibody, including the activation of the complement system, and combining with specific cell surface receptors on basophils, neutrophils, lymphocytes and macrophages.

TABLE 4-1. IMMUNOGLOBULIN ISOTYPES (Human)

Isotype	Heavy chains[a]	Heavy chain subclass	Additional chains	Formula[a]	Number of monomers[b]	Subclass	Valence	MW[c]	Half-life (days)	Serum level (mg/dl)	Percent	Stick figure
IgM	μ			2 Hμ[d] 2L	1		2	180,000				
		μ	J chain	5 [2 Hμ 2L] + J	5	IgM	10	900,000	1	45–150[e]	5–8	
IgG	γ			2 Hγ 2L	1		2	150,000	23	720–1500[e]	75–85	
		γ1		2 Hγ1 2L	1	IgG1	2	150,000	23	430–1050		
		γ2		2 Hγ2 2L	1	IgG2	2	150,000	23	100–300		
		γ3		2 Hγ3 2L	1	IgG3	2	150,000	8	30–90		
		γ4		2 Hγ4 2L	1	IgG4	2	150,000	23	15–60		
IgA	α			2 H α 2L	1		2	170,000	5.8	90–325	10–16	
		α1		2 H α1 2L	1–serum	IgA1	2	170,000	5.8	80–290		
			J chain & SC[f]	2 [2 Hα1 2L] + J + SC[f]	2–external[g] upper body and GI	sIgA1	4	390,000	na	na		
		α2		2 Hα2 2L	1–serum	IgA2	2	170,000	5.8	10–35		
			J chain & SC	2 [2 H α2 2L] + J + SC	2–external[g] lower GI	sIgA2	4	390,000	na	na		
IgD	δ			2 Hδ 2L	1		2	180,000	2.8	3	<1	
IgE	ε			2 Hε 2L	1		2	190,000	2.5	0.03	<1	

[a] All monomers contain two identical heavy (H) and two light (L) chains; light chains are κ–κ or λ–λ

[b] The number of monomeric subunits expressed on the surface of the B cell is always 1 or in the form secreted by plasma cell.

[c] Molecular weight.

[d] The carboxyl-terminal cytoplasmic tail portion of the μ chain of the surface-bound IgM monomer differs significantly from the μ chain present in the pentameric secreted form of IgM.

[e] Serum level for all members of this class.

[f] Secretory component.

[g] The dimeric form is transported across specialized epithelial cells to the external environment. sIgA1 is found in tears, nasal secretions, saliva, and breast milk. sIgA2 is found in the gastrointestinal system.

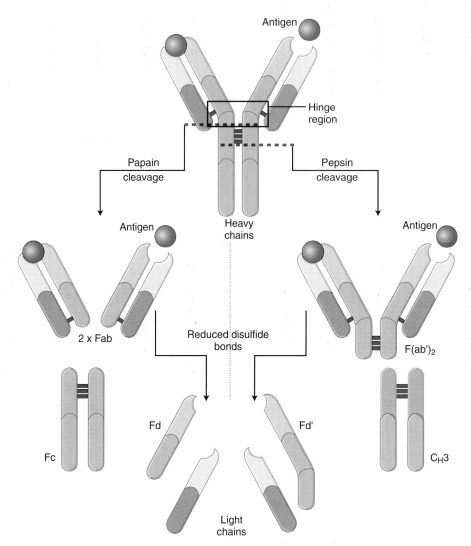

FIGURE 4-2. Landmarks of the immunoglobulin molecule. The basic structure of an immunoglobulin monomer is defined by the fragments formed following enzymatic cleavage or by interchain disulfide bond reduction. Pepsin cleavage results in the production of two fragments with antigen-binding or Fab activity, each of which contains an intact light chain (V_L, C_L) and a partial heavy chain (V_H, C_H1). Papain also produces a crystallizable or constant fragment called Fc containing two heavy chain fragments (C_H2, C_H3, and, sometimes, C_H4) linked by a disulfide bond. Reduction of the Fab interchain disulfide bonds results in an intact light chain (V_L, C_L) and a so-called Fd fragment (V_H, C_H1). Pepsin cleaves the immunoglobulin monomer heavy chains below the disulfide bonds to create an F(ab')$_2$ fragment, so-named because it has an antigen-binding valence of two and each Fab fragment has several extra amino acids, denoted by the prime mark (Fab', for something extra) linked by disulfide bonds. Pepsin digests a large portion of C_H2 and, sometimes, C_H3 and C_H4. Further reduction of F(ab')$_2$ interchain disulfide bonds produces intact light chains and an Fd' fragment (an Fd with extra amino acids).

- *Fd* is the heavy chain (V_H, C_H1) portion of an Fab fragment, resulting from papain cleavage.
- *Fd'* is a heavy chain (V_H, C_H1) portion of Fab. The prime (') mark denotes extra amino acids due to a pepsin cleavage site.
- *F(ab')$_2$* is a dimeric molecule produced by pepsin cleavage. It is composed of two identical light chains and two identical Fd' fragments linked by disulfide bonds.

Variable region

Immunologists estimate that each person has the ability to produce a range of individual antibodies capable of binding a total of well over 10^{10} **epitopes**, the smallest definable molecular structures that can be recognized by the immune system (Chapter 1). According to the **germline theory**, a unique gene encodes each antibody. Unfortu-

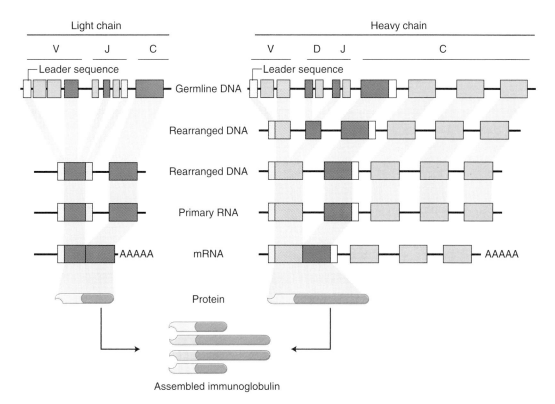

FIGURE 4-3. **Synthesis of immunoglobulin heavy and light chains.** Diversity in the variable portion of immunoglobulin molecules results from a process known as DNA chromosomal rearrangement. A series of genes for κ (chromosome 2) or λ (chromosome 22) light chains or for all heavy chain isotypes (chromosome 14) form the basic building blocks. To generate a light chain, one of 30 to 40 variable (V_Lκ or V_Lλ) gene segments recombines with one of four or five joining (J) segments and a single constant (C_L) segment. To generate a heavy chain, one of 65 heavy chain variable (V_H) gene segments recombines with one of several diversity (D_H) and joining (J_H) gene segments and a single constant region (C) gene segment. The rearranged DNA is then transcribed into primary RNA, intervening sequences are edited out of messenger RNA (mRNA), and polypeptides are produced and assembled in the Golgi apparatus.

nately, for this theory the number of antibody genes would need to be one hundred to one thousand-fold greater than the entire human genome! An alternative theory, the **somatic mutation theory,** holds that a single germline immunoglobulin gene undergoes multiple mutations that generate immunoglobulin diversity. This scheme, however, requires an unimaginable mutation rate. The immune system has developed a much more elegant solution—the **chromosomal rearrangement** of separate gene segments, which employs some elements of the germline and somatic mutation theories (Fig. 4-3). Each light and heavy immunoglobulin chain is encoded by a series of genes occurring in clusters along the chromosome. In humans, the series of genes encoding the κ light chain, λ light chain, and heavy chains are located on chromosomes 2, 22, and 14, respectively. When a cell becomes committed to the B-lymphocyte lineage, it rearranges the DNA, encoding its light and heavy chains by cutting and splicing together some

of the DNA sequences, thus modifying the sequence of the variable region genes.

How does the immune system utilize chromosomal rearrangement? Some simple arithmetic is in order.

SIDEBAR 4.2 GENERATION OF V_L REGION OF κ AND λ LIGHT CHAINS

For a κ V_L region, one of 40 V ("variable") gene segments recombines with one of five J ("joining") gene segments ($40 \times 5 = 200$). For a λ V_l region, one of 30 V gene segments recombines with one of four J gene segments ($30 \times 4 = 120$). Because the combinations are apparently generated at random, this process can generate up to 320 different light chain variable regions (sum of the κ and λ light chains).

Since the antibody-binding site is composed of both the V$_L$ and V$_H$ portions of the immunoglobulin molecule, up to 3.4×10^6 ($10,530 \times 320$) be generated by recombination alone. This variation is increased further by junctional diversity.

Constant region

You have already seen that there are five different primary types of heavy chains (μ, δ, γ, α, and ε). Normal individuals express all five different immunoglobulin classes or isotypes. All immunoglobulins are composed of at least a single four-chain monomer. Monomers are divalent, having two identical antigen binding sites. Different immunoglobulin **classes** or **isotypes** are determined by their heavy chain characteristics. Some isotypes are composed of multiple copies (dimers or pentamers) of identical immunoglobulin monomers; for example, multimeric forms of IgA and IgM have four and ten antigen-binding sites, respectively (Table 4-1).

IgM is the heaviest isotype, with a molecular weight approaching 1,000,000 daltons. It is found as either a cell-surface-bound monomer (2 H (μ), 2 L) or as a secreted pentamer (five monomers, each containing 2 H (μ), 2 L) for a total of 10 H and 10 L chains, linked by disulfide bonds and a J ("joining") chain (Table 4-1). IgM comprises approximately 6% to 8 % of the serum immunoglobulins.

IgG exists as both surface and secreted monomeric (2H (γ), 2L) molecules (Table 4-1). Human IgG can be divided further into four subclasses—*IgG$_1$, IgG$_2$, IgG$_3$,* and *IgG$_4$.* Heavy chains for these subclasses are designated as γ_1, γ_2, γ_3, or γ_4, respectively. Approximately 72% to 80% of total serum immunoglobulin is IgG.

IgD has a monomeric structure (2H (δ), 2L) similar to that of IgG. IgD has a very low serum concentration (less than 1%) and is found almost exclusively on B cell surfaces (Table 4-1).

IgA is found in both monomeric (2H (α), 2L) and dimeric forms (Table 4-1). IgA is usually associated with mucous membranes and their secretions. Two subclasses, IgA$_1$ and IgA$_2$, have been identified and either subclass can be found in monomer or dimeric form. Secretory IgA (sIgA) is composed of two monomers bound by a joining or J chain to form a dimer (Table 4-1). Epithelial cells synthesize the secretory component polypeptide. **Secretory component** (SC) is thought to facilitate passage of sIgA through specialized epithelial cells into mucous secretions, as well as protecting sIgA from proteolytic attack. The secretory dimeric form is more resistant to enzymatic degradation than is the monomeric form. This is important for sIgA's function in fluids such as saliva, tears, breast milk, and gastric secretions. The monomeric subclass, IgA$_1$, accounts for almost 90% of the IgA found in serum. The secretory form of IgA$_1$, sIgA$_1$, is predominantly found in secretions above the diaphragm, including saliva, tears, lung and nasal secretions, and milk. The IgA$_2$ subclass accounts for approximately 10% of serum IgA. Its secretory form, sIgA$_2$, accounts for the majority of IgA found in the lumen of the lower portion of the gastrointestinal system. Approximately 13% to 19% of serum immunoglobulin is IgA. However, large amounts of IgA are synthesized and secreted daily at the mucosal surfaces of the GI

Patient Vignette 4.1

John C., a 30-year-old man, was admitted to the hospital following a severe car accident. He had lost a significant amount of blood and required an immediate blood transfusion and fluid replacement. The patient has a known history of IgA deficiency.

What precaution(s) should be taken?

The two most common B-cell immunodeficiencies are IgA and IgG deficiencies. The most common selective immune deficiency is selective IgA deficiency. Patients with IgA deficiency are at increased risk of a severe reaction from a blood transfusion. These patients may have IgE or IgG4 anti-IgA antibodies, which can cause anaphylaxis. They should only be given blood from IgA-deficient patients or washed packed red blood cells.

tract. More IgA is produced per day than all the other isotypes combined.

IgE is present in relatively low concentration in serum. Less than 0.001% of the serum immunoglobulin is IgE. Its basic structural formula (for both B-cell-surface and secreted forms) is 2H(ε) 2L, and each heavy chain contains one variable and four constant region domains (Table 4-1). Atopic individuals, those people susceptible to allergic reactions, often show elevated concentrations of IgE. IgE is **homocytophilic** (i.e., it is passively acquired by mast cells or basophils). Basophils and mast cells have FcRε receptors for the Fc portion of free IgE molecules. Subsequent crosslinking, by antigen, of IgE on mast cell surfaces triggers mast cell degranulation and the release of histamine and other inflamatory mediators, leading to immediate hypersensitivity (allergic) responses (Chapter 8).

Additional degrees of immunoglobulin variation

The generation of diversity can account for the variable regions that recognize a great portion of the antigenic universe. An individual B cell syn-thesizes immunoglobulin of only a single specificity (one particular combination of V_l and V_H). However, B cells have the ability to change the class or isotype of the immunoglobulin they produce, a process known as **isotype switching** [Fig. 4-4]. Since an immune response is the body's way of waging war against what it perceives as foreign, immunoglobulins can be considered the "missiles" of the immune system. The variable regions or antigen-binding portions of the molecules are similar to the warheads on the missiles. A single B cell can manufacture only one particular warhead. However, this warhead can be placed on any of a number of rockets (or constant regions). The B cell's production apparatus is such that, once activated, it can only produce one isotype at a given time. However, since each isotype is specialized for interactions with other molecules and cells of the immune system, the isotype switch permits antibodies that bind to the same epitope to trigger a variety of different types of immune responses. The mechanism by which the isotype switch is accomplished is discussed later in this chapter.

Additional variations also increase the diversity of antibodies produced by the body. When B cells are initially stimulated (primary response),

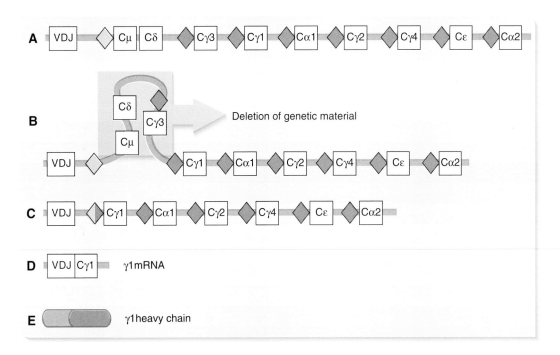

FIGURE 4-4. **Isotype switching.** T cell cytokines (e.g., IL-4, IFN-γ, IL-5, etc.) signal B cells to switch immunoglobulin isotypes. **(A)** In this representation of the human DNA constant region gene order (not to scale), rectangles indicate genetic loci and diamonds indicate switching sequences or regions. **(B)** Intervening DNA region between the first switch region (Sμ) and Sγ1 (in this example) forms a loop and is deleted. **(C)** The two DNA switch regions (Sμ and Sγ1, in this example) are joined. **(D)** Messenger RNA (mRNA) is transcribed. **(E)** The mRNA is translated into an IgG1 heavy chain.

not all of them become plasma cells, synthesizing and secreting Ig until they burn out and die. Some of the stimulated B cells are held in reserve for future exposures to antigen. These are termed **memory B cells.** When stimulated by subsequent exposures to the same antigen, memory B cells undergo isotype switches and also accumulate small mutations in the DNA encoding their light and heavy chain V regions during their rapid proliferation. This process, **somatic hypermutation,** provides additional variation that "fine-tunes" the antibody responses to antigens that are frequently or chronically present. This fine tuning leads to a process termed **affinity maturation,** which is discussed in later in this chapter.

We can summarize the basic variations among immunoglobulin molecules as follows:

- An **isotype** class or subclass of immunoglobulin is common to all members of that species encoded by all alleles at a given genetic locus. All isotypes (and subtypes such as IgG_1, IgG_2, etc.) are determined by the C_H regions of the heavy chains and are produced by all healthy individuals.
- An **allotype** is determined by different alleles (inherited variants) at a given isotype locus for both immunoglobulin heavy and light chains. For instance, while ten different alleles may exist for a locus within a particular population, any one individual can express only a maximum of two allelic forms, one inherited from the father and one from the mother.
- An **idiotype** is a structural determinant on a specific antibody, characteristic of that antibody and different from others even of the same isotype and allotype. Idiotypes are usually located in or near the antigen-binding site. Conventionally, idiotypes are identified by the production of an antibody directed against the variable region of another specific antibody. The basic rule for all B cells is *one cell, one idiotype.*

Allelic exclusion

Although an individual inherits both maternal and paternal alleles for immunoglobulin loci, a single B cell can express only one V_L and one V_H allele to the exclusion of all others. Both must be on the same member of the chromosome pair— either maternal or paternal. The restriction of V_L and H_L expression to a single member of the chromosome pair is termed **allelic exclusion.** The presence of both maternal and paternal allotypes in the serum reflects the expression of different alleles by different populations of B cells.

Antibody-antigen reactions

Interaction of antibody (Ab) with antigen (Ag) is one of the most specific noncovalent biochemical interactions known; it can be represented by the simple formula

$$Ag + Ab \xrightleftharpoons{} AgAb$$

Notice that the reaction is driven to the right. A basic tenet of this reaction is that *antigen-antibody interactions are reversible.* The strength of interaction (i.e., how far to the right it is driven) is termed its *affinity.* By applying the Law of Mass Action, affinity equilibrium is derived:

$$K = \frac{K_a}{K_d} = \frac{[AgAb]}{[Ag] \cdot [Ab]} \qquad Where \; \frac{K_a}{K_d} = \frac{K_{association}}{K_{dissociation}}$$

The average equilibrium constant (K), expressed as (liters/mole), can be calculated:

$$K = \frac{1}{[Ag_{free}]}$$

It is this equilibrium constant (K) that immunologists refer to as affinity. Immunoglobulins show a wide range of affinity (10^{-4} to 10^{-14}), with most antibodies falling in the 10^{-5} to 10^{-7} range. The forward (association) reaction for binding an epitope is one of the fastest biochemical reactions known, only ten times less than the theoretical limit of 10^9 liters/mole/sec for diffusion-limited reactions. **Valence** (the number of antigen-binding sites on an immunoglobulin molecule) varies from two for monomeric forms of all isotypes to four (secretory IgA), and ten (for pentameric IgM). The term *avidity* is often used to describe the collective affinity of multiple binding sites on an antibody molecule.

The **precipitin reaction** is the term applied to the interaction of soluble antigen with soluble antibody, resulting in a precipitate. Although discovered in the late nineteenth century, not until the 1930s were scientists able to quantify the amount of antibody present in serum using this reaction. In order to understand antigen-antibody reactions, you must understand the **quantitative precipitin reaction.**

In the classical experiment by Heidelberger and Kendall (1935), capsular polysaccharide from *Streptococcus pneumoniae* was used as antigen and serum from an immunized animal was the antibody source (an antiserum). Varying amounts of antigen (in a constant volume) were mixed with an equal, constant volume of antiserum and incubated (Fig. 4-5). Precipitate formed in several tubes and was separated (by centrifugation) from the supernatant. Heidelberger and Kendall then determined the amount of total nitrogen in the precipitate. Since the antigen is a polysaccharide and does not contain nitrogen, any nitrogen detected must be of antibody (i.e., protein) origin. This experiment demonstrated that *antibody is a protein* and that antigen and antibody react in a *predictable* manner. The degree of antigen-antibody cross-linking results in lattice formation and can be used to describe the three distinct zones of the quantitative precipitin curve.

- *Zone of antigen excess.* The antigen-antibody complexes formed are too small to precipitate.

- *Equivalence zone.* Optimal precipitation occurs in this area of the curve. Large, visible precipitating complexes are formed. It is this property, the formation of a visible precipitate, that is the basis for many immunological tests.
- *Zone of antibody excess.* Not enough antigen is present to form a precipitate. The net result is formation of soluble complexes.

The principles of the quantitative precipitin curve apply to all antigen-antibody reactions and form the basis for many modern clinical diagnostic tests. In some instances, responses are directly mediated by immunoglobulin; in others, antibody-binding serves as a "tag" to focus and facilitate actions by other elements of the immune system. Immunoglobulin isotypes are important in determining the ultimate outcome of an antibody-antigen reaction. Isotypes of large size (e.g., IgM) are confined to the bloodstream, while those

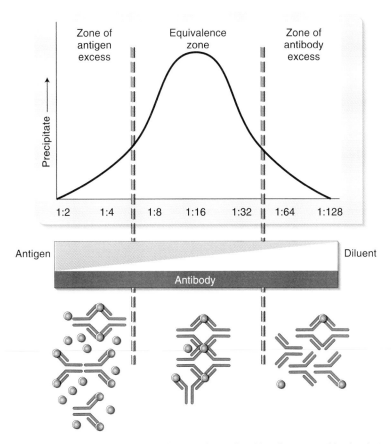

FIGURE 4-5. Quantitative precipitin curve. Antigen (indicated in red) is diluted using a mild salt solution (diluent) in a test tube and is expressed as a reciprocal dilution of antigen or ratio (1:2, 1:4, etc.). Identical amounts of antibody are added to each tube. Following a brief incubation period, precipitation is seen in some of the tubes. Optimal precipitation (the equivalence zone) occurs in tubes where antigen and antibody react to form large lattice-like complexes. Much smaller complexes, too small to precipitate, are formed where there is a relative abundance of antigen to antibody (zone of antigen excess) or of antibody to antigen (zone of antibody excess).

of lower molecular weight (IgG and IgE) can leave the vasculature and enter the tissues. IgG is the only isotype that can cross the placenta and enter the fetal circulation. Maternally derived IgG provides the primary immunologic protection for newborns until their own immune systems become sufficient at about six months of age. IgA can dimerize, and specialized secretory epithelial cells can internalize dimeric IgA, transport it across the cell, and release it to the exterior in saliva, tears, breast milk, and mucous secretions. Secreted IgA (sIgA) is extremely important in immunologic functions involving the alimentary and respiratory tracts, and can also provide some immunologic protection to nursing infants.

Direct effects of antibody

Agglutination

Agglutination is the binding together of multiple cells or particles by antibody-mediated crosslinking of epitopes on their surfaces (Appendix A). This action can inhibit the movement and normal activity of those cells (e.g., bacteria) and render them more susceptible to destruction and removal by phagocytic cells. Agglutination is most effectively achieved by isotypes with larger numbers of binding sites, such as secretory IgA (four binding sites) and IgM (ten binding sites).

Neutralization

Sometimes, antibody attachment to soluble antigens or microbes affects their structure so that the antigen is prevented from binding to a cell [Fig. 4-6]. This binding interferes with the attachment of toxins and microbes to cell surfaces, preventing them from entering the cell or harming it in some other way. This process is known as **neutralization**. IgG and secretory IgA are particularly efficient at neutralization.

Indirect effects of antibody

Often, antibody does not agglutinate or neutralize antigen, but acts as a signal for the activation of other molecules, such as complement, or the activation of cells, such as phagocytes, NK cells, or mast cells.

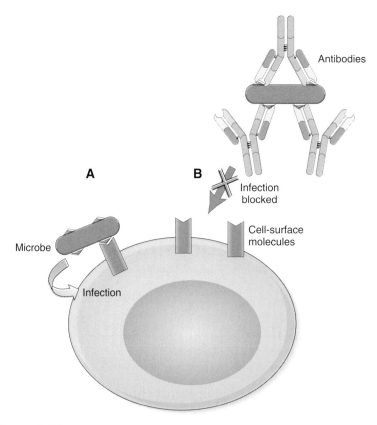

FIGURE 4-6. **Neutralizing antibody. (A)** Binding of surface molecules on microorganisms (red triangles) to surface molecules on cells of the body leads to infection. **(B)** Neutralizing antibodies directed against microbial surface molecules effectively block their binding to host cells, thus preventing infection.

Patient Vignette 4.2

Vera N., a 50-year-old woman with a history of hypothyroidism and chronic diarrhea, presents with recurrent sinusitis and respi-ratory infections. Last year she was hospitalized for pneumonia due to *Streptococcus pneumoniae.***

What is the possible underlying problem?

This patient may have common variable immunodeficiency disorder. Symptoms of this disease usually develop in adulthood. These patients may have recurrent sinusitis and pulmonary infections. The most common causes of infections in these patients include encapsulated bacteria such as *Haemophilus influenza* or *Streptococcus pneumoniae*. In addition, individuals with common variable immunodeficiency disorder may have associated symptoms of malabsorption and autoimmune disease and lymphomas. Most have normal B cells in the peripheral blood; however, they may not have plasma cells in the bone marrow and, therefore they have few or no antibodies. In addition, affected individuals may have impaired T cell function. The T cells produce less IL-2 and IFN-γ than those of healthy people.

Complement activation

Antibodies of the IgG and IgM isotypes bound to antigen may trigger the **classical complement pathway** by interacting with the complement component C1 (Fig. 4-7). IgA, IgD, and IgE cannot interact with C1, and are unable to activate complement via the classical pathway. The C1 component of the serum complement system binds to the conformationally altered Fc region of antigen-bound IgG_1, IgG_3, or IgM. In the case of IgG, C1 must bind and crosslink two IgG molecules in order to be activated. Pentameric IgM, however, can activate C1 because it contains five Fc regions available for C1 binding. The binding of C1 triggers the classical complement pathway, which uses components similar to those we have already seen for the mannan-binding lectin (MBL) complement pathway (Chapter 3).

Antibody (IgG_1, IgG_3, or IgM) recognizes and binds to antigen via the Fab portion of the immunoglobulin molecule, causing a conformational change in the Fc portion near the hinge region. The first component of the classic pathway, C1q, binds directly to the antigen-induced altered immunoglobulin hinge region and becomes activated. In the presence of Ca^{2+}, C1q

$$Antigen + Antibody \rightarrow AgAb$$

$$AgAb + C1q \rightarrow AgAb\overline{C1q} \xrightarrow{Ca^{2+}\ C1r,\ C1s} \begin{array}{c} Ag\ Ab\overline{C1qrs} \\ or \\ AgAb\overline{C1s} \end{array}$$

catalyzes the binding and activation of C1r and C1s to form a C4/C2 convertase (Fig. 4-7).

- *Activation of C4.* The $\overline{C1qrs}$ (usually designated $\overline{C1s}$) complex cleaves C4 into a small fragment (C4a) and a larger fragment (C4b). C4b binds to the membrane.
- *Activation of C2.* The $\overline{C1s}$ complex cleaves C2 into a small fragment (C2a) and a larger fragment (C2b) and C2b binds to C4b.
- *Activation of C3.* $\overline{C4b2b}$, a C3 convertase, is formed by the activation of C4 and C2 and readily cleaves C3 into C3a and C3b. Although some of the C3b binds to the $\overline{C4b2b}$ complex, much of the C3b does not combine with $\overline{C4bC2b}$, but binds directly to the microbial cell surface. The C3 convertase acts as an amplification loop, generating additional chemoattractant fragments (C3a) and cell-membrane-adherent (C3b) fragments. C3b acts as an opsonin, tagging the microbial cell for ingestion by phagocytic cells bearing receptors for membrane-bound C3b.
- *Activation of C5.* The combination of $\overline{C4b2b}$ and C3b forms $\overline{C4b2b3b}$, a C5 convertase.

These enzymes and fragments facilitate destruction of microbes by leading to the assembly of the **membrane attack complex** (MAC, Chapter 3) on the microbial surface and also by increased opsonization due to elevated levels of C3b bound to the microbial surfaces.

Opsonization

Attachment of complement fragment C3b to microbial surfaces can lead to increased phagocytosis of those microbes by interacting with complement receptors (CRs) on the surfaces of the phagocytes. This ability to destroy and remove infectious organisms and cellular debris is an essential part of the body's defenses. Antibody binding to antigen facilitates the uptake and phagocytosis of the cell or material to which it is bound, a process known

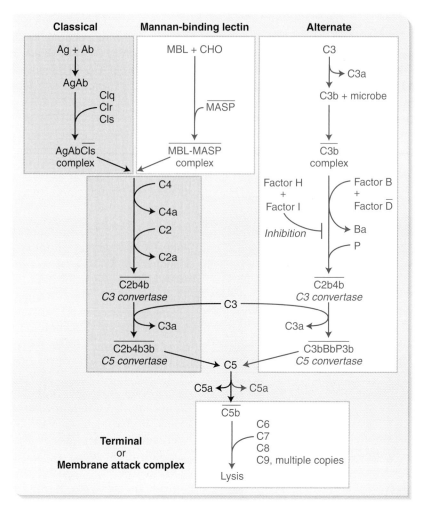

FIGURE 4-7. Classical complement pathway. Proteins of the classical complement pathway are assigned letters and numbers (C1, C2, etc.) that either combine or cleave upon activation. A horizontal bar above the component(s) indicates enzymatic activity (e.g., C1s) and subcomponents or cleavage products are indicated by lowercase letters (e.g., C1q, C1r, C1s or C3a, C3b, etc.). The classical complement pathway is initiated by the interaction of antibody (Ab) with antigen (Ag). A conformational change in the Ab molecule triggers C1q binding, followed by binding of C1r and C1s. The AgAbC̄1s̄ complex cleaves both C4 and C2, forming a C̄2b4b̄ complex that acts as a C3 convertase. This C3 convertase cleaves the native form of C3 into a number of fragments, two of which are shown here. The smaller fragment, C3a, has chemoattractant activity and the larger, C3b, combines with C̄2b4b̄ to make a C5 convertase, C̄2b4b3b̄, that cleaves C5 into two smaller fragments—C5a (another chemoattractant) and C5b that initiates the terminal or lytic pathway of complement.

as **opsonization** (Chapter 3). When an antibody binds to an antigen via its antigen-binding region(s), a conformational change occurs in that antibody's Fc region. Macrophages, other phagocytes, and B cells bear receptors (FcRs) on their surfaces that recognize and bind the "altered" Fc region of immunoglobulin molecules that have already bound to an antigen (Fig. 4-8). The inability of most FcRs to recognize the Fc regions of free unbound Ig prevents them from being distracted by the uptake and degradation of Ig that has yet to bind to anything. When FcRs are bound, the cell ingests and degrades the material initially identified and bound by the immunoglobulins, and, in doing so, becomes activated. Upon activation, phagocytic cells become even more active and increase the rate at which they locate and ingest material. IgM and IgG_1 are the immunoglobulins that most efficiently promote opsonization.

T CELL RECEPTORS

The antigen-specific cell receptor (TCR) is a heterodimer composed of either an αβ or a γδ

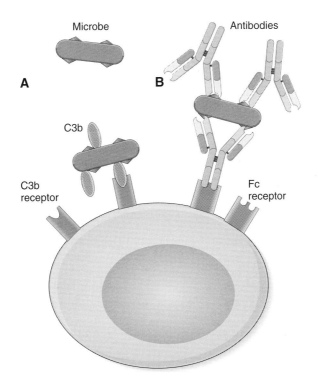

FIGURE 4-8. **Opsonization.** A microbe recognized by either the innate (complement) or the adaptive immune system (antibody and complement) may escape lysis because of the nature of its cell wall. Opsonins such as C3b and antibodies bound to microbial surfaces greatly enhance phagocytosis. Think of this a fail-safe mechanism for the immune system. **(A)** A microbe is recognized by the complement system (alternate, MBL, or classical pathways) and the microbe is decorated with C3b (depicted as blue ovals). Complement receptors (CR1, CR2, CR3, or CR4) on the surfaces of a variety of cells (Table 3-3) bind the C3b attached to the microbial surface, the microbe is internalized, and is destroyed by the phagolysosome. **(B)** Similarly, microbe-bound antibodies may serve as opsonins. Upon antigen binding, a conformational change takes place in the Fc portion of an antibody molecule. Cell-surface Fc receptors recognize and bind the conformationally altered antibody Fc and internalize the microbe-antibody complex for destruction by the phagolysosome.

polypeptide pair (Fig. 4-9). Each polypeptide contains variable and constant domains encoded by genes (and chromosomes) distinct from those responsible for genetically coding immunoglobulins. A T cell expresses either an αβ or a γδ pair. The choice of expressed heterodimer pair is made early in T cell development.

Basic structure

A membrane-bound αβ or γβ TCR heterodimer forms the basic T cell antigen receptor. In addition, it is associated with several other transmembrane molecules that are responsible for stabilization of the interaction of the TCR with its respective ligand (CD4 or CD8) and for signal transduction once a variable region of the TCR is engaged (CD3 complex). CD3 is always associated with the TCR. Unlike antibodies that can readily bind free antigen, a TCR cannot bind soluble antigens, but only enzymatically cleaved

fragments of larger peptides presented as peptide-MHC (pMHC) complexes.

Variable region

The TCR is a member of the Ig supergene family and is composed of two polypeptide chains, an α or δ chain and a larger β or γ chain. Each polypeptide chain of the heterodimer pair contains a variable and a constant region domain. The Vα and Vδ regions are encoded by V and J gene clusters. The Vβ and Vδ regions are encoded by V, D, and J gene clusters, the D gene cluster providing an additional source of variation. The gene clusters undergo DNA rearrangement, similar to that already described for immunoglobulins, to synthesize αβ dimers (Fig. 4-9) or γδ dimers (not shown). As with immunoglobulins, the constant domains of the α and β or γ and δ chains are encoded by constant region genes (Cα and Cβ or Cγ and Cδ). T cell receptors do not

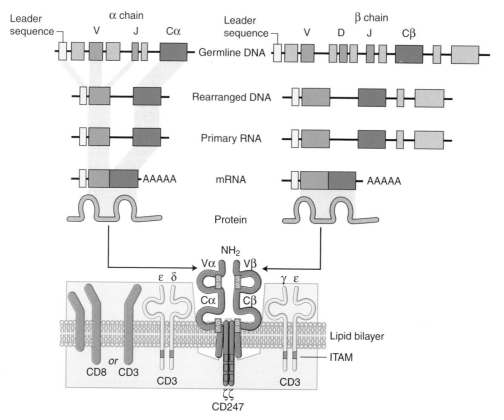

FIGURE 4-9. T cell receptor (TCR) complex and gene rearrangement. The T cell receptor (TCR) complex is composed of an αβ or γδ pair of polypeptides along with associated CD3 (γ, δ, and ε), CD247 (ζ homodimer) and CD4 or CD8 molecules (shaded area). A variable (V) region DNA gene segment combines with a joining (J) segment and a constant (Cα) that is transcribed into messenger RNA (mRNA) and translated into a polypeptide α chain. Recombination of β chain DNA is similar, with the exception that one additional gene segment for diversity (D) is included. The α and β polypeptide TCR is assembled in the endoplasmic reticulum (Chapter 5), where a peptide fragment is loaded into antigen-binding NH₂ portion of the TCR. The fragment-loaded TCR is transported to the cell surface in association with two CD3ε, one CD3γ, one CD3δ, and two CD247 (or ζ chain) molecules (shaded area). The short cytoplasmic tail of the TCR lacks signaling sequences or immunoreceptor tyrosine activation motifs (ITAMs). These are supplied by the CD3 and CD247 molecules. In addition, CD4 or CD4 molecules are associated with the TCR.

undergo any subsequent changes equivalent to the isotype switch, and somatic mutation, important to generating diversity of immunoglobulins, does not occur in T cell receptors.

MAJOR HISTOCOMPATIBILITY COMPLEX MOLECULES

A cluster of closely linked genetic loci comprise the **major histocompatibility complex (MHC)** encoding molecules important to immune functions. While every vertebrate species examined thus far has an MHC, the two most intensely studied are the **human leukocyte antigen (HLA)** complex in humans (chromosome 6) and the **histocompatibility-2 (H2) complex** in mice (chro-

mosome 17). Although we will limit our discussion to humans, the MHCs of these two species are very similar in the nature and number of genes included. This similarity allows us to transfer what is learned in one species to the other.

The MHC can be grouped into five main categories of loci (Table 4-2). Classically, the MHC is considered to include the class I, II, and III loci (Fig. 4-10). Small proteolytic cleavage peptides are loaded by the cell into class I and/or class II molecules for display on its surface. Class I molecules are expressed on the surfaces of all nucleated cells, while class II molecules are normally expressed only by dendritic cells, macrophages, and B lymphocytes. The display of MHC-peptide complexes is "scrutinized" by TCRs on T cells and is crucial for the initiation of adaptive

TABLE 4-2. THE MAJOR HISTOCOMPATIBILITY COMPLEX[a]

Class	Nomenclature	Found on	Functions
I	HLA-A, -B, -C	All nucleated cells	Presentation of intracellularly derived antigens
II[b]	DPα, DPβ, DQα, DQβ, DRα, DRβ1, DRβ2, DRβ4	Dendritic cells, macrophages, B cells, and some activated T cells	Presentation of extracellularly derived antigens
III	C2, C4, Bf	Secreted, not expressed on cell surfaces	Some components of the complement system

[a] The human major histocompatibility complex is also known as the human leukocyte antigen (HLA) system.
[b] Class II molecules α and β are encoded by the α and β loci, respectively. Thus, DPA encodes the DPα chain, DPB the DPβ chain, DQA the DQα chain, etc.

immune responses. Class III molecules include some of the elements of the serum complement system. Recently, several genes have been found within the MHC whose products are important to the functions of the MHC class I and II molecules. These include enzymes, cytokines, and molecules involved in antigen processing and presentation.

Class I molecules

Found on the cell surfaces of all nucleated cells, **MHC class I molecules** are 45-kDa, single-chain glycoproteins that form a complex with 12-kDa

β_2 microglobulin (Fig. 4-10). Co-dominantly expressed genes at each of the three distinct "classical" class I loci, *HLA-A, -B,* and *-C,* are highly polymorphic with over 100 possible alleles at each locus. Up to six different class I molecules, two for each locus, are displayed on the surface of each nucleated cell. All MHC class I molecules fold to produce a cleft that holds a peptide of eight to nine amino acids, although the three-dimensional configurations of the cleft are somewhat variable. Some peptides load into clefts of some MHC class I molecules better than others and, as we will see, this has major implications in the

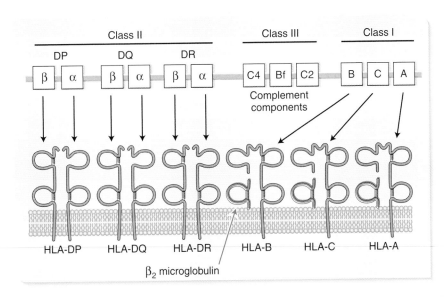

FIGURE 4-10. Major histocompatibility complex (MHC) genes and molecules. Three classes of genes are found within the MHC. Three MHC class I loci, called A, B, and C, encode 45-kDa polypeptides that, together with 12-kDa β2 microglobulin (the blue looped structure), are expressed on all nucleated cells and are known as human leukocyte antigen(s) HLA-A, HLA-B, and HLA-C. MHC class II polypeptides are called HLA-DP, -DQ, and–DR. Each is a heterodimer containing both a 32- to 38kDa α and a 29- to 32-kDa β polypeptide chain. MHC class II molecules are expressed by dendritic cells, macrophages, B lymphocytes, and sometimes by activated T lymphocytes. As members of the immunoglobulin supergene family, MHC class I and II molecules have a looped domain-like structure, often containing an intrachain disulfide bond (blue bar). MHC class I and II molecules encoded on both chromosomes are expressed. MHC class III loci encode several complement components. Unlike MHC class I or II, class III molecules are secreted and not expressed at the cell surface.

nature of the immune response. In addition, a number molecules encoded by "non-classical" class I loci adjacent to the MHC (e.g., HLA-E,-F, -G, -H) are structurally similar to "classical" MHC class I molecules, but are of much more limited variability and tissue distribution. The functions of nonclassical MHC class I molecules are not yet fully clear, but in some cases they present carbohydrate as well as peptide fragments to γδ T cells.

Class II molecules

Unlike Class I molecules, *MHC class II molecules* are normally expressed by only a small number of cells—dendritic cells, macrophages, and B cells. Class II molecules are also expressed on some epithelial cells of the thymus and by some activated T cells. Class II molecules are encoded genes within the *DP, DQ,* and *DR* regions of the human HLA complex (Fig. 4-10). Contained within each region are α and β loci (DPα, DPβ, DQα, DQβ, etc.). After synthesis, MHC class II α and β chains associate only with others encoded within the same region (e.g., DPβ associates only with DPβ, but never with DQβ or DRβ). In combination, the 32- to 38-kDa α and 29- to 32-kDa β chains form a molecular complex that is very similar to that of

the class I complex, with a binding groove available for holding short peptides. The ends of the binding grooves of class II molecules are more open than in class I molecules and can accommodate peptides of 18 to 20 amino acids or more in length. Like class I molecules, class II molecules are highly variable, and numerous allelic forms exist for each locus (except DRα, which appears to be invariant). Keep in mind that each APC simultaneously expresses all of its class II and class I genes. Genetic variation among class II molecules creates a range of subtly varying binding grooves for which antigen fragments compete.

An additional form of variation is available to class II molecules because of their heterodimeric structure. Termed **cis-trans complementation,** this diversity stems from the fact that class II α and β chains combine after synthesis. Thus, a DPα chain derived from a paternal chromosome may combine with either a DPβ chain derived from a paternal or a maternal chromosome (Fig. 4-11). Therefore, individuals heterozygous for both DPα and DPβ (a common situation, given the high level of variation in these genes) can produce a greater range of class II dimer combinations than if they were homozygous at DPα or at DPβ or at both. As we see later, the range of

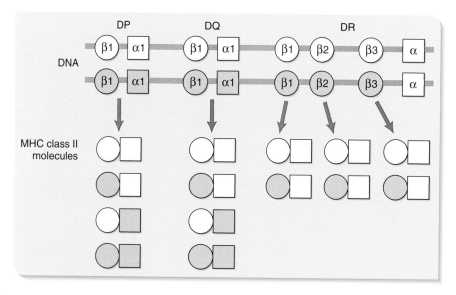

FIGURE 4-11. MHC class II heterogeneity. Each MHC class II molecule is composed of two polypeptide chains, termed α and β, encoded by genes within the DP, DR, and DQ regions. After synthesis, class II α and β chains can only pair with those from the same region (e.g., DPα of one chromosome associates only with the DPβ encoded by either chromosome). The DR region contains three β loci (β1, β2, and β4) and DRα appears to be invariant in human populations. Assuming different alleles at each of the loci, 14 different MHC class II molecules are expressed by each antigen-presenting cell and by some activated T cells.

different MHC I and MHC II molecules expressed can affect the overall immune capacity of an individual.

Class III molecules

Class III molecules are a subset of the components of serum complement. The C2 and C4 components, as well as the regulatory factor B (Bf) are encoded within the complex (Fig. 4-10). The various components of complement are synthesized by a variety of cells.

CLUSTER OF DIFFERENTIATION MOLECULES

Cluster of differentiation (CD) molecules are cell surface molecules that indicate the functional capacities of lymphocytes and other cells. To date, over 250 CD molecules have been identified and many are important in distinguishing lymphocyte subsets. We will introduce CD molecules on a "need to know" basis. For a more complete listing, see Appendix B.

CD3

The **CD3 complex** is comprised of several molecules associated with the T-cell antigen receptor (Fig. 4-9). It is composed of six polypeptides (2 CD3ε + 1 CD3γ + 1 CD3δ + 1 CD247 ζ–ζ homodimer) and is found on all T cells. It provides support for the TCR and is involved in transmembrane signaling when the TCR is filled.

CD4

CD4 is a 55-kDa molecule belongs to the Ig supergene family with four immunoglobulin-like domains. A cell-surface molecule, CD4 is found in association with the TCR on approximately two-thirds of mature T cells (the T-cell subset known as helper T (Th) cells). CD4 molecules recognize the lateral, nonpeptide-binding portion of MHC class II molecules. The TCRs of CD4$^+$ T cells are "restricted" to the recognition of MHC class II-peptide complexes.

CD8

CD8 is a two-chain cell-surface complex containing 32- to 34-kDa polypeptides that are expressed either as a homodimers ($\alpha\alpha$) or heterodimers ($\alpha\beta$) by approximately one-third of mature T cells. CD8$^+$ T cells are also called **cytotoxic** *T* (Tc) and **suppressor** *T* (Ts) cells to reflect their function. CD8 molecules associate with the TCR and recognize MHC class I-peptide complexes. Mature $\alpha\beta$ T cells express either CD4 or CD8. However, during an early developmental stage, $\alpha\beta$ T cells express both CD4 and CD8. The $\gamma\delta$ T cells, on the other hand, often express neither CD4 nor CD8.

CLINICAL APPLICATION

CD molecules are important features in the definition and diagnosis of B and T cell neoplasms. For example, low-grade lymphoma of the T cell type has CD3$^+$ and CD56$^-$ markers and the NK type has CD3$^-$ and CD56$^+$ or CD56$^-$ markers.

CYTOKINES AND CHEMOKINES

Cytokines are low-molecular-weight soluble proteins used for cellular communication. Cytokines are involved in all aspects of the innate and adaptive immune response, including cellular growth and differentiation, inflammation, and repair. Originally, cytokines were called **lymphokines** and **monokines** to reflect lymphocytic or monocytic origin. We now recognize that these substances are produced by a wide variety of leukocytes and nonleukocytes. A large number of cytokines have been identified, although the roles of many of them are not yet fully understood. Many cytokines are crucial in regulating lymphocyte development and the types of immune responses evoked by specific responses. Low-molecular-weight cytokines known as **chemokines** (chemoattractant cytokines) stimulate lymphocyte movement and migration. Cytokines and chemokines most basically involved in common immune responses are listed in Appendix C. These molecules and their functions will be discussed in detail as we consider the various immune responses in which they are involved.

ADHESION MOLECULES

Adhesion molecules provide stable cell-to-cell contact. While this is a seemingly simple activity, the ability of cells to examine the surface of other cells and to establish stable contact with them is vital. A variety of surface molecules enable adhesion and are classified into two major categories.

Some adhesion molecules are needed to provide basic stable contact. For cells to communicate and for cell-surface receptors and ligands to interact, the cells must be able to establish and maintain close surface-to-surface contact for some minimal period of time. **Integrins** are found on the surfaces of a wide variety of cells and can interact with other molecules that are based on the Ig superfamily motif, which is also found on a wide variety of cells, and with extracellular matrix. These interactions initiate the adhesion of many types of cells so that additional interactions can then develop to build stable interactions. They might be thought of as a cellular form of Velcro™.

Other adhesion molecules are more limited in their tissue distribution and are designed to identify particular tissues and to facilitate the interactions of particular cells (Fig. 4-12). These molecules include the **selectins** and the **addressins**. For example, newly differentiated lymphocytes need to migrate to lymph nodes to undergo their next stage of development. This is accomplished by interactions between specialized molecules found on the lymphocytes such as *CD62L* (also known as L-selectin) and other molecules (e.g., GlyCAM-1, an addressin) located on the endothelium of blood vessels passing through lymph nodes. Interactions between these molecules signal the lymphocyte that it has found a lymph node and then facilitate movement of the lymphocyte out of the vessel and into the node. Other selectins and addressins as-

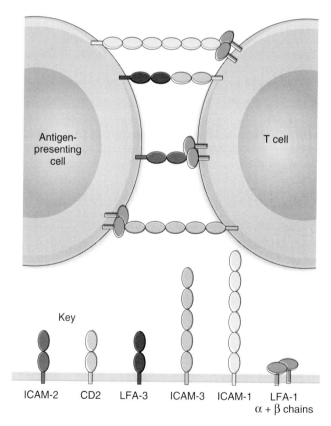

FIGURE 4-12. **Cell adhesion molecules.** Cell adhesion molecules stabilize contact between cells. Leukocyte functional antigen-1 (LFA-1) is a heterodimer containing α and β polypeptide chains with cytoplasmic tails and is expressed by a variety of leukocytes; it may bind to intercellular adhesion molecules-1, -2, or -3 (ICAM-1, -2, -3). Leukocyte functional antigen-3 (LFA-3) interacts with CD2.

sist in the movement of lymphocytes and other cells to the gut, epithelium, and sites of tissue inflammation.

CLINICAL APPLICATION

Leukocyte adhesion deficiency 1 is due to the absence of an adhesion molecule. Since the leukocyte cannot adhere, chemotaxis cannot occur and the leukocyte cannot migrate. Because the leukocyte cannot migrate to the site of inflammation, an inflammatory response is absent. Affected individuals have histories of delayed separation of the umbilical cord, increased white blood cell counts, and recurrent infections of skin, mucous membranes, and gastrointestinal tract. They will also have potentially life threatening bacterial and fungal infections.

Summary

- Molecules of the adaptive immune system include immunoglobulins, T cell receptors, cell determinant or cluster of differentiation (CD) molecules, major histocompatibility (MHC) molecules (in humans, the human leukocyte antigen or HLA molecules), cytokines, and complement.
- The basic **immunoglobulin** monomer contains two identical light (L) and two identical heavy (H) glycoprotein chains linked by disulfide bonds.
- Both heavy and light chains may be divided into regions or **domains,** homologous portions of an immunoglobulin chain, each composed of approximately 110 amino acids and containing an intradomain disulfide bridge.
- Light chains contain two regions, a **variable** (V_L) and a *constant* (C_L) domain. Heavy chains contain a single variable (V_H) and multiple constant domains (C_H1, C_H2, C_H3, and sometimes C_H4).
- Normal individuals express all five immunoglobulin **classes** or **isotypes.** IgM is the heaviest isotype. Human IgG can be divided further into four subclasses: IgG_1, IgG_2, IgG_3, and IgG_4. IgD has a very low serum concentration (less than 1%) and is found almost exclusively on B cell surfaces. IgA is usually associated with mucous membranes and their secretions. Atopic individuals (those susceptible to allergic reactions) often show elevated concentrations of IgE.
- The antigen-specific **T cell receptor** (TCR) is a heterodimer composed of either of an $\alpha\beta$ or a $\gamma\delta$ polypeptide pair.
- Genes of the **major histocompatibility complex** (MHC) encode molecules important to immune functions. The MHC includes class I, II, and III loci. **Class I molecules** are expressed on the surfaces of all nucleated cells, while **class II molecules** are normally expressed only by dendritic cells, macrophages, and B lymphocytes. **Class III molecules** include some of the elements of the serum complement system.
- **Cluster of differentiation** (CD) molecules indicate the functional capacities of lymphocytes and other cells. The **CD3** complex is composed of several molecules associated with the T cell antigen receptor. **CD4** is found in association with the TCR on approximately two-thirds of mature T cells, called helper T (Th) cells. CD8$^+$ T cells are also called cytotoxic T (Tc) and suppressor T (Ts) cells to reflect their function. **CD8** molecules associate with the TCR and recognize MHC class I-peptide complexes.
- Complement activation is another important immune response in which immunoglobulins "tag" cells and molecules for destruction. IgG_1, IgG_3, and IgM antibodies, once bound to antigen, can trigger the **classical complement pathway** by interacting with component C1 of the classical pathway.
- **Opsonization** refers to an increase in uptake and destruction of antigen by phagocytic cells using a variety of receptors.
- *Cytokines* are low-molecular-weight soluble proteins used for cellular communication.
- Some **adhesion molecules** are needed to provide basic stable contact. These molecules include the **integrins,** the **selectins,** and the **addressins.**

Suggested readings

Gellert M. Recent advances in understanding V (D) J recombination. *Adv Immunol* 1997;64:39.

Poljak RJ. Structure of antibodies and their complexes with antigens. *Molec Immunol* 1991;28: 1341.

Review questions

DIRECTIONS: Each of the number items or incomplete statement in this section is followed by answers or by completions of the statement. Select ONE lettered answer or completion that is BEST in each case.

1. Which of the following isotypes is found as a pentamer in the serum?
   (A) IgA
   (B) IgD
   (C) IgE
   (D) IgG
   (E) IgM

2. Activation of the classical complement pathway involves:
   (A) binding of antigen by IgE.
   (B) factors B and P.
   (C) interaction between mannan and mannan-binding lectin (MBL).
   (D) binding of antigen by IgM or IgG.
   (E) binding of antigen by C3b.

3. Antibody idiotype is determined by the:
   (A) antigen-binding region.
   (B) Fc region.
   (C) light chain constant region.
   (D) hinge region.
   (E) heavy chain constant region.

4. Which of the following isotypes is homocytophilic?
   (A) IgA
   (B) IgD
   (C) IgE
   (D) IgG
   (E) IgM

5. An important function of TNF is to:
   (A) induce isotype switches in B cells
   (B) increase body temperature
   (C) induce expression of IL-2 receptors on Th1 cells
   (D) induce apoptosis in infected target cells
   (E) induce degranulation of mast cells

6. Adhesion molecules
   (A) are important in stabilizing the interactions between leukocytes.
   (B) are important in agglutination reactions.
   (C) are involved in the quantitative precipitin reaction.
   (D) do not play a significant role in the immune response.
   (E) are responsible for "joining" immunoglobulin monomers into pentameric forms of IgM.

7. Cluster of differentiation (CD) molecules are found
   (A) exclusively on T cells.
   (B) exclusively on B cells.
   (C) only on erythrocytes.
   (D) exclusively on leukocytes.
   (E) on every cell of the body.

8. Chemokines are:
   (A) CD molecules on steroids.
   (B) another name for chemoattractant cytokines.
   (C) adhesion molecules.
   (D) complement receptors.
   (E) native (not activated) components of the classical complement pathway.

9. Which isotypes promote opsonization?
   (A) IgA and IgM
   (B) IgD and IgA
   (C) IgE and IgG
   (D) IgG and IgM
   (E) IgM and IgA

10. The predominant antibody isotype within the oral cavity is:
    (A) IgA_1
    (B) IgG_3
    (C) IgA_2
    (D) IgG_2
    (E) IgE

11 A 36-year-old woman has a known history of selective IgA deficiency. She is scheduled for an elective surgery within the next several weeks that may require blood transfusion. What should the patient be cautioned about?
    (A) Patients with IgA deficiency have an increased risk of anaphylactic reactions to blood transfusion.
    (B) Patients with IgA deficiency have an increased risk of anaphylactic reactions to general anesthetics.
    (C) Patients with IgA deficiency have an increased risk of adverse reaction to antibiotic therapies.
    (D) Patients with IgA deficiency have an increased risk of anaphylactic reactions to all drugs.

The Adaptive Immune Response

Chapter Outline

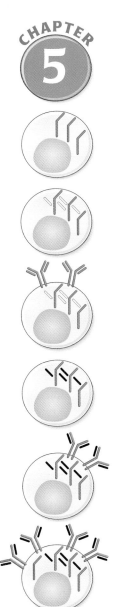

Introduction The **adaptive immune** system recognizes antigens using randomly generated B-cell and T-cell surface receptors (BCRs and TCRs). On antigen encounter, the small number of lymphocytes bearing the appropriate antigen-specific receptor must clonally expand, making enough cells to deal with the antigenic insult. Consequently, adaptive immune responses to an initial encounter with an antigen develop rather slowly compared with those of the innate system. Adaptive immune responses to subsequent antigenic encounters are rapid and robust, often stopping microbial invasion with a speed that rivals or exceeds that of innate immune responses. The ability to recall previous antigenic exposure and respond appropriately is termed **memory** and is a hallmark of the adaptive immune system.

Because the adaptive system can make receptors that recognize nonpathogenic antigens, adverse immune reactions such as autoimmunity, graft rejection, transfusion reactivity, and allergic responses may occur. The adaptive system uses a variety of checks and balances to minimize potential self-destruction and relies on the collaboration between different cell types for recognition, regulation, and effector function. T cells play a pivotal role as antigen-specific regulators and sometimes as effector cells. Because of their central role in adaptive responses, the manner in which T cells recognize and are activated by antigen is highly regulated. Antigen-specific TCRs do not recognize soluble antigens, but recognize only **peptides bound to major histocompatibility complex** (pMHC) molecules. In addition, co-stimulatory signals are required for the activation of T cells in addition to the recognition of pMHC fragments. Induction of most adaptive immune responses requires that T cells interact with **antigen-presenting cells** (APCs)—dendritic cells, macrophages, or B cells. Dendritic cells and macrophages actively sample their environment. APCs enzymatically break down and display (to T cells) peptide fragments of cells and molecules they encounter. APCs also provide appropriate co-stimulatory molecules necessary for the activation of T cells. Depending on the nature of the signals encountered, antigen-specific T cells will either initiate an immune response or remain unresponsive. Here, we explore the nature of the interactions that result in adaptive immune responses.

INITIATION OF AN ADAPTIVE IMMUNE RESPONSE

In contrast to the innate immune system, the adaptive immune system uses specific receptors generated randomly by deoxyribonucleic acid (DNA) rearrangement. Many more receptor specificities are generated than an individual will ever encounter during her or his lifetime. The limited occurrence of an appropriate epitope-specific receptor expressed by lymphocytes requires clonal cell proliferation to develop sufficient numbers of lymphocytes to adequately deal with the antigenic insult. Expansion of antigen-specific cells requires time, typically 18 to 24 hours per generation, a rate that is 50 times less than the doubling time for many microbes. In general, the adaptive immune response, once established, is deadly for the microbe.

The innate immune system is the gateway to the adaptive immune response. Adaptive immune responses are initiated by cells of the innate system, resulting in the clonal expansion of antigen-specific T cells, and effector responses often end with the utilization of cells and/or molecules of the innate system. On crossing the skin or mucosal barrier, both microbial and soluble antigens encounter phagocytic cells of the innate immune system, where they are (hopefully) destroyed. The proteolytic fragments are loaded into MHC molecules and displayed on the cell surface in a process called **antigen presentation.**

Antigen presentation

Microbes enter the body at their own peril. The skin and mucous membranes offer protective barriers against microbial invasion. However, cuts, abrasions, or hypodermic injections break this barrier. Initial microbial encounter often results in the invader's destruction by chemical means (e.g., complement-mediated lysis) or by phagocytosis followed by enzymatic degradation. Phagocytic leukocytes (dendritic cells, macrophages, and polymorphonuclear cells) located throughout the body are responsible for the removal of cellular debris produced by cells that have died through natural or hostile causes and for the phagocytosis of microbes.

Specialized cells located in the skin and mucous membranes, known as dendritic cells, act as sentinels of the immune system. These cells actively engulf self and nonself molecules, as well as foreign cells, dying cells, and cell fragments. The internalized material is proteolytically degraded into peptide fragments, and some peptides are loaded onto MHC class I and II molecules and displayed on the APC cell surface. Cells that display peptides bound by MHC class II molecules are known as **professional APCs** and are primarily dendritic cells, macrophages, and B cells. Occasionally, other cells such as intestinal epithelial cells can also act as APCs.

The role of dendritic cells in the initiation of adaptive immune responses

Dendritic cells are heterogeneous and widely distributed throughout the body. In the skin, a subset of dendritic cells is known as **Langerhans cells**. Although dendritic cells are most abundant in the skin and mucous membranes, they comprise less than 1% of the cells in these tissues. Immature dendritic cells are actively phagocytic, engulfing and degrading both self and nonself molecules and cell fragments, but are not effective APCs. Despite active degradation of the ingested cells and molecules, few peptides are displayed on

the cell surface as pMHC complexes. On encounter with a microbe, dendritic cells rapidly mature and are transformed into efficient APCs that can activate previously unstimulated T cells. Although their phagocytic capacity decreases, maturing dendritic cells have an increased number of pMHC complexes and co-stimulatory molecules displayed on their cell surfaces. They are also capable of migration. Mature dendritic cells are the most efficient APCs and efficiently activate previously unstimulated T cells. Other APCs such as macrophages are far less efficient and are usually only capable of restimulating T cells.

Antigen uptake

Immature dendritic cells capture microbes, infected cells, dead cells, or their molecules either by receptor-mediated phagocytosis or by macropinocytosis. Phagocytosis involves cell-surface receptors associated with specialized regions of the plasma membrane called **clathrin-coated pits** (Fig. 5-1). These receptors include Fc (FcγRII, FcαR), complement (CR3 and CR4), heat shock proteins (hsps), and low-density lipoprotein-binding scavenger receptors (SR). Receptor engagement induces actin-dependent phagocytosis, receptor internalization, and the formation of small, uniform size (approximately 100 nm) intracellular vacuoles.

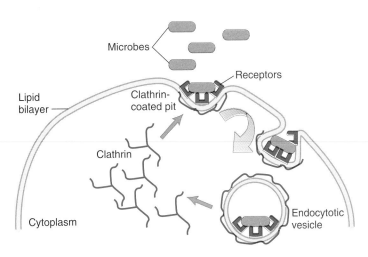

FIGURE 5-1. Clathrin-coated pits. Phagocytosis involves the capture of cells, particles, or molecules by specialized receptors associated with special regions of the cell membrane called clathrin-coated pits. Clathrin is a trimeric cytoplasmic protein that forms polyhedral lattice structures that cause further invagination of the cell membrane, which eventually pinches off to form an endocytotic vesicle.

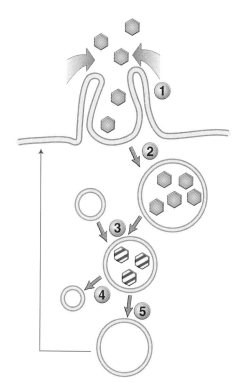

FIGURE 5-2. Macropinocytosis. Macropinocytosis is endocytosis accompanying cell-surface ruffling that does not rely on clathrin-coated pits. 1. Cytoplasmic ruffles of the cell membrane enclose the microbes, particles, or molecules. 2. A cytoplasmic vesicle is formed. 3. Enzyme-containing cytoplasmic vesicles fuse with the endocytic vesicle and the ingested material is degraded. 4. Degraded material is transported to other regions of the cytoplasm. 5. The empty vesicle is recycled to the cell surface.

Dendritic cells also sample large amounts of soluble molecules present in the fluids by **macropinocytosis**. In contrast to phagocytosis, macropinocytosis does not rely on clathrin—associated receptors. Instead, the plasma membrane forms a ruffle that folds back on the cell surface to form relatively large (up to 5 μm) intracellular vesicles (Fig. 5-2).

Maturation and migration

Immature dendritic cells voraciously ingest both soluble and particulate matter from their environment. This activity results in the enzymatic destruction of the ingested material. To initiate an adaptive immune response, dendritic cells must mature. Direct or indirect sensing of an impending or ongoing infection results in dendritic cell maturation. **Direct sensing** occurs through engagement of **pattern-recognition receptors** (PRRs) expressed

on dendritic cells that recognize **pathogen-associated molecular patterns** (PAMPs) on viruses, bacteria, fungi, and protozoa. **Indirect sensing** occurs through the engagement of **toll-like receptors** (TLR), in addition to those recognizing PAMPs, cytokine receptors, tumor necrosis factor (TNF) receptor family molecules, **receptor for the Fc-portion of immunoglobulin** (FcR), or cell death sensors. Which PRRs are engaged conveys the nature of the microbe to the cell, and this assists the dendritic cell to determine the nature of the immune response.

Although the physiological mechanisms of dendritic cell maturation remain to be clarified, part of the maturation process requires dendritic cell migration. Either direct or indirect sensing changes the adhesive properties of dendritic cells, resulting in migration of dendritic cells from the tissues to draining lymph nodes. The final stage of maturation appears to require localization of dendritic cells to the T-cell—rich zones of secondary lymphoid organs where dendritic cells interact with T cells. Mature dendritic cells characteristically have enhanced levels of antigenic pMHC complexes and co-stimulatory and adhesion molecules, and they secrete chemotactic cytokines, and chemokines are expressed to attract naïve T cells.

Macrophages

Nonactivated resting **macrophages** and **monocytes** are far less efficient than dendritic cells in stimulating naïve T cells. Like dendritic cells, macrophages are actively phagocytic. Unlike dendritic cells, resting (not activated) macrophages do not express cell-surface MHC class II molecules. On activation, stimulated macrophages appear to lack the migratory capacity characteristic of dendritic cells and also are far less efficient than dendritic cells in stimulating naïve T cells. Activated macrophages, however, rapidly express cell-surface MHC class II molecules and efficiently restimulate previously activated T cells.

Antigen processing and presentation

Antigen-specific adaptive immune responses require the proteolytic processing of protein antigens to generate short peptides that then can be bound by MHC molecules on the surface of an APC. Adaptive immune responses result from the interaction of T-cell receptors with pMHC.

Whether a peptide fragment is loaded into a MHC class I or II molecule depends, in large part, on the origin of the protein. Exogenous proteins—those that originate outside of the cell, such as bacteria and proteins found in the extracellular tissues and fluids—are loaded into MHC class II molecules. Endogenous proteins, those synthesized within the cell's cytoplasm, such as viral proteins, are loaded into MHC class I molecules.

MHC class II and exogenous proteins

Extracellular protein molecules and cells, whether bound by cell-surface receptors associated with clathrin-coated pits or by macropinocytosis, are internalized into phagocytic cells by the formation of acidified intracellular vesicles or **phagosomes** (Fig. 5-3A). One or more enzyme-laden vesicles or **lysosomes** then fuse with the phagosome, forming

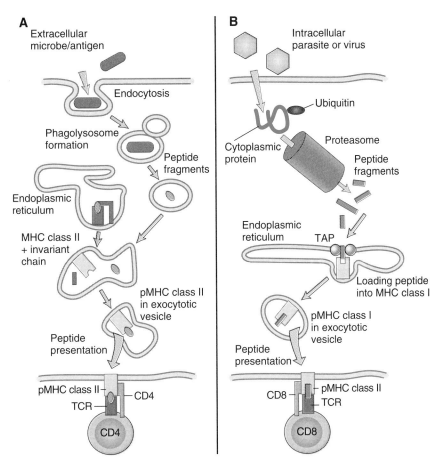

FIGURE 5-3. Pathways for antigen presentation. How antigen enters an antigen-presenting cell strongly influences the outcome of the immune response. **(A)** Antigens present in the extracellular fluid enter the cell by phagocytosis or macropinocytosis. Antigens are contained within cytoplasmic phagocytic vesicles that fuse with lysosomal vesicles to form phagolysosomes in which the ingested material is enzymatically degraded into short peptides. MHC class II α–β polypeptide complexes together with an invariant chain are assembled within the endoplasmic reticulum. Vesicles bud off from the endoplasmic reticulum and fuse with the peptide-containing phagolysosomes. The invariant chain disintegrates on the decrease in pH and the peptide may then occupy the peptide-binding groove in the MHC class II molecule. The vesicle containing the pMHC class II complex is transported to the cell surface for display and recognition by a TCR on a CD4+ T cell. **(B)** Some antigens such as parasites or viruses circumvent phagocytic vesicles and directly enter the cellular cytoplasm. Many of these proteins, marked by the covalent attachment of ubiquitin, are subject to degradation by the proteasome enzyme complex. Small peptide fragments produced by proteasome degradation enter the endoplasmic reticulum by a gatekeeper heterodimer known as the transporter associated with antigen processing, or TAP. TAP transports peptides into the endoplasmic reticulum and loads them into MHC class I molecules. Exocytotic vesicles containing pMHC class II molecules bud off from the endoplasmic reticulum and are transported to the cell surface. pMHC class I complexes are displayed for recognition by the TCR of CD8+ T cells.

a **phagolysosome** that proteolytically cleaves the extracellular proteins into small peptides. Enzymatic cleavage of cells or proteins into peptides is called **antigen processing**. Within the endoplasmic reticulum, MHC class II molecules are synthesized and associated with an **invariant (Ii) chain**. The Ii chain's purpose is to keep the peptide-binding cleft of MHC class II molecules free of the cell's own peptides, until peptides of exogenous origin are available. **Exocytotic vesicles** (vesicles that export material out of the cell) containing MHC class II-Ii complexes bud off from the endoplasmic reticulum and fuse with peptide-containing phagolysosomes. Proteolytic enzymes within the fused exocytotic–phagolysosome vesicle cleave Ii so that only a 24-amino acid peptide known as **class II-associated invariant chain peptide (CLIP)** remains in the peptide-binding cleft of the class II molecule. Also present within the fused vesicle is a nonpolymorphic molecule known as **human leukocyte antigen-DM** (HLA-DM) that does not associate with Ii. HLA-DM facilitates CLIP removal and makes the MHC antigen-binding cleft available for binding of exogenous peptides. Vesicles containing newly loaded pMHC class II complexes

are transported and displayed on the cell surface. HLA-DM is not displayed on the cell surface.

MHC class I and endogenous proteins

Not all pathogens come in through the "front door" of phagocytic vesicles. Some pathogens avoid phagocytes altogether. Pathogens such as viruses and intracellular microbes directly enter the cytoplasm of cells. Cytoplasmic proteins are constantly degraded in all nucleated cells. **Ubiquitin**, a highly conserved 76-amino acid protein, covalently attaches to proteins destined for destruction (see Fig. 5-3B). Although the mechanism(s) by which proteins are targeted for destruction is not yet understood, the binding of one or more ubiquitin molecules is essential for protein destruction by a large protein complex within the cytoplasm known as the **proteasome**. Postproteasome peptides are transported to the endoplasmic reticulum. A heterodimer known as **transporter associated with antigen-processing** (TAP) serves as a gatekeeper to the endoplasmic reticulum. Postproteasome peptides of six to 25 amino acids in length are transported from the cytoplasm into the endoplasmic reticulum by the TAP dimer. Newly synthesized MHC class I molecules bind to the chaperone protein **calnexin** within the endoplasmic reticulum. The calnexin–class I polypeptide (also called Iα) complex allows β_2 microglobulin to associate with class Iα. On formation of the Iα:β_2 complex, calnexin is replaced with **calreticulin** and **tapasin** chaperone proteins. Tapasin associates the nascent class Iα:β_2 complex with the TAP dimer to allow the loading of peptides into the MHC class I:β_2 complex (Fig. 5-4). Peptide loading stabilizes the MHC I:β_2 complex; without a peptide, the complex rapidly disintegrates. Peptide–class I complexes are transported by specialized structures (exocytotic vesicles) that export molecules to the cell surface for display.

T-lymphocyte development

Fundamentally, the immune system distinguishes between "self" and "nonself." We can view the range of epitopes to which the adaptive immune system can respond as its "repertoire." As you might imagine, in the random process of generating diversity, a variety of TCR specificities would be generated for peptides that you may never encounter during your lifetime. Three distinct categories of TCR specificities can be identified; those that recognize peptides that will never be encoun-

---

Patient Vignette 5.1

A 2-month-old infant from North Africa presents with chronic diarrhea and gastrointestinal, pulmonary, upper respiratory and urinary tract infections. The recent blood cultures reveal *Pseudomonas* bacteria. He also has cytomegalovirus infection.

What is the possible clinical situation?

This infant may have a form of **severe combined immunodeficiency disease** (SCID). The presenting clinical signs and symptoms are consistent with **bare lymphocyte syndrome type II**. The defect is caused by lack of class II antigens. The B- and T-cell lymphocytes are normal but the CD4$^+$ cells are significantly reduced. Most children with severe combined immunodeficiency disease have very poor T-cell function, low immunoglobulin levels, and antibody responses that are significantly reduced. The treatment for this disease is bone marrow transplantation. Bare lymphocyte syndrome is one of the rarest forms of SCID.

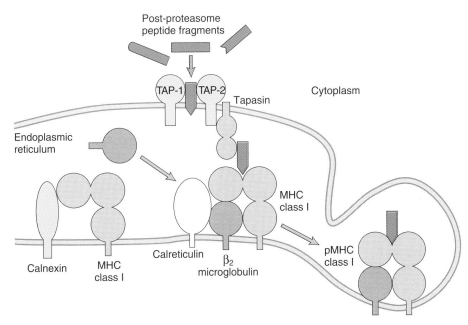

FIGURE 5-4. Transporter associated with antigen-processing (TAP). Proteins are enzymatically degraded by the proteasome into peptides, which are transported to the endoplasmic reticulum. A gatekeeper heterodimer known as the transporter associated with antigen processing (TAP-1 and TAP-2) transports peptides into the endoplasmic reticulum. Calnexin or Iα, a chaperone molecule, binds to newly synthesized MHC class I molecules. Calnexin allows the placement of β_2 microglobulin to form a MHC class I:β_2 complex. Calnexin is replaced by another chaperone, calreticulum. A third chaperone, tapasin, associates with TAP for loading peptide into the MHC class I:β_2 complex. If peptide is not loaded, the MHC class I:β_2 complex rapidly disintegrates.

tered, those that recognize peptides produced by potential pathogens or peptides of foreign origin, and those that recognize peptides that are produced by our own cells. Reaction against "self" peptides by the immune system would place the body's cells and tissues under constant attack by the very system whose role it is to protect and defend. Fortunately, the adaptive immune system has evolved an elegant solution against this threat—the **positive and negative selection** of T cells within the thymus.

T-cell precursors migrate from the bone marrow to enter the thymus as **thymocytes,** They express neither αβ TCR nor cluster of differentiation 4 (CD4) or CD8 molecules (Fig. 5-5), and are called **double-negative (DN) cells**. DN cells proliferate in the subcapsular region of the thymus and differentiate to express low levels of newly generated αβ TCR, *both* CD4 and CD8, and are called **double-positive (DP) cells**. DP cells move inward to the deeper portion of the thymus, where they are fated to die within 3 to 4 days, unless their TCRs recognize an MHC class I or class II molecule on thymic dendritic cells. This process is termed **positive selection**. Although the mechanism of positive selection

process is yet unclear; partial recognition of class II by CD4 or class I by CD8 molecules must occur. T cells that recognize "self" MHC molecules survive. A DP thymocyte with a TCR that engages MHC class I may become a CD8[+] T cell and a DP thymocyte that recognizes MHC class II may become a CD4[+] T cell.

Class I and class II molecules are not displayed on cell surfaces unless they are loaded with a peptide. Only molecules of "self" origin are available on thymic APCs, and these are presented to the DP thymocytes in the deep or medullary area of the thymus. Thymocytes that show strong interaction with MHC molecules or pMHC complexes undergo apoptosis (programmed cell death), a process known as **negative selection**. Thymocytes that survive both positive and negative selection migrate from the thymus to populate lymphoid tissues and organs as T cells. By applying both positive and negative selection of thymocytes, the adaptive immune system is assured of a population of naïve T cells with TCRs that respond to non-self peptides presented by self-MHC molecules and in which self-reactive T cells have been eliminated.

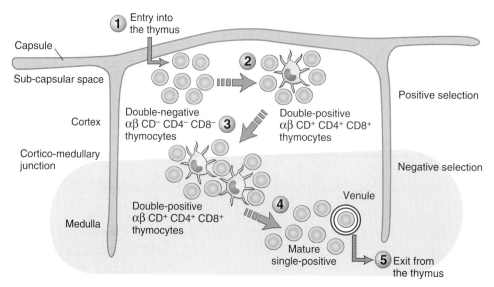

FIGURE 5-5. Positive and negative selection within the thymus. Lymphocyte precursor cells from the bone marrow travel via the circulation to the subcapsular space of the thymus. 1. The newly arrived cells are called double-negative (DN) thymocytes because they do not express a T-cell receptor (TCR), CD3, CD4, or CD8 molecules. 2. DN cells proliferate and differentiate into thymocytes that express a TCR and both CD4 and CD8 molecules. At this stage, they are called double-positive (DP) thymocytes. 3. DP thymocytes die within 3 to 4 days unless they recognize an MHC class I or class II molecule expressed by cortical dendritic cells at the cortico-medullary junction in the thymus. This process is called positive selection. 4. DP thymocytes that show strong interaction with MHC or pMHC undergo programmed cell death (apoptosis), a process known as negative selection. Cells that survive both positive and negative selection and express the TCR and CD4 or CD8 are mature single positive (SP) thymocytes. 5. Mature SP thymocytes cross the endothelium of a venule and exit the thymus as T cells.

Antigen-specific recognition by T lymphocytes

The adaptive immune response is in large part directed by T cells. Unlike cells of the innate system, the antigen-specific T-cell receptor cannot recognize soluble molecules, only those bound to MHC molecules. The nature of the T-cell response to antigen is strongly influenced by the nature of the presentation. The interface between APC and naïve T cell is sometimes called the **immunologic synapse**.

Recognition: the immunologic synapse

The first step in building the immunologic synapse occurs when the TCR recognizes antigenic peptides bound by the peptide-binding cleft of an MHC molecule (Fig. 5-6). The weak bond between the pMHC and TCR is stabilized by interaction with either CD4 or CD8 molecules. CD4 molecules bind with the nonpeptide-binding portion of MHC class II molecules, and CD8 molecules bind with the nonpeptide portion of MHC

class I molecules. Recall that mature T cells express either CD4 or CD8, not both. Therefore, responses by CD4$^+$ T cells are generally directed toward antigens of extracellular origin, and CD8$^+$ T-cell responses are generally against antigens of intracellular origin.

Interaction of the pMHC–TCR–CD4 or pMHC–TCR–CD8 complex provides a signal to the T cell. Yet, this first signal, although necessary, is not sufficient to stimulate naïve T cells to proliferate and differentiate. A **costimulator molecule** must provide a second signal. One of these is CD45 or common leukocyte antigen (Fig. 5-7). It is thought that CD45, acting through its cytoplasmic phosphatase domains, dephosphorylates and activates kinases such as Fyn. Inositol triphosphate kinase (IP$_3$K) in association with CD28 and Fyn activates the guanine–nucleotide exchange factor (GEF) Ras. Ras activates the **mitogen-activated protein** (MAP) kinase cascade, ultimately leading to the activation of AP-1, a family of factors that initiate transcription of a number of specific genes. Without co-stimulation, T cells either become selectively unresponsive, a state

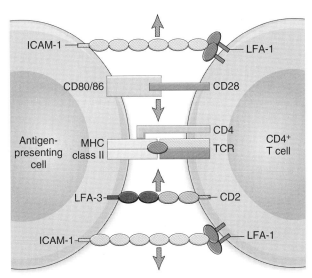

↓ ↑ Indicates direction of movement of molecules in the membrane relative to the TCR.

FIGURE 5-6. Immunologic synapse. The T-cell receptor (TCR) recognizes peptide bound in MHC (pMHC). The weak binding between TCR and pMHC class II is stabilized by the CD4 molecule on the T cell interacting with the nonpeptide-binding portion of MHC class II and provides an initial stimulatory signal to the T cell. In addition, cell-to-cell adhesion by leukocyte function antigen-1 (LFA-1) expressed by T cells interacts with immune cell adhesion-1 (ICAM-1) molecules on the antigen-presenting cell and functions to keep the cells in close proximity. The LFA-1–ICAM-1 complexes move laterally away from the pMHC–TCR–CD4 interact. At the same time, co-stimulator complexes such as CD80/86 on the APC interact with CD28 on the CD4+ T cell and move toward the pMHC–TCR–CD4 complex. Co-stimulator molecules provide a second signal necessary for T-cell activation.

called **anergy**, or die by apoptosis. Mature dendritic cells or activated macrophages express high levels of **B7-1 (CD80)** and B7-2 (**CD86**) and may interact with **CD28** expressed by naïve T cells to provide a second co-stimulatory signal to the T cell (Fig. 5-7). Other molecules may also serve as either co-stimulators or amplifiers of the immunologic synapse; among these is the interaction of APC-expressed CD40 with T-cell expressed CD154 (also called CD40 ligand or CD40L). Engagement of the TCR by pMHC induces expression of CD154, which engages the CD40 present on mature dendritic cells and activated macrophages. The CD40–CD154 interaction stimulates the expression of CD80/CD86 by APCs. In addition, both mature dendritic cells and activated macrophages may increase their expression of adhesion molecules, such as **immune cell adhesion molecule-1** (ICAM-1) that interacts with its ligand **leukocyte function antigen-1** (LFA-1) on T cells. Resting T cells express an isoform of CD45 (leukocyte common antigen) known as CD45RA. On activation, T cells express the alternative isoform of CD45, called CD45RO, that as-sociates with the TCR to make the T cell more sensitive to low concentrations of pMHC complexes.

T-cell signal transduction

The immunologic synapse functions to stabilize noncovalent interactions between the APC and T cell and to move T-cell molecules into close proximity, forming a cluster. The close proximity of cytoplasmic tails of certain T-cell molecules leads to the activation of protein tyrosine kinases and adapter proteins through **immunoreceptor tyrosine-based activation motifs** (**ITAMs**). The basic ITAM contains two tyrosines separated by approximately 13 amino acid residues. Although the TCR recognizes and binds to the pMHC complex, it cannot signal to the cell interior that this event has occurred because the cytoplasmic portions of the $\alpha\beta$ or $\gamma\delta$ chains that comprise the TCR lack ITAMs. Instead, a complex of ITAM-bearing invariant molecules, collectively known as **CD3**, associates with the TCR and are responsible for signaling.

The CD3 complex is composed of six polypeptides (2 CD3ε + 1 CD3γ + 1 CD3δ + 1 CD247

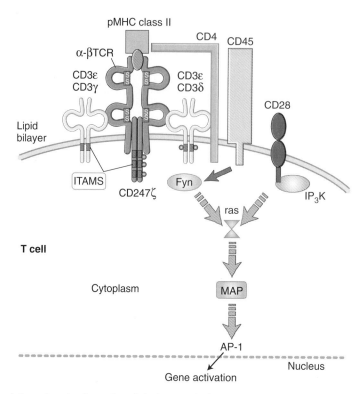

FIGURE 5-7. Co-stimulatory signals. Formation of the immunologic synapse sets the stage for a number of cytoplasmic signals leading to T-cell activation by costimulatory molecules. Common leukocyte antigen (CD45) dephosphorylates and activates Fyn kinase. Both CD28 and Fyn associate with inositol triphosphate kinase (IP₃K) and activate the *rat sarcoma* (Ras) protein, setting off a cascade of events that initiate gene transcription.

ζ-ζ homodimer) (see Figs. 3-3 and 4-10). The cytoplasmic portion of each ζ polypeptide chain contains three ITAMs, and each of the other chains contains a single ITAM. As the immunologic synapse is formed, CD4 (or CD8) engages the MHC class II (or class I) as part of the pMHC–TCR complex, and this activates a Src family tyrosine kinase, Lck, on the cytoplasmic tail of CD4 (or CD8) (Fig. 5-8). Activated Lck phosphorylates the ITAMs in the CD3 complex that are close together in the cluster formed. Phosphorylation of multiple ζ-chain ITAMs results in the binding of the **cytoplasmic tyrosine kinase, ZAP-70** (70-kiloDalton [kDa] ζ-associated protein). ITAM-bound ZAP-70 is also phosphorylated and activated by Lck. Activated ZAP-70 then phosphorylates the remaining ITAMs on the ζ chain, as well as a number of other molecules. Among these are **phospholipase C-γ (PLC-γ)** and the **linker of activation for T cells (LAT)**. **Phosphatidylinositol 4,5-biphosphate (PIP₂**, a membrane phospholipid) is cleaved by PLC-γ to form **inositol triphosphate (IP₃)**

and **diacylglycerol (DAG)**, which function as secondary messengers. PLC-γ activation increases intracellular divalent calcium (Ca²⁺) activating calineurin, a Ca²⁺-dependent phosphatase, which, in turn, dephosphorylates cytoplasmic **nuclear factor of activated T cells (NFAT)** required for the activation of cytokine genes such as **interleukin-2** (IL-2) and IL-4. DAG, in the presence of Ca²⁺, activates **protein kinase C (PKC)** that, in turn, phosphorylates the **inhibitor of NF-κB (IκB)** that is complexed with *nuclear factor κB* (**NF-κB**), a 50-kDa and 75-kDa heterodimeric nuclear transcription factor. Once IκB is phosphorylated, NF-κB migrates from the cytoplasm to the nucleus, allowing the activation of a number of cytokine genes. ZAP-70 also phosphorylates an adapter protein, the so-called **linker of activation for T cells (LAT)**. LAT activates small **guanine-nucleotide exchange factors (GEFs)**, such as *rat sarcoma* (Ras) and *ras*-related *C3* botulinum toxin substrate (Rac) proteins. These proteins activate a cascade of intracellular enzymes through either the MAP kinase

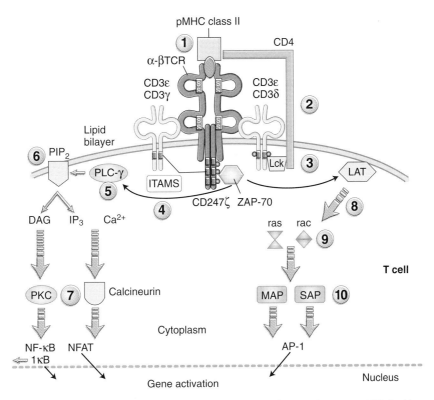

FIGURE 5-8. **T-cell signal transduction.** 1. The T-cell receptor (TCR) complex contains an α–β TCR (in this example) that has engaged a peptide–MHC class II complex (pMHC class II). Six polypeptides of the CD3 complex (2 CD3ε + 1 CD3γ + 1 CD3δ + 2 CD247ζ) contain one to three immunoreceptor tyrosine-based activation motifs (ITAMs, red rectangles). 2. As the immunologic synapse is formed, CD4 engagement of the pMHC class II activates Lck tyrosine kinase. 3. Lck phosphorylates multiple ITAMs on the CD3ε,γ,δ chains (blue dots) and CD247ζ chains resulting in binding of the cytoplasmic tyrosine kinase, ZAP-70. 4. ZAP-70 phosphorylates the remaining CD247ζ ITAMS, and a number of additional molecules are activated, including phospholipase C-γ (PLC-γ) [5] and the linker of activation for T cells (LAT) [6]. 7. Activated PLC-γ cleaves phophatidylinositol 4,5-biphosphated (PIP$_2$) to form inositol triphosphate (IP$_3$) and diacylglygerol (DAG) to function as secondary messengers. 8. IP$_3$ and calcium influx activates calcineurin to activate nuclear factor of activated T cells (NFAT) to activate cytokine genes within the nucleus. DAG activates protein kinase C (PKC) that phosphorylates the inhibitor of nuclear factor-κB (NF-κB), which is complexed with NF-κB. NF-κB then migrates from the cytoplasm to the nucleus to activate a number of cytokine genes. 9. ZAP-70 also phosphorylates LAT, which in turn activates the guanine–nucleotide exchange factors (GEFs), Ras and Rac. 10. Rac and Ras activate MAP kinase or SAP kinase, leading to the activation of AP-1, a family of factors that initiate transcription of a number of specific genes.

or **stress-activated protein (SAP)** kinase pathways that ultimately lead to the activation of the **activator protein-1 (AP-1)** family of transcription factors and the initiation of transcription of specific genes. The activation of transcription factors leads to the synthesis of a number of cytokines and receptors, as well as T-cell proliferation and differentiation. The nature of the resulting immune response depends on a number of factors that are as yet poorly understood.

Activated or effector T cells

The nature of the initial interaction of naïve T cells is important in the development of the adaptive

immune function. Initial recognition of antigen by naïve T cells, called **priming**, is crucial for the proliferation and further differentiation of T cells. We have already seen that CD4$^+$ T cells recognize exogenous peptides associated with class II molecules and that CD8$^+$ T cells recognize endogenous peptides associated with class I molecules. Primed CD4$^+$ T cells, called T **helper** or **Th** cells because they "help" other cells, respond to an antigenic insult, and might develop along one of two pathways. One developmental pathway results in the differentiation of **Th1 cells** that generally respond to intracellular pathogens by recruiting and activating macrophages and monocytes. The second results in the differentiation of **Th2 cells** that generally respond to extracellular pathogens by stimulating B cells to differentiate into plasma cells and secrete antibody. APCs and other cells are influential in determining whether a Th1 or Th2 effector response ensues. Primed CD8$^+$ T cells are functionally defined as cytotoxic T (Tc) cells or as suppressor (Ts) cells. Cytotoxic T cells are responsible for the lysis of virus-infected cells, tumor cells, and most grafts of foreign tissue. Suppressor T cells are responsible for the down-regulation of immune responses.

CD4$^+$ Th1 cells

CD4$^+$ Th1 cells develop in response to intracellular pathogens or intracellular antigenic insults.

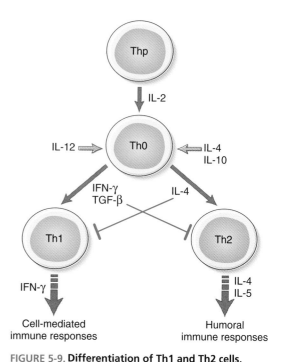

FIGURE 5-9. **Differentiation of Th1 and Th2 cells.**
Naïve CD4$^+$ T cells before activation are known as T-helper precursors (Thp). On activation, Thps secrete interleukin-2 (IL-2) and express an IL-2 receptor, causing the cell to proliferate as a pathway-uncommitted Th0 CD4$^+$ T cell. Influence by cytokine signals produced by antigen-presenting cells (APCs) or other leukocytes, such as the Th0 cell, will differentiate along the Th1 or Th2 pathway. If Th0 cells encounter APC-secreted IL-12, it will differentiate into a Th1 cell that secretes IFN-γ and TGF-β. Th1 cells are important mediators of cell-mediated immune responses. If Th0 cells encounter IL-4, they will differentiate along the Th2 pathway, producing cells that secrete IL-4 and IL-10. Animal models have shown Th2 cells to be polarized mediators of humoral immune or antibody responses. Although human Th1 and Th2 cells show polarization in cytokine secretion, polarization of Th1–Th2 immune function is less apparent. Several cytokines produced by Th1 and Th2 are cross-inhibitory; IFN-γ (Th1) inhibits development of the Th2 pathway and IL-4 and IL-10 inhibit the Th1 pathway.

> **SIDEBAR 5.1 INTRACELLULAR PATHOGENS**
>
> *I just read that the TCRs of CD4$^+$ T cells recognize pMHC class II complexes of exogenous origin. How can a peptide derived from an intracellular pathogen that circumvents phagolysosome vesicles to live in the cytoplasm load into a class II molecule?*
> To avoid detection by the adaptive immune system, some pathogens use a "stealth mechanism" by circumventing phagolysosome vesicles altogether. Others may enter the cell in phagosomes but are able to leave them and enter the cytoplasm. But their ruse is not perfect, because some infected cells die, prompting dendritic cells to take up dead cells and cellular debris by either phagocytosis or macropinocytosis. The proteolytic peptides are then displayed in class II molecules. Mystery solved.

Antigen-naïve **CD4$^+$ Th precursor (Thp)** cells activated through the immunologic synapse express a variety of cytokines and cell-surface cytokine receptors. On initial activation, CD4$^+$ T cells secrete **interleukin-2 (IL-2,** formerly known as T-cell growth factor) and express an **IL-2 receptor (IL-2R)** (Fig. 5-9). At this point, these cells are called Th0 cells because they are not yet committed to either the Th1 or the Th2 pathway. Interaction of IL-2 with its receptor (autocrine stimulation) causes the cell to proliferate, therefore increasing the number of antigen-specific T cells. In addition, the nature of the antigenic stimulus influences cytokine secretion by APCs, and these

influence CD4$^+$ T-cell differentiation. If the APC is stimulated by microbe-derived lipopolysaccharide (LPS, a characteristic feature of Gram-negative bacteria), CD155 (the ligand for CD40), and/or interferon-γ (IFN-γ) (produced by **natural killer [NK]** or CD4$^+$ T cells) at the time of antigen encounter, it will also begin to secrete IL-12. Activated, naïve CD4$^+$ T cells express receptors for IL-12, IL-4, and IFN-γ. Engagement of the IL-12R induces CD4$^+$ T lymphocytes to further differentiate into Th1 cells that actively secrete cytokines, such as IFN-γ, TNF, and a variety of chemokines that increase leukocyte recruitment and activation. Adhesion molecule expression, mainly of LFA-1 and **very late antigen-4** (VLA-4), is also greatly increased for activated Th1 cells. As we will see, these molecules are important for migration of Th1 cells to sites of infection. IFN-γ production by Th1 cells serves to further stimulate the production of IL-12 by dendritic cells and activated macrophages, amplifying the differentiation of CD4$^+$ T cells along the Th1 pathway. Conversely, IFN-γ serves as a negative signal for CD4$^+$ Th2 cells by inhibiting their proliferation.

CD4$^+$ Th2 cells

Activation of naïve CD4$^+$ T cells through the immunologic synapse may result in their development into Th2 cells. As we have seen, activation through the immunologic synapse results in the expression of a variety of cytokines and cell-surface cytokine receptors by the CD4$^+$ T cell. If **IL-4** is present at the time of T cell activation, **IL-4 receptors** (**IL-4R**) on the CD4$^+$ T cells stimulate production of more IL-4 and IL-4R (see Fig. 5-9). There are several possible sources of IL-4; NKT cells (a specialized subset of CD4$^+$ T cells that have characteristics more like an NK cell of the innate system than CD4$^+$ T cells of the adaptive system), mast cells, and pre-existing CD4$^+$ Th2 cells in the vicinity. Little is known about what prompts NKT and mast cells to secrete IL-4. Some immunologists believe that CD1 molecules engage bacterial lipids, resulting in the secretion of IL-4 by NKT cells. Like IL-2, the interaction of IL-4 with the IL-4R functions as autocrine stimulation for cell-cycle entry and proliferation that result in increased numbers of antigen-specific T cells. IL-4 is a potent inhibitor of Th1 differentiation. IL-4 also stimulates Th2 cells to produce and secrete additional cytokines such as **tumor-growth factor-β** (TGF-β), IL-5, and IL-10. IL-5 stimulates the growth and differentiation of eosinophils. IL-10 inhibits IL-12 and co-stimulatory molecule production by APCs. TGF-β inhibits T-cell proliferation and macrophage activation. In addition to its role in Th2 differentiation, IL-4 is a potent stimulus for antibody production and the principal cytokine responsible for stimulating isotype switching by B cells.

CD8$^+$ T cells

Some pathogens, such as viruses, use a stealth mechanism for infecting cells that involves entering and replicating within the cytoplasm and thus avoiding contact with phagocytic vesicles entirely. Fortunately, the adaptive immune system has also evolved several mechanisms to detect and destroy these would-be stealthy invaders.

Sometimes dendritic cells or activated macrophages also become infected as they scavenge cellular debris caused by infectious organisms. Some of the infecting pathogen's proteins are ubiquinated within the cytoplasm of the APC, enzymatically degraded by proteasomes, transported to the endoplasmic reticulum, and displayed on the APC surface as pMHC class I complexes. In addition, phagocytically acquired peptides from the pathogen are displayed on the APC surface by MHC class II molecules. Interaction of naïve CD4$^+$ T cells with the pMHC class II on the APC results in the development of Th1 cells that secrete both IL-2 and IFN-γ. Naïve, antigen-specific CD8$^+$ T cells recognize pMHC class I on the surface of the APC (Fig. 5-10). Expression of CD80 or CD86 by the peptide-presenting APC serves as one possible co-stimulator as it engages the CD28 molecule on the CD8$^+$ T cell. Secretion of IL-2 and/or IFN-γ by adjacent Th1 cells may also provide co-stimulation for the naïve CD8$^+$ T cell. In addition, CD40 expression by the APC and its interaction with CD154 (CD40 ligand) may stimulate CD8$^+$ T-cell differentiation. Activation of CD8$^+$ T-cells results in their rapid proliferation and differentiation into effector cells with cytolytic functions called **cytotoxic T lymphocytes** (**CTL**). The costimulatory role for CD4$^+$ T cells in the generation of CTL is not absolute. This fact is derived from the experimental observation that mice lacking CD4$^+$ T cells nevertheless make near-normal numbers of CTLs. Fully differentiated CTLs contain two types of granules: one type contains **perforin**, a pore-forming protein, and the other **granzymes**, or serine proteases.

T-cell anergy and regulatory T cells

There are occasions in which T-cell responses would be a distinct disadvantage to the body. Immune responses to foreign antigens in the respiratory and alimentary tracts may inhibit gas exchange and nutrient uptake. Self-antigens that arise after T cells have been seeded into peripheral organs, such as gene products synthesized only after puberty, also have the potential to attack. Prevention of post-thymic, self-reactive T

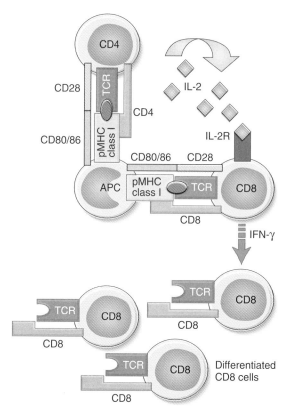

FIGURE 5-10. CD8$^+$ T-cell activation. Antigen-presenting cells (APCs) present pMHC class II to the TCR of naïve CD4$^+$ T cells, and engagement of CD28 with CD80/86 stimulates IL-2 secretion by the CD4$^+$ T cells. Simultaneously, APCs present pMHC class I to the TCR of naïve CD8$^+$ T cells, and engagement of CD28 with CD80/86 provides a second stimulatory signal. The secondary signal prompts the expression of IL-2R and secretion of IFN-γ, which in turn stimulates the proliferation and activation of the CD8$^+$ T cell. CD8$^+$ T cells mature and differentiate into cytotoxic T lymphocytes (CTL).

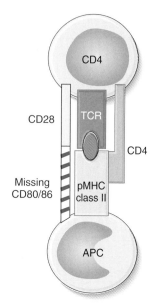

FIGURE 5-11. Anergy. Absence of CD80 or CD86 results in antigen unresponsiveness by the naïve T cell, which is also called anergy. Anergic cells fail to proliferate and differentiate in response to what would otherwise be a normal stimulatory signal.

cells and antigen unresponsiveness is called **peripheral tolerance**. Several mechanisms of peripheral tolerance are known. One mechanism of peripheral tolerance relies on the absence of a costimulatory signal. We have seen that T-cell activation requires engagement of both the TCR and co-stimulators. Recognition of the pMHC complex by TCR without co-stimulation results in a T cell that is unresponsive. These T cells remain refractory even on restimulation by an APC that expresses both pMHC complex and costimulatory molecules (Fig. 5-11). Such refractory T cells are said to be in a state of **anergy**, in which partially stimulated T cells fail to proliferate and differentiate in response to what would be a normal stimulatory signal. In addition, the co-stimulatory signal can also be viewed as a sur-

vival stimulus. Repeated activation of T cells without co-stimulation results in apoptotic death of those T cells.

A second method of peripheral tolerance induction occurs by prolonged and constant stimulation of recently activated T cells. In this case, excessive restimulation by pMHC complexes and a specific co-stimulatory molecule induces T-cell apoptosis.

A subpopulation of CD4$^+$CD25$^+$ T cells has been described that actively assure peripheral tolerance of aggressively self-reactive T cells. These so-called **T regulatory**, or **Treg**, cells inhibit effector CD4$^+$ T cells by either contact-dependent suppression or the production of immunosuppressive cytokines, such as TGF-β and IL-10. In addition, a subpopulation of CD8$^+$ T cells distinct from CTLs has been defined that suppress CD4$^+$ T cell responses. These are termed **suppressor T (Ts)** cells. The physiologic processes of Treg and Ts are, as yet, poorly understood.

Antigen recognition by B cells

The cells and molecules with which antibodies interact must be able to distinguish between free antibodies and bound antibodies (those that have "tagged" antigens for destruction). On binding of the Fab portion of the antibody molecule to an appropriate antigen, a conformational change occurs in the antibody that results in the exposure of particular sites in the Fc portion of the molecule. The exposure of these sites makes them available for detection and binding by molecules such as the C1 component of complement and by the Fc receptors of phagocytes and other cells.

B-cell activation and signal transduction

Unlike the TCR, the antigen-specific **B-cell receptor** (BCR or surface-bound immunoglobulin) recognizes epitopes on soluble molecules without involvement of other cells or molecules. The BCR complex on a naïve, mature B cell is composed of membrane-bound IgM and IgD and is associated with invariant **Igα** and **Igβ** molecules (Fig. 5-12A). Like ζ chains of the T-cell CD3 complex, cytoplasmic tails of Igα and Igβ contain ITAM motifs. Antigen-induced cross-linking of BCRs clusters Igα and Igβ molecules and leads to ITAM phosphorylation by **sarcoma (Src) kinases** (*e.g.*, **Lyn**, **Blk**, or **Fyn**). Recall that B cells express immunoglobulin of *only one specificity*, meaning that all the BCRs on a single cell have identical variable regions. In other words, a single B cell expresses only one idiotype specificity. Therefore, an antigen must contain multiple identical epitopes that can cross-link BCRs on a single cell. The phosphorylated ITAMs provide a docking site for the **Syk** tyrosine kinase, a B-cell

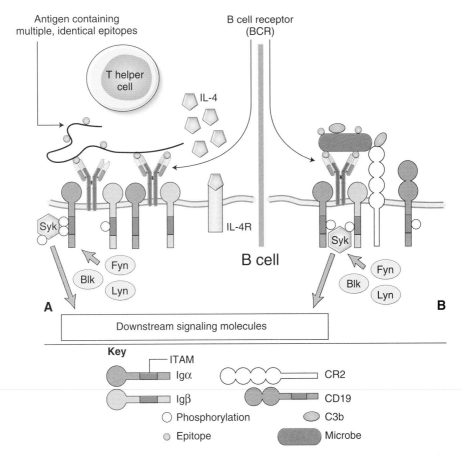

FIGURE 5-12. B-cell activation. B cells recognize epitopes on molecules without antigen presentation. Surface immunoglobulin serves as the B-cell receptor (BCR). The signal for BCR antigen engagement is through invariant Igα- and Igβ-associated molecules. **(A)** Naïve B cells require a second signal for activation that is provided by CD4⁺ T cells through cytokines, such as IL-4. Antigen-induced BCR cross-linking causes ITAM phosphorylation by Src kinases (Lyn, Blk, or Fyn). Phosphorylated ITAMs allow Syk tyrosine kinase to dock and begin the downstream signaling cascade. **(B)** Microbes recognized by complement may also activate specific B cells. The BCR recognizes epitopes on the microbe and a complement receptor (CR2) recognizes C3b bound to the microorganism resulting in the phosphorylation of ITAMs on Igα, Igβ, and CD19. Phosphorylated ITAMs allow Syk tyrosine kinase to dock and subsequent downstream signaling cascade.

equivalent of T cell ZAP-70. Syk phosphorylates itself and a number of downstream signaling molecules, including PLC-γ and adapter proteins. Plasma membrane PIP_2 is cleaved by PLC-γ into IP_3 and DAG. IP_3 increases cytoplasmic Ca^{2+} and DAG induces enzymes such as PKC to activate transcription factors, including NFAT, NK-κB, Myc, and AP-1. In addition, PKC phosphorylates serine–threonine residues. BCR cross-linking results in the Ras phosphorylation and leads to the activation of MAP kinase.

> ### CLINICAL APPLICATION
> ### HYPER-IGM SYNDROME
>
> **Hyper-IgM syndrome** is an X-linked disease that is caused by a CD154 (CD40 ligand) abnormality. CD154 of affected individuals, normally expressed by T cells, is unable to interact with the CD40 on B cells. Without proper CD154:CD40 interaction, B cells are unable to switch isotypes. Consequently, affected individuals have elevated IgM and low IgG and IgA levels. Hyper-IgM is usually diagnosed in infancy. Infants with the disease have infections of the lungs, ears, sinus, and pharynx; they may also have chronic diarrhea and opportunistic infections. These patients are also usually susceptible to malignancies.

B cells may also be activated by the interaction of the BCR and **complement receptor 2 (CR2)**. CD19, a member of the immunoglobulin supergene family, has a cytoplasmic tail with ITAM motifs and is associated with CR2 on the B cell surface (Fig. 5-12B). Recall that complement components, especially C3b, as part of the innate immune system, recognize and bind to microorganisms. Engagement of the microbe by the BCR and of microbe-bound C3b by CR2 results in ITAM phosphorylation of Igα, Igβ, and CD19, and subsequent B-cell activation.

BCR-bound antigens are internalized by endocytosis, enzymatically degraded, and displayed on the B-cell surface as pMHC class II complexes. Activated B cells enter the cell cycle and increase their expression of CD80/86, IL-2R, IL-4R, and anti-apoptotic proteins. They now await a T-cell signal. Communication between B and T cells determines what antibodies will be generated against the appropriate antigen. Activated B cells express both pMHC class II and CD80/86. The $CD4^+$ T-cell rec-

ognizes both pMHC class II by the TCR and CD80/86 by CD28. These two signals stimulate the T cell to express CD154 (CD40 ligand) and to secrete cytokines. The T-cell cytokines induce B-cell CD40 expression. CD40:CD154 signaling causes B-cell proliferation and differentiation. The T-cell cytokines serve to stimulate B-cell proliferation and differentiation into **plasma cells** and to promote isotype switching.

Isotype switch

The isotype of the antibody that binds antigen strongly influences the ultimate nature of the humoral immune response. The isotype determines whether the antibody activates complement, and whether the antibody remains within the body or is secreted into a lumen or mucous membrane, or whether the tissues of the body immobilize it. Cytokines secreted by T cells influence B-cell proliferation, the isotype produced (including isotype switching), and B-cell differentiation into plasma cells (Table 5-1).

B-lymphocyte development

Only B cells and their terminally differentiated form, plasma cells, synthesize immunoglobulins. B cells are derived from pluripotent hematopoietic stem cells in the liver before birth and/or from the bone marrow thereafter. B cells comprise two major lineages, B-1 and B-2 cells. B-1 cells are so named because they are the first to develop and are a self-renewing population that predominates in the peritoneal and pleural cavities. Although much of the function of B-1 cells is unknown, we know that they constitutively secrete IgM antibodies of limited diversity that react strongly with carbohydrates and poorly with proteins. A large proportion of serum IgM antibodies found in normal individuals are of B-1 origin. In contrast, B-2 cells, also called conventional B cells, arise after birth, are continuously replaced from the bone marrow, and are widely distributed throughout the lymphoid organs and tissues. Because of more extensive somatic gene rearrangements, B-2 cells display a broader repertoire of immunoglobulin specificities and affinities. Unlike B-1 cells, resting B-2 cells produce low levels of immunoglobulins that increase only on their activation by helper T cells, causing them to differentiate into antibody-secreting cells. The following section describes the development of conventional B-2 cells.

TABLE 5-1. T-CELL CYTOKINES THAT INDUCE B-CELL DIFFERENTIATION AND PROMOTE THE ISOTYPE SWITCH

Cytokines that induce B cell proliferation	Cytokines that promote isotype switching	Isotype	Location
IL-2, IL-4, IL-5	IL-2, IL-4, IL-5	IgM	Serum
IL-2, IL-4, IL-5	IL-4, IL-6, IL-2, IFN-γ	IgG	Serum
IL-2, IL-4, IL-5	IL-5, TGF-β	IgA	Mucosal surfaces
IL-2, IL-4, IL-5	IL-4	IgE	Decorating basophils and mast cells

Once committed to the B-cell pathway, B-2 cell precursors pass through several stages that involve changes in gene activity to provide the appropriate enzymes and structural molecules necessary for mature B-2 cells. In many cases, the changes in gene activity are induced by molecules, such as IL-7, produced by the stromal cells of the bone marrow. Among the changes defining the developmental progression of the B-cell lineage are those involving the ability to synthesize and express immunoglobulin molecules on the cell surface.

- **Pro-B cells** initiate the production of enzymes such as **recombination activation genes**, *Rag-1* and *Rag-2*, and other molecules necessary for the construction of an immunoglobulin molecule, including the chromosomal rearrangement of V, D, and J genes to form the variable V_H domain. The first component synthesized is the μ immunoglobulin heavy chain, which remains confined to the cytoplasm (Fig. 5-13A).
- **Early-stage pre-B cells** are characterized by the cytoplasmic presence of a transitional or surrogate light chain. This chain is neither a true λ or κ light chain. It serves as a temporary substitute capable of interacting with the μ heavy chains present in the cytoplasm to permit assembly of a monomer-like structure (2 heavy chains, 2 surrogate light chains) that can be transported to the membrane for surface expression (see Fig. 5-13B). **Late-stage pre-B cells** synthesize either a κ or λ light chain that replaces the transitory light chains, resulting in the expression of true IgM molecules on the cell surface. Again, this includes the chromosomal rearrangements necessary for formation of the V_L domain. With the formation and expression of IgM, the pre-B cell becomes an **immature B cell**. Because the IgM has not yet bound to its antigen, immature B cells are also called **naïve B cells**.

- **Immature** or **naïve B cells**, with their surface antigen receptors now in place, undergo a selective process to remove any that may be self-reactive (see Fig. 5-13C). If their surface immunoglobulin finds and binds to epitopes within their bone marrow environment, they undergo apoptosis. Those B cells that survive this test leave the bone marrow and enter the circulation. On leaving the bone marrow, immature B cells have a short half-life and must quickly find their way to a lymph node. Once there, they receive additional signals from the lymph node stromal cells that enable them to continue developing. Among the critical steps that new B cells undertake after entering a lymph node is further modification of their immunoglobulin expression by beginning to synthesize δ heavy chains so that they can simultaneously express both IgD and IgM molecules (with identical antigenic specificity) on their cell surface (see Fig. 5-13C). The ability to produce both IgD and IgM with identical antigen-binding regions is accomplished by a mechanism involving alternative splicing of the mRNA encoding the heavy chains (Fig. 5-14). With the expression of both IgD and IgM, the immature B cell becomes a **mature B cell**, even though it may not yet have bound antigen.
- **Mature B cells**, co-expressing IgD and IgM, are ready for activation. In the overwhelming majority of cases, activation requires the binding to surface immunoglobulin to antigen and an interaction with T cells (see Fig. 5-13D).
- **Plasma cells** are immmunoglobulin-producing and secreting cells derived from B cells. These terminally differentiated, oval cells have a relatively short lifespan of less than 30 days and are immunoglobulin-producing "factories." They are characterized by a basophilic cytoplasm and large, nonstaining Golgi apparatus. Although they secrete large quantities of immunoglobulin, very little is displayed on their cell surfaces (see Fig. 5-13E).

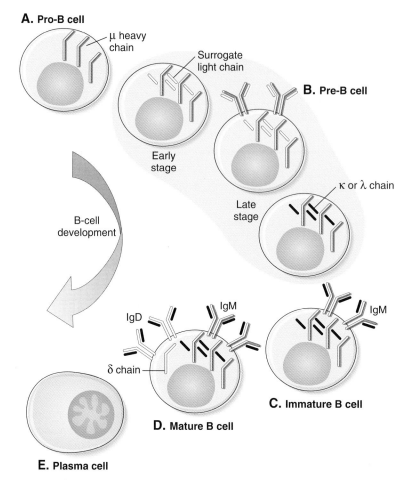

A. Pro-B cell
μ heavy chain

Surrogate light chain

B. Pre-B cell

Early stage

κ or λ chain

B-cell development

Late stage

IgM

IgD

IgM

δ chain

C. Immature B cell

D. Mature B cell

E. Plasma cell

FIGURE 5-13. **Stages of B-cell development.** The developmental pathway of B-2 cells from pro-B cell to plasma cell reflect changes in gene activity within the cell and the ability to synthesize and secrete immunoglobulin molecules. **(A)** A pro-B lymphocyte represents the early stages of B-cell development in which V, D, and J gene segments combine to form an immunoglobulin μ heavy chain that is confined to the cytoplasm. **(B)** The maturation to pre-B cells (shaded area) begins with the cytoplasmic expression of a surrogate light chain (early stage) followed by surface expression of both μ and surrogate light chain monomers. In the late stage of pre-B cell development, κ or λ light chains are seen in the cytoplasm in addition to μ heavy chains. **(C)** Immature B cells express IgMκ or IgMλ monomers on their surface membranes. **(D)** Mature B cells express both IgM and IgD on their cell surfaces. **(E)** Plasma cells are the end stage of differentiation of B-cell lineage. Plasma cells are "factories," synthesizing and secreting large amounts of immunoglobulin.

EFFECTOR FUNCTIONS OF THE ADAPTIVE IMMUNE SYSTEM

We have seen that the adaptive immune system often relies on cells and molecules of the innate immune system to initiate a response, and that T and B lymphocytes amplify in number in response to antigenic stimuli to produce mature activated T and B cells. The cells and molecules of the adaptive system in turn often use cells, such as macrophages and neutrophils, and molecules, such as complement, of the innate system

to focus and delivery a fatal blow to an invader. One way of looking at the role of the adaptive system would be to see it as ultimately amplifying and intensifying the innate system's effector functions.

The terms *cellular* and *humoral* adaptive immune responses are actually misnomers. All immune responses have a cellular basis. However, not all immune responses require antibody for effector function. For the majority of adaptive immune responses, T cells play a critical role. Cell-mediated immune (CMI) responses are di-

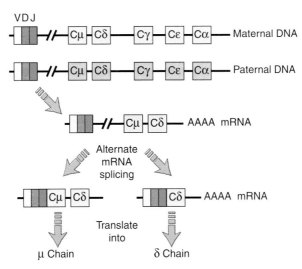

VDJ

Maternal DNA

Paternal DNA

AAAA mRNA

Alternate
mRNA
splicing

AAAA mRNA

Translate
into

μ Chain   δ Chain

FIGURE 5-14. Alternate mRNA splicing in B cells. B cells produce immunoglobulin of only one isotype at a time (see Fig. 4-14). Mature, unstimulated B cells are the exception to this "rule." Mature B cells (see Fig 5-13D) express both IgM and IgD. This is accomplished by a mechanism of alternative splicing of the mRNA encoding the heavy chains.

rected by T cells (hence are T-dependent responses) and mediated by cells (*e.g.*, macrophages or neutrophils). With one exception (ADCC), antibody is not involved. You will see a parallel between the cellular and humoral systems in cell–cell interactions.

Cell-mediated immune responses

Think of cell-mediated immune responses as hand-to-hand combat. T cells act as field lieutenants directing other leukocytes (mostly macrophages) to sites of infection and urging them to kill the infectious foe or the human cell in which the foe is hiding. Other T cells, cytotoxic T-lymphocytes, act as samurai and actively engage in cell-to-cell combat, directly killing their infectious opponent or the human cell in which it is hiding.

Delayed hypersensitivity reaction

In 1890 Robert Koch observed that intradermal injection of tubercle bacillus (*Mycobacterium tuberculosis*) into sensitized hosts (those who previously had encountered the bacillus) resulted in a localized skin reaction within 24 to 48 hours that reached a maximum by 72 hours. Because this **hypersensitivity** reaction to the bacillus is *delayed*, taking 24 to 48 hours for the reaction to become apparent, and has been termed the **delayed**

(-type) **hypersensitivity** (DTH, also called **type IV reaction**, see Chapter 8) reaction (Fig. 5-15). The DTH reaction is localized to the immediate area surrounding the site of injection. The reaction is characterized by localized induration or edema (swelling), may lead to localized necrosis and ulceration, and is followed by a decrease in the swelling and/or healing of the lesion.

> **CLINICAL APPLICATION**
> **ASSESSMENT OF CELL-MEDIATED IMMUNE FUNCTION**
>
> Common antigens for delayed (-type) hypersensitivity skin testing include *Candida albicans, Trichophyton species* (fungi that cause hair, skin, and nail infections), tetanus (*Clostridium tetani*), *and* mumpsvirus (a paramyxovirus). A positive test indicates an intact T-cell function.

Both DTH and the related reaction, **contact sensitivity** (CS, also called **contact dermatitis**), are T cell-mediated responses to intracellular antigenic insults. In these reactions, antigen-specific CD4[+] Th1 cells recruit macrophages and monocytes to the site of antigen or infection. At the site of

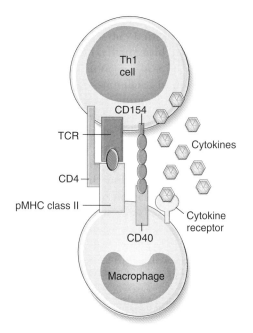

FIGURE 5-15. Delayed (-type) hypersensitivity. A localized cell-mediated immune reaction is known as delayed (-type) or type IV hypersensitivity. Recognition of pMHC class II and the interaction of CD40 ligand (CD154) with CD40 results in cytokine secretion (primarily IFN-γ) by CD4$^+$ Th1 cells. Cytokine receptors signal macrophages to activate and secrete IL-1, IL-12, and TNF-α, and to increase MHC class II expression, degradative enzymes, and reactive oxygen species. The activated macrophage is a killing machine destroying everything that comes within its "grasp."

infection or antigen repository, the Th1 cells activate these phagocytes into a killing frenzy in which they destroy both infected and normal cells. An excessive hypersensitivity reaction can often lead to gross tissue damage and even death. In the process of affecting a cure, the immune system can inflict unnecessary damage to the body—a classic case of overkill.

Leukocyte migration

Activated Th1 cells, showing increased levels of cell-surface integrins, namely LFA-1 and VLA-4, are found in the circulation. Phagocytes within the tissue at the site of antigen or infection respond by secreting TNF. TNF signals nearby epithelial cells to increase the levels of selectins and ligands for LFA-1 and VLA-4 on their lumenal surfaces. Interaction of adhesion molecules and their ligands allows activated Th1 cells to localize at the epithelium overlying the site of inflammation. The Th1 cells migrate through the epithelium and are retained at the site of inflammation.

Macrophage activation

On arrival at the inflammation site, Th1 cells interact with macrophages. Successful recognition of the pMHC class II complex by the Th1 TCR assures antigen specificity and causes the Th1 to express CD154 (CD40 ligand) and secrete IFN-γ. Stimulation of the macrophage by the CD154:C40 interaction and IFN-γ activates the macrophage. The activated macrophage up-regulates CD80/86 molecule expression; secretes IL-1, IL-12, and TNF; increases class II expression; and increases the production of degradative enzymes and **reactive oxygen intermediates (ROI)**.

Function of activated macrophages

The activated macrophage is a killing machine. With increased phagocytic capacity, the macrophage also increases its production of lysosomal enzymes and **reactive oxygen intermediates (ROIs)**. The secretion of TNF, IL-1, and chemokines attracts **polymorphonuclear cells** (PMNs or neutrophils) to the site, hallmarks of a classical inflammatory response. The activated macrophages and PMNs remove cellular debris, infected cells, and even some normal cells. Activated macrophages also stimulate tissue repair by secretion of platelet-derived growth factor, TGF-β, and fibroblast growth factor, which stimulate both scar formation and angiogenesis or blood vessel formation. Within 6 to 12 hours after introduction of antigen into the dermis of a sensitized individual, the area surrounding the injection site begins to show **erythema** or reddening of the skin because of the increase in blood flow and vascular permeability. Initial erythema is accompanied by progressive tissue **induration** or tissue swelling, again because of increased blood flow and vascular permeability, a reaction that peaks at 24 to 72 hours after antigen is introduced.

> **CLINICAL APPLICATION**
> **CHRONIC GRANULOMATOUS DISEASE**
>
> **Chronic granulomatous disease (CGD)** is an inherited phagocyte disorder. The disease is caused by the inability of neutrophils and monocytes to produce superoxide anions, rendering them incapable of killing ingested

(continued)

organisms. Individuals with CGD have recurrent infections in the lung, liver, and bone, and have draining lesions of the lymph nodes in the neck and axilla. They are prone to infection with catalase-positive organisms such as *Staphylococcus aureas* but not catalase-negative organisms such as *Streptococcus pneumoniae*. Catalase-negative organisms provide the phagocyte with the missing hydrogen peroxide and thus contribute to their own destruction.

Cytotoxic T-cell responses

A cytotoxic T lymphocyte's (CTL) function in life is to bring death to infectious organisms such as viruses and to the cells that harbor these invaders. Before the immune system gives CTLs the license to kill, several well-defined steps must occur so that the cells targeted for destruction are properly recognized. CTLs are unique in the adaptive immune system, because once they are activated they have the autonomy to kill a target cell without assistance by another leukocyte.

Target cell recognition

Most viruses, as well as some bacteria, replicate within the cytoplasm of a host cell. What happens if the organism replicates in a cell that does not express MHC class II? Intracellular pathogens replicate in the host cytoplasm, where the proteasome, a large protease complex, degrades ubiquinated cytoplasmic proteins. Cytoplasm-derived peptide fragments are transported by the **transporter associated with antigen presentation (TAP)** complex into the endoplasmic reticulum, where they are loaded into MHC class I molecules, then transported to the "target" cell surface to await recognition and cell contact by CD8$^+$ CTL. A differentiated CTL needs to only recognize pMHC class I to deliver a fatal blow. Target cell binding by the CTL is enhanced by both CD8 and LFA-1 integrin binding.

Coup de grace

The initial TCR binding to a target cell by a CTL is followed by the engagement of addition TCRs that localize at the CTL–target cell junction and up-regulation of **Fas ligand (FasL)** (Fig. 5-16). Contact between the CTL and target cell lasts only a few minutes, during which a fatal hit is de-

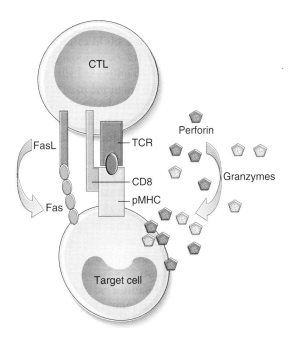

FIGURE 5-16. Killing by CD8$^+$ T cells (CTL). On recognition of pMHC class I by the TCRs of an activated CD8$^+$ CTL, the CTL up-regulates its cell-surface expression of the Fas molecule (CD95) for engagement with Fas ligand (FasL or CD178). Although CTL–target contact lasts only a few minutes, a fatal "kiss of death" has been delivered to the target cell by perforin granules (in black) and granzymes (in blue). Perforin granules polymerize to form pores in the cell membrane, through which granzymes enter, activating caspase-triggered programmed cell death or apoptosis of the target cell.

livered to the target cell. The perforin- and granzyme-containing cytoplasmic granules of the CTL co-localize with the TCRs and are released to contact with the target cell. Perforin granules polymerize within the target cell membrane to form a pore, creating an osmotic imbalance that ultimately leads to the lysis of the target cell. Granzymes also enter through the perforin-created pores and activate caspases, intracellular cysteine proteases that in turn activate a biochemical cascade leading to apoptotic lysis of the cell. Interaction of FasL on the CTL with Fas on the target cell also induces apoptosis. The effector T cell protects itself against the effects of it own weaponry by modifying its membrane (in the region of contact with the target cell) to be resistant to the effects of the perforin and granzymes.

Humoral immune responses

Antibody, once secreted by plasma cells, can mediate a variety of different antigen- or epitope-specific responses. Antibody specifically reacts with epi-

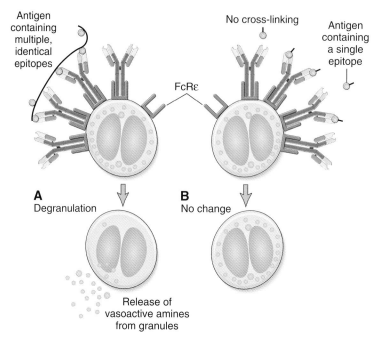

FIGURE 5-17. Mast cell degranulation. Mast cells and basophils have cell-surface receptors for the Fc portion of the IgE molecule (FcRε). IgE produced by plasma cells binds to the FcRε before an encounter with an antigen. Mast cell-bound IgE molecules specifically bind epitopes. **(A)** Binding of multiple epitopes on complex molecular structures cross-links IgE leads to mast cell or basophil degranulation and the release of vasoactive amines. **(B)** Binding of univalent epitopes does not cross-link the cell-bound IgE and degranulation does not occur.

topes on soluble antigens, which, in some cases, leads to the production of **immune complexes** (antigen–antibody complexes). Immune complexes can be either soluble or precipitate, causing a **precipitin reaction**. **Immune complex disease** (*e.g.*, **serum sickness**) is a severe manifestation of antigen–antibody complex formation. Antibodies can also bind to and cross-link cells or particles causing an aggregate formation in a reaction known as **agglutination**. In addition, antibody that specifically recognizes cell surface antigen may activate the classical complement pathway, resulting in opsonization and/or lysis of the target cell. Antigen–antibody reactions are also used for diagnosis (Appendix A).

Antibody-dependent cell-mediated cytotoxicity

Antibodies often recognize and bind to cell-surface antigens, such as those on parasitic pathogens. Eosinophils and NK cells recognize alterations in the Fc portion of the bound antibody and kill the antibody-decorated cell by a process known as **antibody-dependent cell-mediated cytotoxicity** (**ADCC**). Unlike opsonization, ADCC does not in-

volve phagocytes. Receptors on eosinophils and NK cells recognize and bind the Fc regions of immunoglobulin (usually IgG) bound to cell surfaces (see Fig. 3-3A). On making contact, eosinophils and NK cells kill the antibody-tagged cells by damaging their membranes.

Mast cell degranulation

Mast cells and **basophils** contain cytoplasmic granules composed of a variety of chemical mediators (*e.g.*, histamine, serotonin, platelet-activating factor) involved in the generation of inflammation (Chapter 8). The surfaces of mast cells are covered with specialized receptors (FcεRI) that bind the Fc domains of IgE molecules (Fig. 5-17). However, unlike the Fc receptors on phagocytes, NK cells, and the like, mast cell receptors are designed to bind free IgE that has not yet combined with antigen. Thus, mast cells "adsorb" IgE from the serum (hence the low serum levels of IgE) and use it as a surface receptor for antigen. When an appropriate antigen binds and cross-links the IgE molecules on mast cell surfaces, the mast cells **degranulate** and the mediators, such as vasoactive amines (*e.g.*, histamine), contained within their

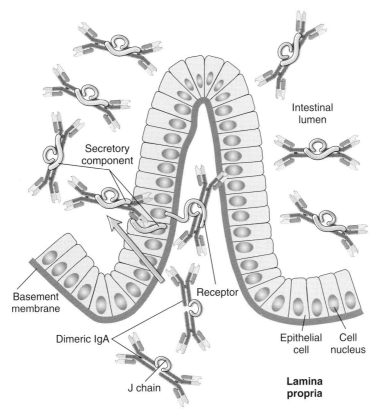

Intestinal
lumen

Secretory
component

Basement
membrane

Receptor

Dimeric IgA

Epithelial   Cell
cell   nucleus

J chain

**Lamina
propria**

FIGURE 5-18. **Secretory IgA as it crosses the mucous membrane.** Specialized epithelial cell receptors lining the mucous membranes have a specialized receptor that binds dimeric IgA at the basement membrane. These receptor molecules are responsible for the transport of dimeric IgA to the lumenal surfaces of the epithelium. A portion of the receptor, known as the secretory component, remains with the secreted dimeric IgA and adds protection from enzymatic degradation of IgA in the external environment.

cytoplasmic granules, are released to initiate an inflammatory response. Inflammation generated via IgE in this manner is referred to as **type I hypersensitivity** or, more commonly, an **allergic response** and is discussed further in Chapter 8.

Fetal protection

The adaptive immune system of the mother provides passive protection to the fetus. This protection is accomplished by the passive transfer of IgG across the placenta. No other immunoglobulin isotype or complement can cross the placenta to enter the fetal circulation. Recall that the half-life for most IgG is 23 days (see Table 4-1). Because maternal antibody levels in fetal circulation approach that of the mother, the newborn can expect 6 to 9 months of passive immunity acquired from the mother. Passively acquired antibodies are the predominant immunologic protection of the newborn while its own immune system becomes sufficiently functional to provide its own

protection. Defects in the infant's immune system, if present, most often become apparent at 6 to 9 months of age when passive maternal protection is lost.

Protection of mucosal surfaces

Specialized epithelial cells in the salivary and lacrimal glands, respiratory tract, small intestine, and breast tissue bind dimeric IgA (either IgA_1 or IgA_2) at their internal surfaces using a specialized receptor. Dimeric IgA is transported through the cell and released at its external surface. A portion of the receptor remains with the secreted IgA molecule (Fig. 5-18). The receptor remnant, known as the **secretory component**, gives the secreted IgA additional protection against degradation in the external environment. Secretory IgA_1 is released into the saliva, the tears, and breast milk, and secretory IgA_2 is released into the intestinal lumen, where it acts as an effective neutralizing antibody.

RECIRCULATION AND HOMING OF ADAPTIVE IMMUNE SYSTEM CELLS

Initiation of adaptive immune responses requires that the small number of available antigen-specific T cells identify and bind to relatively small numbers of specific pMHC complexes found on APCs. This is a formidable challenge for the adaptive immune system—how to bring together a specific TCR with the appropriate pMHC. The induction of an immune response is greatly facilitated by the continuous migration of naïve T cells through the lymphoid organs and tissues where they have the opportunity to "look" at a wide variety of peptides displayed on MHC molecules.

Naïve T cells encounter pMHC complexes by recirculating through the peripheral lymphoid organs. Specialized postcapillary venules are found within lymph nodes and mucosal lymphoid tissues, but not the spleen. The epithelia of these postcapillary venules are thicker than other epithelia and are termed **high-endothelial venules** (**HEV**). HEVs express addressins that are bound by L-selectin (CD62L) expressed on naïve T cells. After initial CD62L:L-selectin–mediated attachment, the T cells migrate through the endothelial junctions into the lymph node, a process known as **diapedesis** (Fig. 5-19). HEVs are located in the deep cortical regions of the lymph nodes, and it is here that naïve T cells may or may not encounter specific antigens. Encounter with the appropriate self-MHC molecule ensures the T cell's post-thymic survival, and it migrates toward the medulla of the lymph node to the draining lymphatic vessel. The lymphatic vessels eventually join the thoracic duct, where leukocytes are returned to the circulation. If, however, the naïve T cell encounters the appropriate pMHC on an APC, the T cell proliferates through several generations and differentiates into an effector T cell. Activated effector T cells then migrate through the medulla to be returned to the circulation via the lymphatic vessels and the thoracic duct.

Adjuvants or substances used to enhance the immune response and inflammatory stimuli cause dendritic cells within the draining lymphoid organ to secrete cytokines and chemokines that attract T cells. In addition, dendritic cells express adhesion and costimulatory molecules, as well as cytokines that influence the duration of APC–T-cell interaction and ultimately the differentiation of effector T cells.

Unlike their naïve counterparts, effector T cells leave the lymphoid organs on activation by as yet unknown mechanism(s), having acquired the capacity to migrate into nonlymphoid organs. Activated T cells show a decrease in L-selectin and increases in both CD44 and integrin expression. On activation, some T cells lose expression of the β-chemokine (also called CC chemokine for adjacent cysteine residues on the molecule) receptor CCR7, but increase their expression of CCR1, CCR2, CCR5, and other chemokine receptors that mediate T-cell migration to inflammatory sites (Fig. 5-20).

It is key that not all activated cells acquire effector function and migrate into the peripheral

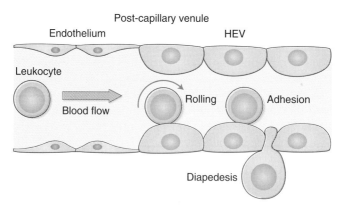

FIGURE 5-19. High-endothelial venules (HEV) and diapedesis. Specialized postcapillary venules are found in the peripheral lymphoid organs. The cells lining the venules are thickened and are called high-endothelial venules (HEV). Adhesion molecules or addressins expressed by HEV bind to L-selectin (CD62L) expressed by naïve T cells. The binding slows lymphocytes, causing them to roll along the epithelium and temporarily adhere to the HEV. The T cells migrate through endothelial junctions into the lymphoid organs by a process known as diapedesis.

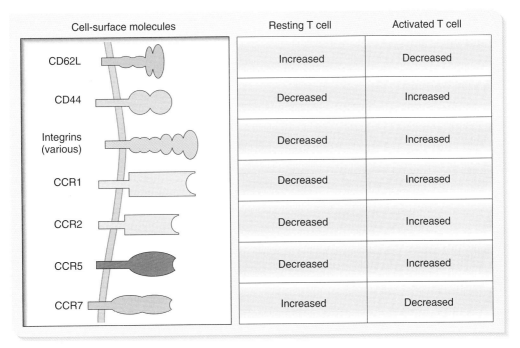

Cell-surface molecules	Resting T cell	Activated T cell
CD62L	Increased	Decreased
CD44	Decreased	Increased
Integrins (various)	Decreased	Increased
CCR1	Decreased	Increased
CCR2	Decreased	Increased
CCR5	Decreased	Increased
CCR7	Increased	Decreased

FIGURE 5-20. Changes in selectin molecules in activated versus resting T cells. T-cell activation causes alteration in the expression of a variety of cell-surface molecules that affect cell trafficking. Activation down-regulates the expression of L-selectin (CD62L) and the b-chemokine receptor CCR7 (CC indicates adjacent cysteine residues on the chemokine), but up-regulates the expression of CD44, CCR1, CCR2, CCR5, and a variety of integrins.

tissues. Some activated cells retain CCR7 expression and retain their capacity to migrate within lymphoid tissues. These cells are thought to be **memory T cells**, those that rapidly become activated on re-introduction of antigen. Memory cells are crucial for adaptive immune responses to re-introduced antigen or re-infection, allowing rapid mobilization, migration, and increase effector responses at peripheral sites.

PROTECTION FROM SUBSEQUENT INFECTION OR ENCOUNTER WITH ANTIGEN

The adaptive immune system, although relatively slow to respond to an initial antigenic encounter, responds much more rapidly on subsequent encounters with the same antigen. Both cell-mediated and humoral adaptive immune responses gradually decline after an antigen or infectious organism is cleared. Re-encounter with the same antigen or infectious organism within weeks of the original antigenic insult leads to a rapid clearance of the antigen or organism. This protective process is called **protective immunity**. Re-encounter with anti-

gen or infectious organism at much later times, even years after the initial antigenic insult, again results in rapid antibody and T cell-mediated immune responses. The long-lasting ability to recall an immune response is called **memory**.

Immunologic memory

A hallmark of the adaptive immune system is **immunologic memory**. Simply put, once an infectious organism stimulates an adaptive response, subsequent encounters with that organism produce mild or even unapparent effects because of the rapid and enhanced action of antibodies or effector T cells. Perhaps the most outstanding characteristic of the adaptive immune response is also its least understood. Antigen-specific cells that have been clonally expanded and have undergone some activation during previous encounter with antigen can be rapidly mobilized, thus shortening the response time to antigen. This rapid response and, in the case of antibodies, increase in antibody affinity quickly remove and destroy the antigen. To permit these accelerated responses, several of the "rules" governing the activation of naïve cells have been relaxed for those that are already activated.

Antigen presentation

All antigen presentation requires at least partial antigen degradation. Presentation to previously activated antigen-specific CD4$^+$ T cells requires stimulation by the same pMHC class II and co-stimulatory signals. Unlike antigen-naïve CD4$^+$ T cells, effector T cells do not need to undergo several rounds of division. In addition, B cells are effective antigen presenters to Th2 cells by mechanisms discussed below. Differentiated CD8$^+$ T cells only need to recognize pMHC class I and *do not require co-stimulation*. Essentially, activated CTLs have been given license to kill without any further consultation by another leukocyte.

Secondary T-cell responses

The initial activation of antigen-naïve T cells increases their numbers by more than 1000-fold. Many of these cells will undergo apoptosis once the antigenic threat is removed from the body. Yet a number of effector and/or memory T cells will persist at levels 10- to 100-fold greater than their antigen-naïve predecessors. Because effector

T cells and long-lived memory T cells have very similar, if not identical, surface molecules, it has been difficult to distinguish one from the other experimentally. The most notable surface phenotypic change that distinguishes effector/memory T cells from antigen-naïve T cells is the surface expression of CD45. **Common leukocyte antigen** or **CD45** is a transmembrane tyrosine phosphatase that is expressed as two different isoforms created by alternative splicing of CD45 RNA. The greater molecular weight isoform CD45RA is found on the surfaces of antigen naïve T cells. The lower molecular weight isoform CD45RO is expressed in greater density by effector/memory T cells.

Secondary B cell responses

The initial humoral or antibody response after infection or immunization can be divided into four distinct phases: a lag period, log phase, plateau, and decline (Fig. 5-21). During the initial or **lag phase**, antibodies are not detectable. It is at this stage that B cells are undergoing initial expansion in cell number induced by both antigen and T cells. During the **log phase**, antibody titer against the inductive antigen exponentially

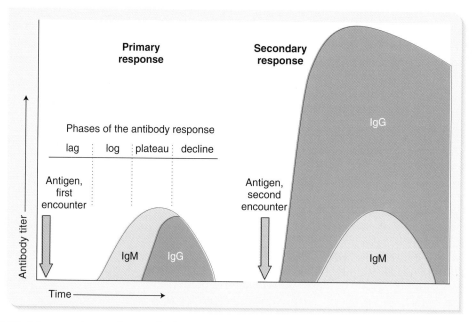

FIGURE 5-21. **Primary and secondary antibody responses.** On initial antigen encounter, the primary immune response goes through four distinct phases: lag, log, plateau, and decline. IgM antibodies dominate the primary antibody or humoral immune response. The secondary antibody response occurs on subsequent exposure to the antigen. The lag, log, plateau, and decline phases are altered compared to a primary response. IgG antibodies predominate, with a greatly foreshortened lag phase and a more intense log phase. The IgG titer at the plateau phase is much greater than that seen for a primary response, and the decline phase is prolonged for several weeks or months. The kinetics of the IgM response on second antigenic is the same as seen for the first antigenic encounter.

increases. The **plateau phase** is the peak of the curve, where maximal amount of antibody is detected. During the **decline phase**, antibody production and titer decreases. In general, the period from infection or immunization to the plateau phase is 7 to 10 days, with a lag period of 5 to 7 days. Relatively low-affinity IgM antibodies predominate in the primary response (Table 5-2). The length of time required to attain the plateau phase depends greatly on the nature of the immunizing antigen, the quantity of antigen or severity of the infection, the route by which the antigen is introduced, the relative epitope complexity of the immunogen, and the persistence of the antigen. In contrast, secondary B-cell responses have a greatly reduced lag phase, an accelerated log phase, and a plateau phase in which antibody titers can easily be 1,000- to 100,000-fold greater than those of the primary response. Although the half-life of the antibody is unchanged, the decline phase is prolonged because far greater quantities of antibody are produced. Secondary antibody responses are dominated by IgG antibodies; IgM antibodies tend to be at the same level as seen in the primary response. Depending on the nature of the infection or immunization, IgA and/or IgE antibody responses may also be found in large quantity. In responding to a secondary antigen insult, B cells undergo hypermutation of their immunoglobulin variable regions, producing ad-

ditional variation and effectively fine-tuning the "fit" of the antibody to a particular antigenic epitope. This is process called **affinity maturation** and is discussed further in Chapter 6.

LIMITATIONS OF THE ADAPTIVE IMMUNE SYSTEM

Strange as it may seem, the strengths of the adaptive immune system are also at the root of its primary weaknesses. For every individual, the adaptive immune response is an act of creation. Antigen-specific receptor molecules, TCR and BCR, must be generated before encountering an antigen. As we have seen, the receptor generation, although elegant, is random. Receptors for certain epitopes may be generated in relative abundance, but for others no receptor may be generated. Immunologists refer to this as "**the hole in the repertoire.**" Fortunately, most immunogens contain a variety of epitopes, and if a receptor for one epitope is not generated, there is a good possibility that receptors for other epitopes on the immunogen will be present.

Presentation of pMHC complexes by APCs serves to restrict T cells from responding to soluble antigens. Which peptides can be bound and presented in MHC molecules is determined by the three-dimensional structure of the peptide-binding cleft of the MHC molecule. Slight ge-

TABLE 5-2. PRIMARY AND SECONDARY HUMORAL IMMUNE RESPONSES

	Primary response	Secondary or memory response
Time course	Adaptive immune responses are T cell-dependent. Antigen is processed and presented by APC and both B and T cells must clonally expand to the stimulus. This requires time. The antibody response proceeds in 4 phases; lag, log, plateau, and decline phase.	T-cell and B-cell clonal expansion occurred during the primary response and some of these became memory cells. Memory cells "sit on the shelf" ready to act on a second encounter with antigen. Therefore, the immune system acts much faster and the immune response persists longer.
Titer	Titer is a term used for relative quantity. Relatively small quantities of antibody are produced in a primary response, compared to a secondary response (see column, right).	A greater titer (quantity) of antibody is produced relative to a primary response.
Isotype	The IgM isotype predominates in a primary antibody response. IgG appears later than IgM.	IgG (or IgA or IgE) predominates. IgM plays a relatively minor role in a secondary response.
Affinity	Affinity means "goodness of fit." Of the 10^6 to 10^7 different possible antibody specificities, some antibodies fit an antigen better than others. Primary responses see little selection for the best affinity, but show a rather wide spectrum of antibody affinity for the immunogen.	Memory T cells with the greatest affinity for pMHC class II molecules are preferentially stimulated. These, in turn, stimulate B cells possessing the highest affinity antigen receptors (BCR). This represents a fine-tuning of the immune response by selecting the most efficient T cells and B cells.

netic variation among MHC molecules among different individuals means that MHC molecules made by one gene may be able to bind a certain peptide better than an MHC molecule encoded by another allele. Ultimately, this means that some individuals have the *genetic predisposition to respond to certain peptides* better than others. This predisposition also points to an underlying genetic basis for certain autoimmune diseases (see Chapter 9) or for immunodeficiency diseases (see Chapter 7).

Compared with the innate system, the adaptive immune system is *relatively slow to respond to first encounter with antigen*. The repertoire of antigen-specific receptors generated is enormous. If each cell expresses a single, antigen-recognition specificity, this means a low initial precursor frequency for B or T cells for any given epitope. To mount an effective adaptive immune response, it is necessary to increase antigen-specific cell numbers by several rounds of cellular proliferation, a process that requires several days. In this same time interval, a pathogen could multiply and produce enormous numbers of progeny. Fortunately, the ability of the adaptive system to establish memory often makes an individual "immune" from recurrence of the infection.

The adaptive immune system responds "by committee" and this sometimes results in **mistaken identity**. For example, we have seen that microbes are engulfed and destroyed by APCs, their products are presented to T cells, and effector Th2 differentiate and help antigen-specific B cells activate, differentiate into plasma cells, and secrete antibody. The T cell-inducing peptide and B-cell specificity need not be identical and they often are not. However, they must be physically linked. Self-reactive TCRs are often eliminated during thymic education, but there is no equivalent for B cells. Consequently, a T cell may recognize a foreign antigen and inadvertently provide help to a B cell with a self-reactive BCR and differentiate into a plasma cell to secrete self-reactive antibody. Chapters 7 through 9 are devoted to the consequences of the inattentiveness and over-reactivity of the adaptive immune system.

INFLAMMATION IN ADAPTIVE IMMUNE RESPONSES

Nearly all effector adaptive immune responses use elements of the innate immune system. With the exception of killing mediated by CD8[+] T cells (CTLs), all adaptive immune responses have the potential to cause injury to bystander tissues. As we have seen for innate responses, inflammation is the immune system's opportunity to throw every bit of weaponry at its disposal at a perceived threat. But why would it want to do this? Perhaps the most important adage for both the innate and adaptive immune systems is pathogen containment and destruction. Delayed hypersensitivity reactions arise from antigen-specific CD4[+] Th1 recruitment of phagocytic cells. Activated phagocytes perform a frenzy of phagocytosis and killing. Friend or foe, it does not appear to matter. What does matter is that the perceived pathogen is contained and destroyed. Antibody–antigen reactions serve to immobilize the antigen by agglutination or render it unable to find its way by neutralization. Some antibodies, when bound to antigen, activate complement that contains and destroys the perceived pathogen by opsonization and/or lysis. However, activated molecules of the complement cascade may "tag" normal tissues for opsonization or lysis. In addition, anaphylatoxins of the complement cascade can act as chemical signals promoting vascular permeability and attracting leukocyte infiltration and activation at the site, further increasing inflammation. Although we may think of the innate immune system as the gateway to the adaptive response, the innate system also often appears to function as the "hit man" of the adaptive response. The adaptive response effectively intensifies and focuses the innate system.

Summary

- Adaptive immune responses require that specific T cells, initially present in low frequency, identify and bind to relatively small numbers of specific peptides bound to MHC (pMHC) complexes found on antigen-presenting cells (APCs).
- **Antigen presentation** is the process in which proteolytic fragments of antigens are loaded into MHC molecules (pMHC) and displayed on the cell surface. APCs efficiently present pMHC leading to T-cell activation and reactivation. In general, cells that display pMHC class II molecules are known as professional APCs, and these are primarily **dendritic cells**, macrophages, and B cells.
- Proteolytic fragments of exogenous proteins, those that originate outside of the cell such as bacteria and proteins found in the extracellu-

lar tissues and fluids, are loaded into MHC class II molecules. Proteolytic fragments of proteins originating within the cell's cytoplasm, such as viral proteins, are loaded into MHC class I molecules.

- Immature dendritic cells capture microbes, infected cells, dead cells, or their molecules either by receptor-mediated phagocytosis or by macropinocytosis.

- By applying both **positive and negative selection** of thymocytes, the adaptive immune system is assured of a population of naïve T cells that have TCRs that can respond to nonself peptides presented by self MHC molecules. Self-reactive T cells are eliminated.

- Naïve CD4$^+$ T cells activated through the immunologic synapse begin to express a variety of cytokines and cell-surface cytokine receptors.

- **Humoral immune responses** are those that involve the actions of immunoglobulins, antibodies, or complement. Only B cells and their fully differentiated form, **plasma cells**, synthesize immunoglobulins. Mature B cells, co-expressing IgD and IgM, are ready for activation.

- T and B cells amplify in number in response to antigenic stimuli to produce mature, activated T and B cells.

- **Delayed (-type) hypersensitivity (DTH) reactions** are localized to the immediate area surrounding the site of injection of antigen. The reaction is characterized by localized induration (swelling), may lead to localized necrosis and ulceration, and is followed by a decrease in the swelling and/or healing of the lesion.

- Eosinophils and NK cells recognize alteration in the Fc portion of the bound antibody. These cells kill antibody-"tagged" cells by a process known as **antibody-dependent cell-mediated cytotoxicity (ADCC)**.

- Mast cells and basophils contain cytoplasmic granules composed of a variety of chemical mediators (*e.g.*, histamine, serotonin, platelet-activating factor) involved in the generation of inflammation.

- The adaptive immune system of the mother provides passive protection to the fetus. This is accomplished by the passive transfer of IgG across the placenta.

- Specialized epithelial cells in the salivary and lacrimal glands, respiratory tract, small intestine, and breast tissue transport **dimeric IgA** (either IgA$_1$ or IgA$_2$) from their internal surfaces to their external surfaces using a specialized receptor that is proteolytically shortened to become **secretory component**.

Suggested readings

Appleman LJ, Boussiotis VA. T cell anergy and costimulation. *Immunol Rev* 2003;192:161–180.

Bradley LM. Migration and T-lymphocyte effector function. *Curr Opin Immunol* 2003;15:343–348.

Carsetti R, Rosado MM, Wardmann H. Peripheral development of B cells in mouse and man. *Immunol Rev* 2004; 197:179–191.

Crivellato E, Vacca A, Ribatti D. Setting the stage: an anatomist's view of the immune system. *Trends Immunol* 2004;24:210–217.

Cyster JG. Lymphoid organ development and cell migration. *Immunol Rev* 2003;195:5–14.

Al-Daccak R, Mooney N, Charron D. MHC class II signaling in antigen-presenting cells. *Curr Opin Immunol* 2004;16:108–113.

van den Elsen PJ, Rudensky A. Antigen processing and recognition. Recent developments. *Curr Opin Immunol* 2004;16: 63–66.

Germain RN, Jenkins MK. In vivo antigen presentation. *Curr Opin Immunol* 2004;16:120–125.

Jacobelli J, Andres PG, Boisvert J, et al. New views of the immunological synapse: variations in assembly and function. *Curr Opin Immunol* 2004;16:345–352.

Jin Y, Fuller L, Ciancio G, et al. Antigen presentation and immune regulatory capacity of immature and mature-enriched antigen presenting (dendritic) cells derived from human bone marrow. *Human Immunol* 2004;65:93–103.

Krogsgaard M, Huppa JB, Purbhoo MA, et al. Linking molecular and cellular events in T-cell activation and synapse formation. *Sem Immunol* 2003;15:307–315.

Krummel MF, Davis MM. Dynamics of the immunological synapse: finding, establishing and solidifying a connection. *Curr Opin Immunol* 2002;14:66–74.

Ruland J, Mak TW. Transducing signals from antigen receptors to nuclear factor κB. *Immunol Rev* 2003;193:93–100.

Pitcher, LA, va Oers, NSC. T-cell receptor signal transmission: who gives and ITAM? *Trends Immunol* 2003;24:554–560.

Schwartz RH. T cell anergy. *Annu Rev Immunol* 2003;21: 305–334.

Starr TK, Jameson SC, Hogquist KA. Positive and negative selection of T cells. *Annu Rev Immunol* 2003;21:139–176.

Review questions

DIRECTIONS: Each of the numbered items or incomplete statements in this section is followed by answers or by completions of the statement. Select ONE lettered answer of completion that is BEST in each case.

1. TAP-1 and TAP-1 molecules are required for
   (A) expression of the IL-2 receptor
   (B) prevention of antigen binding to newly synthesized MHC II molecules
   (C) processing of particulate antigen by phagocytic cells
   (D) loading of antigen into newly synthesized MHC I molecules
   (E) generation of variable regions of the BCR and TCR

2. Negative selection of B cells occurs in the
   (A) thymus
   (B) lymph node
   (C) spleen
   (D) blood vessels
   (E) bone marrow

3. What cells use somatic hypermutation to expand the diversity of antigen receptors?
   (A) B cells and T cells
   (B) T cells, but not B cells
   (C) B cells, but not T cells
   (D) T cells and dendritic cells
   (E) dendritic cells and B cells

4. Which cytokine promotes the differentiation of $CD4^+$ T cells into the effector Th1 pathway?
   (A) IL-4
   (B) IL-12
   (C) IL-5
   (D) IL-10
   (E) TNF

5. Rag-1 and Rag-2 enzymes are required for
   (A) expression of the IL-2 receptor
   (B) prevention of antigen binding to newly synthesized MHC II molecules
   (C) processing of particulate antigen by phagocytic cells
   (D) loading of antigen into newly synthesized MHC I molecules
   (E) generation of variable regions of the BCR and TCR

6. On activation T cells express IL-2 receptors. What is their source of IL-2?
   (A) APC
   (B) T cells
   (C) NK cells
   (D) B cells
   (E) Follicular epithelial cells

7. MHC class I molecules present peptides derived from
   (A) ingested antigens
   (B) the cell's cytoplasm
   (C) scavenger receptors
   (D) opsonized microbes
   (E) protease inhibitors

8. Which cytokine do Th1 cells use to activate macrophages?
   (A) TNF-β
   (B) IL-4
   (C) IL-2
   (D) INF-γ
   (E) IL-12

9. MHC class II molecules present peptides derived from
   (A) ingested antigens
   (B) the cell's cytoplasm
   (C) ζ chain (CD247) processed antigens
   (D) TAP-processed peptides
   (E) protease inhibitors

10. Recirculating lymphocytes identify inflammatory sites through interaction between
    (A) lymphocyte selectins and vascular endothelial addressins
    (B) lymphocyte CD154 and CD40 on vascular endothelium
    (C) lymphocyte LFA-3 and vascular endothelial ICAM-2
    (D) lymphocyte FcR and IgG bound to the vascular endothelium
    (E) lymphocyte FcR and high levels of C3b bound to the vascular endothelium

11. The cells responsible for ADCC killing are
    (A) CTL
    (B) activated macrophages
    (C) NK cells
    (D) mast cells
    (E) B cells

12. Immunoglobulins of this isotype can cross the placenta to the fetus
    (A) IgA
    (B) IgD
    (C) IgE
    (D) IgG
    (E) IgM

13. A 4-month-old infant presents with *Pneumocystis carinii* pneumonia. Immunologic testing reveals low IgG and IgA levels and elevated IgM. What is a possible diagnosis?
    (A) Hyper IgM syndrome
    (B) IgA deficiency disorder
    (C) Bare lymphocyte syndrome
    (D) X- linked agammaglobulinemia

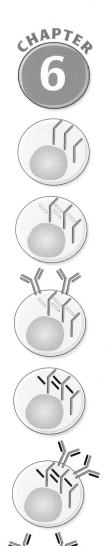

Protective Immune Responses

Chapter Outline

Introduction Whether the immune system responds to an antigen, and how that decision is made or manipulated, is vital for the protection of the body. The immune system is designed to attack infectious organisms that enter the body and these organisms often resist by evading or subverting the immune system. Immune protection can often be enhanced using vaccination as a preemptive strike against invasion by infectious organisms. Often it is important for the immune system not to respond to antigen. The mucosal surfaces are continually bathed in a broad range of nonself molecules and microorganisms in the food and fluids we consume and in the environment we contact. Because most of the antigens encountered by the mucosal surface are not threatening, the immune defenses that protect the mucosal surfaces are able to modulate and diminish responses against such benign antigens.

TYPES OF PATHOGENS

From the human vantage point, the microbial world has four types of citizens: (1) those that do not inhabit humans; (2) those that live on or in the human body to the benefit of one or both partners and harms neither; (3) those that live on or in the human body in a state of truce, causing harm to neither; and (4) those with the potential for causing harm to the human host, termed **pathogens** (the agents of infectious disease). A pathogen's potential for causing disease may vary, depending on circumstances. Some pathogens invade the human body as a necessary part of their life cycle. Others are **opportunistic** pathogens in that they are often present but become a threat when the immune system is weakened. Other pathogens produce products that are life-threatening to the host, such as the *Vibrio cholera* toxin. Humoral immunity against cholera toxin is crucial to protection.

Pathogens encountered by the immune system may range in size from microscopic viruses and bacteria to parasitic worms that may be several meters in length. They may even include **prions**— infectious entities that contain protein, but no nucleic acid, that can invade cells and replicate.

EFFECTIVE IMMUNE RESPONSES TO PATHOGENS

Pathogens or their toxic products vary in the ways that they enter the body (*e.g.*, contaminated food or water, wounds or other breaches in integument, injection by bites of insect vectors) and the environments within the body that they inhabit once they enter. They also vary in the ways that they grow and move about the body and reproduce.

Types of responses to pathogens

All of these factors determine the type of immune response that can most effectively attack and destroy them. Not all immune responses are equally effective against all pathogens. The responses most likely to provide protection are determined by the type and lifestyle of the pathogen in question (Tables 6-1 and 6-2).

TABLE 6-1. SELECTED INFECTIOUS ORGANISMS, CHARACTERISTICS AND ASSOCIATED INNATE RESPONSES

			Effector response for clearance of active infection				
Category	Infection	Representative organism(s)	Phagocytosis [a]	PMN	Complement [a,b]	NK cells [c]	Other [d]
Viruses	Intracellular, cytoplasmic	Influenza					
		Mumps					
		Measles					
		Rhinovirus					
Bacteria	Intracellular	Listeria monocytogenes					
		Legionella spp.					
		Mycobacteria					
		Rickettsia					
	Extracellular	Staphylococcus spp					
		Streptococcus spp					
		Neisseria spp					
		Salmonella typhi					
Protozoa	Intracellular	Plasmodium malariae					
		L. donovani					
	Extracellular	Entamoeba histolytica					
		Giardia lamblia					
Fungi	Extracellular	Candida spp					
		Histoplasma					
		Cryptococcus					

[a] Effective (▪); reduced effectiveness because of bacterial capsules (▪); ineffective except during extracellular transit (▫)
[b] Lysis and/or opsonization
[c] NK cells can be activated by molecules on intracellular bacteria to produce interferon-β which boosts phagocytic cell activity
[d] Mechanical barriers (skin, epithelial sloughing, respiratory cilia), chemical barriers (fatty acids, microcides of the skin and mucous membranes, pH of the stomach), biological barriers (commensal microbes).

TABLE 6-2. SELECTED INFECTIOUS ORGANISMS, CHARACTERISTICS AND ASSOCIATED ADAPTIVE RESPONSES

Representative Organisms	Infection	Effector response for clearance of active infection						Protective neutralizing antibody
		Humoral responses				Cell-mediated responses		
		IgM, IgG, IgA			IgE	CTL	DTH	
		Complement activation	Opsonization	ADCC				
Viruses Influenza, Mumps, Measles, Rhinovirus	Intracellular-cytoplasmic					▓		▓
Bacteria Listeria, Legionella, Mycobacterium, Rickettsia,	Intracellular-phagosomal/cytoplasmic					▓	▓	▓
Bacteria Staphylococcus, Streptococcus, Neisseria, Salmonella	Extracellular	▓	▓				▓	▓
Protozoa Plasmodium, Leishmania, Plasmodium	Intracellular					▓	▓	▓
Protozoa Entamoeba, Giardia	Extracellular		▓					
Fungi Candida, Histoplasma Cryptococcus	Extracellular						▓	
Flatworms Taenia, Schistosoma	Extracellular				▓		▓	
Roundworms Ascaris, Hookworm	Extracellular			▓	▓		▓	

Humoral responses

Soluble effector molecules, namely the complement system and antibodies, are major arms of the **humoral responses** and are involved in combating most infections. Both the mannan-binding lectin and alternative complement pathways are important humoral components of the innate immune system whose different components function as opsonins, anaphylatoxins, and, through the membrane attack complex, may lyse invaders to prevent infectious organisms for establishing an initial beachhead. In the adaptive system, antibodies directed against epitopes on infectious organisms function as guided missiles to "seek and destroy" infectious organisms by neutralizing their ability to bind to host cells or by targeting microbes for destruction by cells or complement. Once formed and secreted, antibodies patrol the tissues and fluids of the body to provide a defensive shield to prevent reinfection (see Chapter 4).

Humoral responses are generally effective only when infectious organisms are present in the body fluids and intercellular spaces or in organisms whose products are expressed on the surfaces of host cells. Microbial products expressed on host cells are available to binding by antibodies that can, in turn, lead to host cell death by **antibody-dependent cell-mediated cytotoxicity (ADCC)** (see Chapters 2 and 5). Some infectious organisms evade host humoral responses by not displaying their products on host cell surfaces, and the ability of antibodies and complement to inhibit their activities is limited to the occasions when they are in transit between cells and thus exposed to the humoral response.

Affinity maturation is a process whereby antibody responses against a repeatedly encountered infectious agent or other antigen can be refined so that, over time, the antibodies produced against the antigen bind to it with increasing affinity

(Fig. 6-1). As memory B cells undergo serial rounds of reactivation in the follicles of the lymph nodes and spleen, the small changes in the binding sites of their B-cell receptors (BCR; surface-bound immunoglobulins) caused by **somatic hypermutation** during replication cause the surface immunoglobulins of some memory B cells to bind the antigen more tightly, or sometimes less tightly, than before. The affinity (strength of interaction between the BCR and an epitope) influences the replication of the B cells. B cells with BCRs that bind with greatest affinity replicate at a faster rate and will become increasingly dominant with each successive exposure or stimulation. As a result, the antibodies produced by B cells after repeated antigen stimulation bind better than those produced by earlier stimulations. Affinity maturation occurs only in B cells. It does not occur in T cells.

Cell-mediated responses

Humoral responses may not be sufficient to prevent infectious organisms from establishing a foothold. Again, both the innate and adaptive immune systems are conscripted to combat the invaders. Unlike humoral responses, cell-mediated responses ultimately involve cell-to-cell contact. And, as we will see, both humoral and cell-mediated adaptive responses are directed by a CD4$^+$ T-cell command staff.

Phagocytic and NK cells

Innate responses against infectious organisms include phagocytic cells that use pattern recognition receptors (PRRs) to identify and bind pathogen-associated molecular patterns (PAMPs) on microbes (see Chapter 3). Natural killer (NK) cells and phagocytes are able to detect signals, such as certain heat shock proteins, released by cells undergoing stress. NK cells can also detect reductions in the amount of surface MHC class I molecules, a condition induced by some infectious organisms. All of these signals can trigger action by the NK cells and phagocytes to begin destruction of infectious organisms and infected cells before the generation of adaptive responses (see Chapter 3).

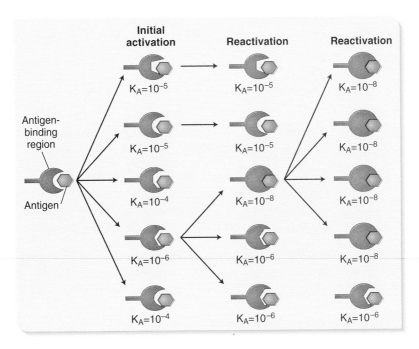

FIGURE 6-1. Affinity maturation. As memory B cells undergo serial rounds of restimulation, the genes encoding their surface antibodies undergo somatic hypermutation in addition to isotype switching. The somatic hypermutation in the genes encoding the antigen-binding sites causes variation in the binding affinity (K_A) between the antibodies and the antigen in question. Those cells expressing antibodies with increased binding affinity for the antibody are induced to proliferate more rapidly and come to dominate the response. Over time, this results in the production of antibodies with increasing binding affinities for the stimulating antigen.

Cytotoxic T lymphocytes

CD8$^+$ **cytotoxic T lymphocytes** (CTLs) bind to and kill infected cells where the infectious organism or its products are located in the cytoplasm. Here, they are degraded by **proteasomes**, transported into the endoplasmic reticulum via transport-associated proteins (TAP), and loaded onto newly synthesized MHC class I molecules for surface presentation.

Viruses infect host cytoplasm and CD8$^+$ CTLs are effective in detecting and eliminating virally infected cells through induction of membrane damage and apoptosis (Fig. 6-2). CTLs secrete perforin, which forms pores in target cell walls to induce their lysis, and granzymes that induce apoptosis. Although most bacteria and protozoa that invade host cells are sequestered in vacuoles within the infected cells, some bacteria such as *Rickettsia* and *Listeria monocytogenes* can escape from the vacuoles and live in the cytoplasm. In addition, antigenic fragments from microbes taken up and destroyed within phagosomes can enter the cytoplasm and the MHC class I presentation pathway. Lytic death of infected cells results in rupture of the cell wall and release of cytoplasmic contents. The additional ability of CTLs to induce infected cells to undergo programmed death by apoptosis provides an additional benefit because it results in the degradation of the genetic material of both the cell and the infectious organisms within, effectively preventing the spread of infection to neighboring cells. Also, apoptotic cell death does not trigger local inflammation, as lytic cell death often does. In comparison with other cellular responses, such as delayed-type hypersensitivity, the action of CTLs is highly discriminating. Although infected cells are destroyed, adjacent uninfected cells are left undamaged.

Delayed (-type) hypersensitivity

The primary cellular response attributed to CD4$^+$ T or Th1 cells is **delayed (-type) hypersensitivity** (**DTH**) (see Chapters 5 and 8 for a detailed discussion of DTH responses). Activated Th1 T cells recognize pMHC class II (peptide presented by MHC class II molecules) cells expressing the appropriate pMHC II combination at sites of

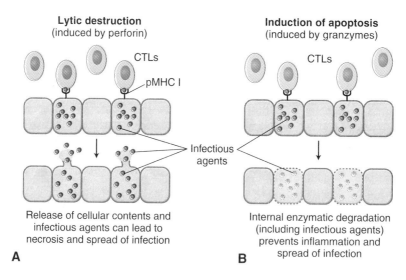

Lytic destruction
(induced by perforin)

CTLs

pMHC I

Infectious agents

Release of cellular contents and infectious agents can lead to necrosis and spread of infection

A

Induction of apoptosis
(induced by granzymes)

CTLs

Internal enzymatic degradation (including infectious agents) prevents inflammation and spread of infection

B

FIGURE 6-2. Lytic and apoptotic destruction of infected cells. (A) Lytic destruction induced by perforins released by cytotoxic T cells and natural killer cells create pores in the infected target cells, leading to osmotic swelling and rupture. The release of cellular contents can induce inflammatory responses, and the release of viable infectious agents can result in the spread of infection to neighboring cells. **(B)** Apoptosis induced by granzymes released by cytotoxic T cells results in an internally driven enzymatic degradation of the target cell. The cell remnants are absorbed by neighboring cells without provoking inflammation. Apoptosis also degrades the nucleic acids within the cell, including that of the infectious organisms within. As a result, spread of the infection is inhibited.

infection, and are stimulated to secrete cytokines that attract and activate macrophages to the site. The activated macrophages produce proteolytic enzymes, oxygen radicals, and other toxic microcidal molecules. They also actively ingest and kill the infectious organisms. Activated macrophages do not discriminate between infected cells and uninfected cells in the vicinity. A great deal of collateral damage and death of uninfected cells occurs from this "friendly fire." As a result, inflammation caused by intense DTH responses may inflict considerable damage on normal tissues while clearing infections that can leave the affected tissues or organs permanently impaired.

SIDEBAR 6.1 CD4$^+$ T CELLS AND CYTOPLASMICALLY DERIVED PEPTIDES

CD4$^+$ T cells can also be activated against fragments of cytoplasmic proteins, such as viral epitopes. Debris from cells destroyed by viral infection is routinely ingested by phagocytic cells. In this way, viral peptides become available for processing and presentation via the exogenous MHC II pathway. Although the activated CD4$^+$ T cells may not play a major role in clearance of virally infected cells, they are important in aiding the proliferation of CD8$^+$ T cells and in activating B cells for production of anti-viral antibodies.

Humans are confronted by a wide range of different infectious organisms. Each of these enters the body, feeds, and reproduces in a particular pattern. Each of the ways in which these invaders inhabit the body has one or more weaknesses that can be exploited by the immune system to resist their growth and hopefully eliminate them.

Viruses

Viruses are obligate intracellular pathogens, regardless of the species infected. Because their genomes are too small to encode all of the molecules needed for replication, they invade cells of other organisms and use the synthetic machinery of the infected cell. In doing so, they often kill the infected cell and spread to adjacent cells to repeat the process. Viruses are typically narrowly restricted to a specific cell type but may travel throughout the body to locate their targets.

Patient Vignette 6.1

 Robert G., a 3 year-old boy, has had six "colds" since he started preschool 10 months ago.

He usually has symptoms of runny nose, nasal congestion, sneezing, and occasional fever of 100°F. He has normal tonsillar tissue and cervical lymph nodes. His symptoms have usually resolved within 1 week. His mother is concerned about the frequent colds.

On the average, children typically have six to ten colds per year and adults have between two and four colds per year. Colds are caused by more than 200 different viruses. The pathogens associated with the common cold are primarily rhinovirus, coronavirus, parainfluenza virus, respiratory syncytial virus, influenza virus, and adenovirus also cause colds. Symptoms usually include runny nose, nasal congestion, sneezing, sore throat, and cough. Other symptoms may include muscle aches, headache, and decreased appetite.

Viral infections trigger both innate and adaptive immune responses. Infected cells synthesize and secrete interferon-α (IFN-α) and IFN-β that not only heighten their resistance to viral replication but also heighten the resistance of neighboring uninfected cells (see Chapter 4). In addition, IFN-α and IFN-β stimulate increased surface expression of MHC class I molecules, making the cells more "noticeable" to CD8$^+$ T cells. NK cells can also recognize and kill virus-infected cells by recognition of stress signals and reduced expression of MHC I molecules. Phagocytic cells, activated by the binding of their PPR to PAMP on viral particles, begin to secrete cytokines that trigger the release of **acute phase proteins** from the liver. These proteins induce a loosening of the junctions between the endothelial cells lining the vasculature to permit freer entry of blood-borne cells and molecules into the infected tissues. They also induce the onset of fever. An increase of body temperature by only a few degrees slows viral reproduction. In addition, some acute phase proteins, such as **C-reactive protein**, are effective opsonins.

After the initial action of elements of the innate immune system, humoral and cellular adaptive responses arise (Table 6-1). Because viruses replicate in the cytoplasm of infected cells, viral products are available for proteasome degradation and presentation in pMHC class I complexes in the same way that fragments of normal cytoplasmic proteins are processed and presented. As a result, virally infected cells display evidence of the pathogen within by displaying pMHC class I on their surfaces for recognition and binding by CD8$^+$ CTLs. Both NK cells and CTLs disrupt the viral "nurseries" by destroying the infected cells and interrupting the replication cycle. On making contact with an infected target cell, NK cells and CTLs secrete **perforin** that creates holes in the target cell membranes, causing lysis by disrupting the osmotic balance. This form of cell death is also called **necrosis**, and induces inflammation. CTLs can also secrete **granzymes** that destroy virus-infected cells by inducing them to undergo **apoptosis**, a process that has additional benefits. When the **caspase** system is induced by granzymes, the target cell begins to enzymatically destroy both its own nucleic acids and those of the viruses and other organisms within the cell, preventing their escape, spread, and replication in neighboring cells. Necrosis does not occur. Instead, postapoptotic cellular "debris" is quietly phagocytosized by neighboring cells in a way that does not attract phagocytic cells and induce inflammation.

During **primary infections** (the first exposures to a particular infectious agent), as cell-mediated responses work to clear the viral infection, B cells generate humoral responses to viral epitopes. The antibodies generated against viruses are not effective in clearing active infections, because the replicating virus is sequestered within cells. However, they can effectively minimize or prevent re-infection. The IgG and IgA isotypes, and IgM to a lesser extent, are efficient at **neutralization**. By blocking the ability of viruses to attach to cells, they inhibit the ability of the infection to spread. In addition, the binding of antibodies to viral particles facilitates the ingestion and destruction of viral particles through opsonization. Where neutralizing antibodies fail to completely inhibit re-infection, the numbers of newly infected cells are generally much lower than in primary infections and clearance proceeds more rapidly, perhaps not even producing clinical symptoms. Cell-mediated responses are again required for clearance, but the necessary level of activity is often insufficient to produce detectable symptoms.

Bacteria

Some bacterial pathogens, termed **extracellular bacteria**, live freely in the body fluids and intercellular spaces, whereas others may enter and reproduce within cells and are called **intracellular bacteria**. These two modes of existence dictate the immune responses that are effective against each type of bacteria.

Extracellular Bacteria

Extracellular bacteria such as *Staphylococci* and *Streptococci* are readily exposed to humoral components of the immune system such as antibodies and complement (see Table 6-1). They are, therefore, susceptible to death and clearance by the innate immune system such as phagocytic ingestion via recognition/binding of PAMPs and by the lectin-binding and alternative pathways of complement activation. Complement activation can lead to increased destruction of bacteria (**opsonization**) through engagement of complement receptors on phagocytic cells and by lysis of bacteria via generation of membrane attack complexes on the bacterial surfaces. Subsequent adaptive responses leading to production of bacteria-specific IgG, IgA, and IgM further trigger

---

SIDEBAR 6.2 HUMORAL RESPONSES TO PNEUMOCOCCAL INFECTIONS

The immune responses to bacteria with polysaccharide capsules, such as *Streptococcus pneumonia*, are exclusively humoral. IgM antibodies bind to the pneumococcal capsular polysaccharides that coat the bacteria and activate the classical pathway of complement and target the bacteria for clearance by opsonization. *S. pneumonia* infections are often fatal for people with C3 deficiencies because they cannot clear the infection.

opsonization through engagement of Fc receptors on phagocytic cells and increase bacterial lysis through the classical pathway of complement activation.

Intracellular Bacteria

Intracellular bacteria include *Mycobacterium tuberculosis*, *Microbacteria leprae*, and *Legionella pneumophila* (causative agents for tuberculosis, leprosy, and Legionnaires disease; see Table 6-1). Although their survival may be threatened by exposure to complement and antibodies en route to their cellular destinations, once inside they are sheltered from humoral responses. In most cases, intracellular bacteria reside within cellular vacuoles called **phagosomes**. Intracellular bacteria avoid destruction within the cell by: (1) physically escaping from phagosomes to live within the cytoplasm (*e.g., L. monocytogenes*); (2) inhibiting formation of **phagolysozomes** by interfering with phagosome–lysosome fusion (*e.g., L. pneumophila* and *M. tuberculosis*); or (3) resistance to the acidic/oxidative environment within the phagolysosome (*e.g., Salmonella spp.*) Intracellular bacteria retard the cell's attempts to destroy them and multiply, sometimes destroying the host cell and escaping to infect other cells.

Turning the tide against intracellular bacteria often requires activation of infected phagocytes by CD4$^+$ T cells. Activation heightens the metabolic activity of phagocytes and production of bactericidal products, allowing them to kill the microbes within the phagosomes. Once activated, the phagocytes also contribute to heightened immune responsiveness through increased phagocytic activity and secretion of cytokines stimulating other cells involved in inflammatory responses. Peptide fragments of internalized bacteria are loaded into MHC class II (pMHC class II; see Chapter 5) and presented on the surface of the infected phagocyte. Previously activated CD4$^+$ T cells with TCR specific for these pMHC class II molecules can recognize and bind them. Chemokines and cytokines such as macrophage chemotactic protein (MCP)-1, tumor necrosis factor (TNF)-α, and TNF-β attract macrophages and facilitate their movement from the vasculature into infected tissues. Also, CD40L (CD154) on the T cells engage CD40 on the phagocyte, and the T cells secrete IFN-γ that binds receptors on the phagocytes. These two signals provide a powerful stimulus for phagocyte activation and generation of DTH. It should be noted that DTH is only effective against cells infected by intracellular bacteria if those cells express MHC class II molecules.

CTL responses can also be generated against intracellular bacteria. For example, as previously mentioned, *L. monocytogenes* and *Rickettsia* can escape phagosomes and live in the cytoplasm. Within the cytoplasm, some of the bacterial proteins are marked by ubiquitin for degradation by proteosomes. The products of degradation occurring within the phagolysosomes are sometimes released into the cytoplasm, again becoming available for loading onto MHC class I molecules for expression on the host cell surface.

Patient Vignette 6.2

 Henry G., a 50-year old man with a history of cancer who is currently receiving chemotherapy, presents with symptoms of fever, chills, headache, and a dry cough lasting for 3 days. Before becoming ill, he attended a convention with his friends and some of them also became ill.

What disease might this patient have?

This patient may have early symptoms of Legionnaires disease, perhaps acquired through exposure to someone with the disease. In addition, he has two risk factors (cancer and chemotherapy) that are potentially immunosuppressive. In 1976, 29 members of the American Legion in Philadelphia died of pneumonia. The pathogen was eventually identified as a Gram-negative intracellular bacterium known as *Legionella pneumophila*. Nineteen species of this bacterium have been identified as the agents of pneumonia in Legionnaires disease. The most common agent is *L. pneumophila*. Affected patients usually have early symptoms of fever, chills, and a dry cough. The disease may spread to other organs, including the gastrointestinal tract and the central nervous system. Infection usually occurs in middle-aged men or immunosuppressed people. The antibiotic most commonly used to treat the disease is erythromycin.

Protozoa

Immune responses to infectious **protozoa** (single-cell, nonphotosynthetic eukaryotic organisms) follow a pattern very similar to those for bacteria. Protozoa that are free-living in the body are susceptible to the actions of complement and antibodies. Many, if not most, pathogenic protozoa (*e.g., Plasmodium spp., Trypanosoma spp.,* and *Leishmania spp.*) spend at least part of their lives within tissues and cells, where some of their reproduction occurs. In this, they are similar to intracellular bacteria. While they are moving to, from, and between cells, they are susceptible to the actions of antibodies and complement. In fact, opsonization caused by bound C3b and antibodies probably provides the greatest protection during these "extracellular" phases. However, once within a cell, cellular responses are required for destruction of the infected cells and the protozoa within. Like immune responses to some intracellular bacteria, CD4$^+$ T cell-mediated responses such as DTH are required for this clearance.

CLINICAL APPLICATION
MALARIA

In 1880, scientists discovered that the parasite *Plasmodium* is the cause of **malaria**, in which the parasite invades and destroys erythrocytes, leading to episodes of anemia. Approximately two decades later, it was discovered that the transmission of malaria occurs via an infected *Anopheles* mosquito bite. Today, malaria is one of the major killers of humans worldwide. Despite the availability of drugs for treatment, approximately 2.7 million people die each year of malaria, and most of them are infants and children in Asia, Africa, and South and Central America.

Fungi

Whereas fungal infections trigger both antibody and DTH responses, it is the latter that are responsible for resistance and clearance. **Fungi** are plant-like organisms that lack chlorophyll and include the yeasts and molds. Normal individuals typically control fungal infections readily, despite the enormous number of fungi in the environment. Only in cases of excessive accumulations (e.g., in the lungs) or some defect in the cellular immune system are significant fungal infections

---

CLINICAL APPLICATION
CANDIDIASIS

Oral thrush or oral candidiasis is a fungal infection of the oropharynx characterized by white plaques or lesions. The diagnosis is made by physical examination and confirmation by microscopic examination with KOH (potassium hydroxide) preparation. *Candida albicans* is normally present in a healthy individual's mouth, gastrointestinal tract, and other parts of the body. The fungus acts as a pathogen when the immune system is altered by diseases such as diabetes, cancer, immunodeficiencies of cell-mediated responses, or immunosuppressive infections such as HIV.

---

seen. Persistent fungal infections are indicators of immune deficiency disease.

The generation of potentially high levels of antibodies, particularly IgG, against fungi is not, however, without its consequences. The simultaneous presence of large amounts of fungi, together with high levels of antibodies specific for that fungi, can trigger a form of inflammatory disease called **immune complex disease** (also called **type III hypersensitivity**) in some individuals. These types of responses are discussed in Chapter 8.

Flatworms and roundworms

Flatworms consist of two major groups—the **trematodes** or flukes and the **cestodes** or tapeworms. Although tapeworms are generally confined to the gastrointestinal tract, different species of flukes preferentially infect a variety of tissues, including the blood, liver, lung, and intestine. Fluke infestations can generate inflammation, mediated by DTH responses that are often directed against the eggs. Many flukes enhance their chances for survival by using mechanisms that inhibit the host's ability to mount immune responses directed against adult and larval forms.

Adult tapeworms attach and anchor themselves to the wall of the intestine and remain there, reproducing while absorbing nutrients from the processed food passing by them. The immune system generates inflammatory responses at the sites where the worms attach to the intestinal wall. Both DTH responses and IgE-mediated inflammatory responses (also known as type I hypersensitivity) can occur, and in some cases cause the worms to detach. Repeated exposures to the same species of tapeworm have been associated with increasing levels of specific IgE and increasing resistance to re-infection.

Pathogenic **roundworms** include organisms such as *Ascaris*, hookworms, and various worms known collectively as **filaria**. Whereas filarial worms generally live in the bloodstream, *Ascaris* and hookworms take up residence in the intestines, where, like tapeworms, they attach and reside for the remainder of their adult lives, reproducing and absorbing nutrients. Like tapeworms, they can trigger cellular and IgE-mediated inflammatory responses that make their local environment less amenable to their remaining. In addition, ADCC contributes to protection. Eosinophils bear receptors that can detect IgG bound to the surfaces of roundworms. These cells bind to the parasite. When large numbers of eosinophils bind, they are capable of killing the worms.

Prions

Prions are associated with several related diseases of the nervous system that occur in several species, including humans. In sheep, they cause a disease known as scrapie; in cattle, they cause bovine spongiform encephalopathy (BSE; commonly called "mad cow disease"); in wild deer and elk, they cause chronic wasting disease; and in humans, they are associated with diseases such as **kuru** and **Creutzfeldt-Jakob disease (CJD)**. No

immunologic defense against prion-related diseases is currently known.

EVASION AND SUBVERSION OF THE IMMUNE RESPONSE

Infectious organisms do not go meekly to their death when confronted by the immune system. After eons encountering their human hosts, they have developed numerous methods for evading, and in some cases damaging or destroying, the host immune system (Fig. 6-3). In military terms, these strategies range from using camouflage to laying mine fields to assassination. Some pathogens cloak themselves in host antigens to fool the immune system into believing that they belong in the body. Others secrete enzymes that destroy immunoglobulins or other defense-related molecules that some near. Yet others, most prominently the human immunodeficiency virus (HIV) that causes acquired immune deficiency syndrome (AIDS), strike at the heart of the immune system by infecting and killing off its most important field generals, the CD4$^+$ T cells.

Camouflage

Blood flukes of the genus *Schistosoma* are masters of disguise. Found world-wide in tropical or semi-tropical regions, schistosomes infect humans

Camouflage
- Donning host antigens
- Hiding within cells
- Reducing expression of antigens
- Programmed switches in expression of genes encoding antigens

Antigenic drift/shift
- Accumulated mutations
- Recombination of microbial or viral genomes

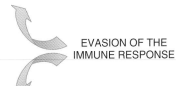

EVASION OF THE
IMMUNE RESPONSE

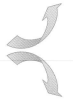

Interference
- Inhibition of phagosome function
- Inhibition of antibody binding
- Cleavage of antibodies/complement
- Directing MHC I molecules into inappropriate cellular compartments
- Altering Th1/Th2 balance

Destruction of the immune system
- Destruction of immune cells

FIGURE 6-3. Evasion of the immune response. Infectious organisms use multiple strategies to evade or inhibit immune responses generated against them by the host immune system.

engaged in aquatic agriculture or other water-related activity. After a swimming larval form (cercaria) enters the body by burrowing through the skin, it metamorphoses and travels to the mesenteric blood vessels where the adult form develops and remains until its death. The larval and adult forms cover themselves with molecules derived from host cells—including MHC molecules and even blood group antigens—so that the host immune system mistakes it as "self." As a result, immune responses against larval and adult forms of the parasite generally do not develop. In experimental animal systems where the parasite was transferred from one host into another, *Schistosoma* was able to replace the "cloaking" molecules of the previous host with those of the new host in less than 15 hours.

Another form of camouflage—invisibility—is used by *Plasmodium ssp.*, protozoa that cause malaria, living and replicating within liver cells and erythrocytes. Erythrocytes, having matured from nucleated reticulocytes, lack nuclei and do not express MHC class I or II molecules or pMHC. Cytotoxic CD8$^+$ T cells searching for infected cells by identifying fragments of pathogen-derived peptides displayed by MHC class I molecules are unable to identify and kill infected cells lacking MHC class I molecules. One might wonder if NK cells could recognize the lack of MHC class I molecules on the infected erythrocytes and kill them. However, recall that erythrocytes lack nuclei and are unable to initiate synthesis of the stress molecules that provide the initial recognition for NK cells. Furthermore, an ability of NK cells to kill infected erythrocytes on the basis of their reduced expression of MHC class I molecules would presumably also extend to uninfected erythrocytes—an undesirable outcome.

Finally, many microbes can alter their antigen expression in a quantitative manner. By reducing the expression of molecules likely to be stimulatory to the immune system, the infectious agents may be able to slip under the immune system's radar.

Antigenic drift/antigenic shift

Many infectious organisms evade the immune response by staying ahead of it in terms of the antigens they express. Bacteria such as *Neisseria gonorrhoeae* and viruses such as influenza, hepatitis C virus, and human immunodeficiency virus (HIV), as well as protozoa such as *Trypanosoma brucei*, periodically change the antigens they express. As a result, previously developed cell-mediated or humoral immune responses may no longer be effective. The immune system must start anew, developing responses to the newly expressed antigens, only to find that by the time they should be sufficient to become effective, the organism has shifted again to yet another new set of antigens.

Changes in antigen expression can be generated in a number of ways. An error-prone transcription, absence of "proofreading" mechanisms to correct potential mutations, rapid replication rate, and genetic recombination can produce significant variation in the antigens expressed by a particular type of microbe, even within a single infected host. Influenza and HIV exploit an error-prone replication process that permits the accumulation of small mutations in the viral DNA, a process termed **antigenic drift** (Fig. 6-4A). As a result, new mutant forms of the genes encoding the antigens are constantly generated, and many of them will be "unrecognizable" to the existing immune response. Other organisms, such as *N. gonorrhoeae*, contain numerous, and slightly varying, copies of the gene(s) encoding their dominant antigenic molecules. Only one of the copies is usually transcribed and expressed at a time, but they are periodically shifted around so that a different copy may suddenly be transcribed and expressed. Such changes may render the existing immune response against the bacteria ineffective and new specific responses must again be generated. A similar, though not identical, strategy is used by *Trypanosoma brucei*, the causative agent of African sleeping sickness, to periodically switch the gene used to produce its major surface antigen and stay one jump ahead of the immune response.

Antigenic shift is a process in which recombination creates major changes in the dominant antigen expressed by the virus (Fig. 6-4B). Antigen shift, as well as antigenic drift, is often seen in the influenza virus and HIV-1, and leads to the introduction of forms of influenza that are able to spread swiftly and with severe consequences. Antigenic shift occurs when viruses from different sources infect the same cell and recombine. For example, a duck-derived virus and a pig-derived virus can coexist in a single cell (for example, in an infected pig) and exchange parts of their genetic material to produce hybrid offspring containing a mix of the two original viruses. These hybrid forms are often so different that individuals with strong immune responses against forms of influenza encountered

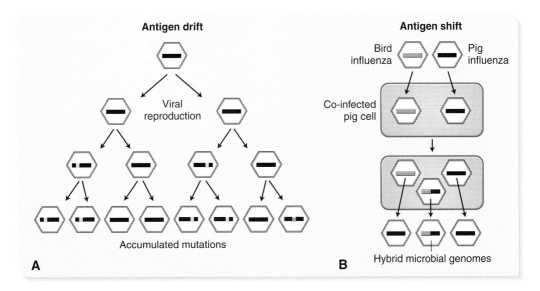

FIGURE 6-4. Antigenic drift and antigenic shift. (A) Antigenic drift occurs as a result of accumulated small mutations that alter antigenic epitopes of the infectious agent. **(B)** Antigenic shift results in sudden large changes in the epitopes of infectious agents as a result of mixture of genomes from different strains of the microbes.

only a relatively short time earlier may find themselves unprotected against the new hybrid forms of influenza generated by antigenic shifts.

Interference

Infectious organisms have developed numerous mechanisms that interfere with the immune responses generated against them. *Chlamydia,* an intracellular bacterium, secretes molecules that interfere with the fusion of the phagosome in which it resides with lysosomes containing the enzymes that can kill and degrade it. Some pathogens such as *Schistosoma* secrete factors that interfere with the ability of local lymphocytes to proliferate. Some bacteria and viruses secrete enzymes that destroy nearby complement molecules or immunoglobulins. Several viruses, including some herpesviruses and adenoviruses, inhibit the loading of peptide fragments into MHC class I molecules.

Finally, some infectious organisms have developed the capacity to mislead the immune system into concentrating on the immune responses that are the least harmful to the organism. Organisms that are susceptible primarily to antibody may induce cellular responses, or vice-versa. Epstein-Barr virus, for example, has a gene that encodes an equivalent of IL-10, a Th2 cytokine that promotes antibody production but inhibits the development of the cellular

immune responses so important in the clearance of viral infections.

Ideally, infections produce a balance of Th1 and Th2 responses. However, because of a variety of environmental and host genetic factors, as well as influences from the pathogen, infections

---

CLINICAL APPLICATION
INFLUENZA

In the United States during the period from 1990 to 1999, influenza viruses have been responsible for an average of approximately 36,000 deaths per year. All age groups are affected, but the rates of serious illness and death are highest in infants, in persons older than 65 years of age, and in patients with chronic medical conditions.

There are two types of influenza viruses that cause the disease: influenza A and B. Influenza A has two surface antigens: hemagglutinin (H) and neuraminidase (N). Because of the antigenic variants that result from antigen drift (*i.e.,* frequent antigenic change during replication), each year's influenza vaccine incorporates one or more virus strains. The strains that are used are based on information gathered from global surveillance of the influenza virus.

can sometimes lead to immune responses that are heavily dominated by either Th1 or Th2 responses. **Hansen disease** (or **leprosy**), caused by *M. leprae*, provides a good illustration of these extremes (as well as a range of Th1/Th2 balances between the extremes). At one extreme (the **tuberculoid** form), some individuals show very strong DTH responses (Th1) against *M. leprae* but generate little or no antibody responses. The DTH response keeps the infectious load of *M. leprae* at a low level, although its intensity often leads to extensive tissue damage. At the other extreme (the **lepromatous** form), patients have little cellular response to the pathogen but high levels of anti-*M. leprae* antibodies develop. Although they do not display the tissue damage associated with the tuberculoid form, they are unable to control the levels of infection, and their tissues often have extremely high infectious loads.

Destruction of the immune response

The ultimate resistance of an infectious organism to the immune system is to bring about its destruction. No infectious agent illustrates this strategy more dramatically than HIV. The ability of HIV to infect and destroy $CD4^+$ T cells strikes at the very heart of the adaptive immune system. $CD4^+$ T cells are critical for the generation of effective adaptive immune responses. $CD4^+$ T cells are essential for the activation and function of the majority of B cells. They are critical in the initiation of $CD8^+$ CTL responses by providing cytokines that facilitate proliferation of $CD8^+$ T cells. And they are the key agent in the recruitment and activation of macrophages for DTH responses. The eventual destruction and depletion of $CD4^+$ T cells leads to the collapse of the host's adaptive immune response, and patients typically die of opportunistic infections. The effectiveness of HIV in subverting the host immune response is even more extraordinary in light of the fact that 10% or more of circulating $CD8^+$ T cells in infected individuals may be specific for HIV in initial infections, and that a great deal of antibody against the virus is also produced against the virus. This provides a devastating example of the ability of microbes to effectively evade the immune system while going on to overwhelm it.

PREVENTION OF INFECTION: VACCINATION

Humans have known of **vaccination**, if not its mechanisms, for thousands of years. Vaccination is an inoculation of nonvirulent or inactivated microbes as a means of inducing specific immunity. Those who survived diseases such as plague, smallpox, and other epidemic diseases were generally safe from the same diseases developing again, even as many others around them might be dying. Not only was their survival a blessing to the survivors but also provided society with a set of individuals able to aid others and perform critical activities in the face of subsequent epidemics.

History of vaccination

The ancient Egyptians and Chinese performed forms of vaccination to attempt to protect themselves against diseases such as smallpox by exposing individuals to powders formed from the crusts and scales of pockmarks on infected individuals. Sometimes mild forms of the disease developed in individuals so treated, or sometimes no visible disease developed at all, but those individuals found themselves protected. In 1794, Edward Jenner demonstrated that intentional inoculation with cowpox (a mild disease in humans caused by a form of vaccinia, a virus that normally infects cattle) conferred protection against smallpox, a potentially fatal human disease caused by a related but more virulent form of vaccinia. At the time, of course, there was no knowledge of the role of microbes in causing such diseases. Jenner called his procedure vaccination, and the word was later adapted to name the viral organism found to be the causative agent. Later, the discovery by Robert Koch of the role of specific microbes in specific diseases stimulated activity in the field. Louis Pasteur advanced the science of vaccination by developing effective vaccines against epidemic diseases of agricultural animals and eventually performed a dramatic demonstration of a rabies vaccine that saved the life of a young boy bitten by a rabid dog.

Since that time, vaccination has revolutionized human and animal health. Routine childhood vaccinations have eliminated much of the misery and occasional permanent crippling or fatal consequences of once commonplace diseases such as measles, diphtheria, and polio. Smallpox, a disease that once killed humans by the thousands, has in turn been practically eliminated and the smallpox virus now exists only in a few protected laboratories.

CLINICAL APPLICATION
SMALLPOX

Smallpox is a highly contagious disease spreading from person to person, often by saliva droplets from the affected person's mouth. Early symptoms are similar to those of influenza and include high fever, headache, fatigue, muscle aches, and vomiting. Approximately 2 to 3 days after the onset of the symptoms, a rash appears. The rash is initially seen on the face and oropharynx; it then spreads to the upper arms, legs, and trunk. The mortality rate is approximately 30%, with death usually occurring during the second week of illness. Treatment for smallpox is mainly supportive, because there is no known effective treatment. Vaccination within 4 days of exposure to smallpox can prevent a fatal outcome and can reduce the severity of the illness.

Thomas Jefferson, in an 1806 letter to Edward Jenner, wrote that, *"Future nations will know by history only that the loathsome smallpox has existed and by you has been extirpated."* Because of a successful worldwide vaccination program, no case of small pox has been reported since 1977. In the United States, routine childhood vaccination for small pox ended in 1972. There is, however, current concern about the potential use of smallpox as a weapon of bioterrorism.

The standard vaccination schedule in the United States is presented in Figure 6-5. The beneficial impact of vaccination has been so widespread that we now face the situation in which many people no longer recognize the dangers that have been overcome. A growing number of parents fail to recognize the need to vaccinate children, and some individuals advocate the elimination of vaccinations because they believe them to be responsible for several, although rare, side effects. As a result, the danger exists that a pool of unprotected individuals may be created that could once again be subject to many of the infectious diseases that once terrorized human populations. It is probably not necessary that every individual in a population be vaccinated. So long as a sufficiently large population is vaccinated, the chances of an infectious agent "finding" an unprotected individual become very small, and the population as a whole remains essentially resistant. This concept is called **herd immunity**. The inherent risk is that if an infectious organism infects a significant number of unprotected individuals, the infection could spread rapidly among them, and ensuing mutations unanticipated by the vaccine could endanger vaccinated individuals as well.

Essential characteristics of vaccines

For vaccinations to be effective in protection of intended populations, several characteristics must be present.

- The vaccine must provide effective protection against the pathogen from which it is derived without significant danger of actually causing the disease or severe side effects.
- The protection provided by the vaccine must be effective over a long period of time.
- The vaccine must stimulate development of those immune responses that are most effective against the pathogen in question (e.g., protective T-cell responses).
- It must stimulate the production of neutralizing antibodies to minimize re-infection.
- It must be sufficiently stable for storage, transport, and use.
- The vaccine must be economically feasible for widespread use.

Types of vaccines

Vaccines may be prepared from pathogenic organisms in a variety of ways.

- **Live vaccines** are those that include organisms capable of normal infection and replication. These vaccines are not used against pathogens causing severe diseases.
- **Attenuated vaccines** are those in which the organisms included are live, but their ability to replicate and cause disease has been damaged by treatment with heat, chemicals, or other means. These vaccines cause only subclinical or mild forms of the disease at worst.

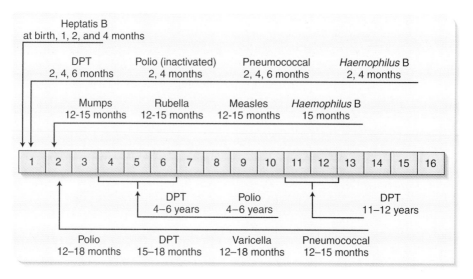

FIGURE 6-5. Currently recommended vaccination schedule in United States. This vaccination schedule is adapted from the 2004 Recommended Childhood and Adolescent Immunization Schedule available on the Centers for Disease Control web site. The scale is given as age (in years). The CDC regularly updates its recommendations, and their site should be consulted for the most current ones available.

- **Killed vaccines** include organisms that have been killed by treatment with physical or chemical agents and may include inactivated toxins (toxoids). They should be incapable of replication or infection but still able to provoke immune responses.
- **Extracts** are vaccines composed of materials derived of materials isolated from disrupted and lysed organisms. These vaccines would be most appropriate for protection against diseases in which the organisms are so virulent that even killed vaccines are not used because of the risk that a few organisms may have survived the treatments intended to kill them.

Modern techniques of molecular biology have permitted two additional forms of vaccines to be generated.

- **Recombinant vaccines** are those in which the organisms have been engineered in the laboratory by the removal of certain genes critical to their ability to actually cause the disease (*e.g.*, the gene encoding a critical toxin) or to reproduce completely. These organisms are typically able to infect host cells and even proliferate but cannot induce the disease they are associated with.
- **DNA vaccines** are those in which the naked genetic material of the organism is injected into the host. The DNA has usually been modified to remove some genes that are critical to

causing disease but includes those whose products will stimulate immune responses. The intent is that host cells will pick up the DNA, incorporate it, and express the gene products from the pathogen. The antigenic stimulus remains intact longer than methods in which the vaccine is rapidly eliminated from the host and the stimulation of the immune system stops.

In general, live vaccines generate the most efficient immune responses, with attenuated vaccines less so, followed by killed vaccines and extracts. Paradoxically, the safer the vaccine, the less effective it may be. Living, replicating organisms may synthesize and express molecules that are highly stimulatory to the immune systems, but those molecules may be absent from vaccines containing only killed or attenuated organisms. The potency of vaccines can be elevated by administering them after mixing them with adjuvants.

Adjuvants

Adjuvants are substances or mixtures that are given together with vaccines to heighten the effectiveness of the vaccination. Adjuvants prolong the period of time that a vaccine persists to stimulate the immune responses, and/or attracts phagocytic cells to the site of application and stimulates their activation so that their antigen presentation to lymphocytes is increased.

Adjuvants are mixtures of bacterial components suspended in some medium such as oil to slow and prolong their dispersal into the tissues. The bacterial material provokes a mild inflammation, attracting phagocytic and other cells to the site. Some vaccine components themselves can serve as adjuvants. In **DTP** (*diphtheria–tetanus–pertussis*) vaccine, the *pertussis* component (from *Bordetella pertussis*, the causative agent of whooping cough) is an effective adjuvant. Other adjuvants include alum and **BCG** (*Bacillus Calmette Guerin*). The latter is not used for human vaccinations in the United States and other countries because it uses material derived from *Mycobacterium* and can cause false-positive indications in persons being tested for tuberculosis.

Difficulties in vaccine development

The development of effective vaccines is not necessarily a straightforward one. Although many dangerous infectious diseases are now prevented or minimized by routine vaccination, many others such as malaria, schistosomiasis, and AIDS still lack effective vaccines. Often the difficulty in developing a vaccine is related to characteristics of the infectious organism. As mentioned earlier, the ability of cells to sequester themselves within certain types of host cells shelters them from the effects of antibodies. If the host is not generating sufficiently effective cellular responses, clearance of the pathogen is difficult. And, as described earlier, some pathogens such as *Plasmodium* enter erythrocytes that do not express MHC class I or II molecules and are essentially invisible to T cells.

In many cases, however, the difficulty lies with the ability of the pathogen to change its antigens so that immune responses generated to that point are ineffective. Perhaps the most dramatic example of this is HIV. The immune system can generate strong antibody responses against certain structures on the viral surface, but because the virus mutates so rapidly during replication, large numbers of new surface structures are constantly being generated that are new to the immune system. These **escape mutants** are free to continue replicating as the immune system tries to catch up. Unfortunately, if and when it does, new generations of new escape mutants have already been generated, and the immune response often plays a hopeless game of catch-up.

MUCOSAL IMMUNITY

The mucosal surfaces of the human body have been estimated to cover an area of approximately 400 square meters that are for the most part in contact with the environment. This area includes the mucosa lining the gastrointestinal (GI) tract (because of our body's tubular design, the lumen of the GI tract is actually external to the body), the respiratory system, the urogenital system, and the surface of the eye. These barrier surfaces are protected primarily by secretory IgA (sIgA) that has been conveyed from the vasculature by specialized epithelial cells underlying the mucus layer that covers the membranes. Although monomeric and dimeric IgA represents less than 20% of serum immunoglobulin (see Table 4-1), sIgA is prevalent in the mucosa. The oral cavity contains approximately 96% $sIgA_1$ and only 4% IgG because of the large amount of sIgA transported into it through the salivary glands. It has been estimated that approximately 75% of human B cells synthesize IgA, and that sIgA comprises approximately 60% to 70% of the total immunoglobulin produced daily.

As an illustration of the importance of the mucosal immune system, we examine the immune response of the GI tract more closely, particularly the intestinal tract. The part of the mucosal immune system related to the intestinal area is often called the **gut-associated lymphoid tissue** (**GALT**). The intestinal wall includes an epithelial lining on the luminal side, an underlying area called the **lamina propria** where most (but not all) of the immune cells serving the intestine are located, and an outer muscular layer (Fig. 6-6A). Within the lamina propria there are clusters of lymphoid tissues called **Peyer patches**, containing follicular structures similar to those seen in the spleen and lymph nodes (see Chapter 5). Peyer patches function similar to lymph nodes and the spleen, with cells entering at the cortical end, intermingling of antigen presenting cells, B cells, and T cells, and the exit of cells at the medullary end. However, unlike the lymph nodes and spleen, approximately 90% of the activated B cells emerging from Peyer patches are committed to production of IgA. They migrate to local lymph nodes and enter the circulation but then usually migrate back to the lamina propria of the small intestine. Those differentiating into plasma cells migrate to the crypts of the villi (Fig. 6-6A) where the dimeric secretory IgA (sIgA) is transported through some of the intestinal

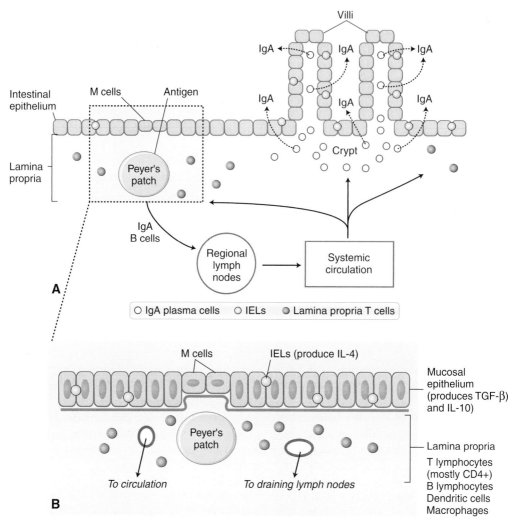

FIGURE 6-6. The mucosal immune system of the gastrointestinal tract. (A) Antigen in the form of microbial fragments or other substances in the intestinal lumen is transported by M cells from the lumen to antigen-presenting cells and lymphocytes in the lamina propria. Activation of B-lymphocytes (predominantly of IgA-producing B cells) occurs in the Peyer patches. T-cell activation occurs primarily in the mesenteric lymph nodes. Activated T and B cells recirculate throughout the body but primarily return to the lamina propria or other sites of mucosal immunity. IgA-secreting plasma cells migrate to the crypts of the villi, where the sIgA they secrete is transported through the intestinal epithelium into the intestinal lumen. **(B)** The intestinal epithelium is interspersed with a variety of lymphocytes that participate in producing a predominantly Th2 environment by secreting several anti-inflammatory cytokines. The intestinal epithelial cells secrete interleukin-10 (IL-10) and T-cell growth factor-β (TGF-β), whereas intraepithelial lymphocytes (IELs) secrete IL-4. The IELs consist of a variety of T cells, mostly CD8[+], with unusual characteristics. The T cells of the lamina propria are predominantly typical CD4[+] T cells with α–β T-cell receptors.

epithelial cells into the mucus layer at the luminal surface. Located in the intestinal epithelium overlying the Peyer patches are cells termed microfold cells or "**M cells**" that are specialized to facilitate the transport of materials from the lumen of the intestine to the underlying lymphoid tissue. M cells can ingest material at the lumen surface and transport it through their cytoplasm to the basal surface where it can be accessed by phagocytic cells and lymphocytes. Current opinion appears to be mixed as to whether M cells are true antigen-presenting cells (APCs) themselves, or only deliver material from the lumen to dendritic cell APCs in the lamina propria and Peyer patches. M cells do, however, appear to be able to discriminate between the beneficial commensal microbes living within the intestine and pathogenic microbes and limit their uptake and transport to the latter.

An additional feature of the GALT lies within its epithelial layer. The epithelial layer is in constant contact with an endless array of nonself antigens derived from ingested food and drink. The potential thus exists for constant and repeated immune stimulation that could eventually lead to inflammation. Fortunately, the GALT has developed mechanisms to prevent being caught up in a never-ending tidal wave of immune responses against nonthreatening substances, and elements of the **intestinal epithelium** play critical roles in this discrimination (Fig. 6-6B). Intestinal epithelial cells can express MHC class II molecules and act as antigen-presenting cells for a specialized subset of T lymphocytes, the **intestinal epithelial lymphocytes (IELs)** that are dispersed among the epithelial cells. Thus, they are able to influence the initial steps in the induction of immune responses. They also secrete IL-10 and TGF-β, both Th2 cytokines, that promote Ig production and inhibit cellular inflammation. Among the IELs, there are several atypical types of T cells, including a subset called the NK-like T cells. These respond rapidly after activation and begin producing large amounts of anti-inflammatory IL-4. Together, the local environment created by these actions is largely a Th2 one, supporting antibody production but minimizing the development of cellular inflammatory responses.

The GALT, together with the mucosal immune systems of the upper and lower respiratory tracts, urogenital tract, and even the secretory tissues of the breast can interact with one another as part of the **mucosal network**. T and B cells activated in the mucosal tissues at one site can often home to other mucosal tissues so that protection generated in one area against particular infectious agents can be transferred throughout the entire mucosal system. For example, during pregnancy, most of the antibodies secreted in breast milk are produced by B cells that have migrated from the GALT to the secretory epithelium of the breast. Thus, the breast milk contains antibodies against gut-associated microbes present in the mother and provides early protection against orally introduced viruses and bacteria.

The ability of GALT to retard potentially harmful responses could potentially be exploited to reduce harmful responses affecting other parts of the body. This approach, the manipulation of the immune response by oral administration of antigen, is discussed further in Chapter 11.

Summary

- **Pathogens** are infectious agents with the potential for causing harm to the human host. Their potential for causing disease may vary. Some pathogens invade the human body as a necessary part of their life cycle.
- **Opportunistic pathogens** are those that are often present but become significant threats only under specific circumstances such as a deficiency in the immune system.
- **Viruses** are obligate intracellular pathogens. Viral infections trigger both innate and adaptive immune responses. During primary infections, B lymphocytes are also exposed to viral epitopes and humoral responses are generated.
- **Extracellular bacterial pathogens** live freely in the body fluids and intercellular spaces, and **intracellular bacteria pathogens** enter and reproduce within cells.
- Immune responses to infectious **protozoa** follow a pattern similar to those for bacteria. Protozoa that are free-living in the body are susceptible to the actions of complement and antibodies. Protozoa that live within host cells require cellular responses for destruction of the infected cells and the protozoa within.
- Although **fungal infections** trigger both humoral and DTH responses, it is the latter that are effective for resistance and clearance.
- **Flatworms** consist of two major groups: the **trematodes** or **flukes** and the **cestodes** or **tapeworms**. Fluke infestations can generate inflammation mediated by DTH responses that are often directed against the eggs. Both DTH responses and IgE-mediated inflammatory responses can occur in response to tapeworm infections.
- Pathogenic **roundworms** include organisms such as *Ascaris*, hookworms, and various worms known collectively as filaria. Roundworms can trigger cellular and IgE-mediated inflammatory responses.
- **Prions** are proteins with no associated nucleic acid that can be transmitted and are responsible for several related diseases of the nervous system in multiple species, including humans.

No immunologic defense against prion-related diseases is currently known.

- Infectious organisms have developed numerous methods for evading, and in some cases damaging or destroying, the host immune system. These strategies include camouflage and periodic change of dominant antigenic molecules through rapid mutation (**antigenic drift**), DNA recombination, or systematic changes in gene expression.
- **Antigenic shift** is a process often seen in the influenza virus in which major changes occur in the dominant antigen expressed by the virus through intermixtures of the genomes of viruses from different sources.
- Infectious organisms have developed numerous mechanisms that interfere with the immune responses generated against them, including destruction of the host immune system.
- **Vaccination** has revolutionized human and animal health. Routine childhood vaccinations have eliminated once commonplace diseases such as measles, diphtheria, polio, and smallpox.
- **Live vaccines** are those that include organisms capable of normal infection and replication. **Attenuated vaccines** are those in which the organisms included are live, but their ability to replicate and cause disease has been minimized by treatment with heat, chemicals, or other means. **Killed vaccines** include organisms that have been killed by treatment with physical or chemical agents.
- **Recombinant vaccines** are those in which the organisms have been engineered in the laboratory by the removal of certain genes critical to their ability to actually cause the disease (e.g., the gene encoding a critical toxin) or to reproduce completely.
- **DNA vaccines** are those in which the naked genetic material of the organism is injected directly into the host for uptake and expression in host cells.
- **Adjuvants** are substances or mixtures that are given together with vaccines to heighten the effectiveness of the vaccination.
- The mucosal surfaces of the human body are protected primarily by **secretory IgA** that has been conveyed from the vasculature by specialized epithelial cells underlying the mucus layer that covers the membranes. The part of the mucosal immune system related to the intestinal area is called gut-associated lymphoid tissue (GALT).

Suggested readings

Iijima H, Takahashi I, Kiyono H. Mucosal immune network in the gut for control of infectious disease. *Rev Med Virol* 2001;11:117–133.

Janeway CA Jr, Travers P, Walport M, Shlomchik P. *Adaptive Immunity to Infection. Immunobiology: The immune system in health and disease*, 6th ed. Philadelphia: Garland Publishing; 2004.

Letvin NL, Barouch DH, Montefiori DC. Prospects for vaccine protection against HIV-1 infection and AIDS. *Annu Rev Immunol* 2002;20:73–99.

Rambaut A, Posada D, Crandall KA, Holmes EC. The causes and consequences of HIV evolution. *Nature Rev Gen* 2004;5: 52–61.

Raupach B, Kaufmann SH. Immune responses to intracellular bacteria. *Curr Opin Immunol* 2001;13:417–428.

Wong P, Pamer EG. CD8 T cell responses to infectious pathogens. *Annu Rev Immunol* 2003;21:29–70.

Review questions

DIRECTIONS: Each of the numbered items or incomplete statements in this section is followed by answers or by completions of the statement. Select the ONE lettered answer or completion that is BEST in each case.

1. The primary defense against fungal infection is
   - (A) complement-mediated lysis
   - (B) cytotoxic T cell activity (CTLs)
   - (C) IgE and eosinophil activation
   - (D) delayed-type hypersensitivity (DTH)
   - (E) IgG-mediated opsonization and complement activation

2. A tapeworm infection develops in a patient after ingestion of raw sushi. What type of immune response(s) will most effectively resist this infection?
   - (A) CD8$^+$ cytotoxic T cells
   - (B) Complement-mediated lysis
   - (C) Natural killer (NK) cell activity
   - (D) Eosinophil activation by IgE
   - (E) Delayed (-type) hypersensitivity (DTH) and IgE-mediated mast cell degranulation

3. *Plasmodium*, the protozoan responsible for malaria, can evade the immune system by

living inside erythrocytes. This evasion is possible because

(A) *Plasmodium* secretes IL-10 that inhibits development of Th1 T cells
(B) erythrocytes lack MHC I and II molecules on their surface
(C) *Plasmodium* disguises itself by adsorbing ABO blood group antigens from erythrocytes
(D) *Plasmodium* converts hemoglobin into a T-cell toxin
(E) erythrocytes do not express B7

4. The most effective vaccines are generally ones made from
(A) purified protein extracts from the pathogen
(B) pathogen DNA
(C) killed pathogens
(D) live or attenuated pathogens
(E) synthetic peptides mimicking those of the pathogen

5. In viral infections, _____ is/are required for clearance of active infections, whereas _____ is/are required to diminish the risk of reinfection.
(A) neutralizing antibodies/cytotoxic T-cell responses
(B) a cytotoxic T-cell response/neutralizing antibodies
(C) an NK cell response/activated macrophages
(D) an IgE response/IgG responses
(E) a DTH response/complement activation

6. Activation of naïve T cells specific for microbial epitopes is initiated by dendritic cells from the site of infection that subsequently migrate to
(A) local lymph nodes
(B) the lamina propria
(C) other sites of inflammation
(D) the bone marrow
(E) the thymus

7. The induction of apoptosis to kill infected cells has what advantage to the immune system over causing necrotic death?
(A) Apoptosis is quicker than necrosis.
(B) Apoptosis degrades DNA within the cell, including that of intracellular infectious organisms.
(C) Apoptotic signals are not delivered by direct contact but can be delivered by soluble molecules.

(D) Cytotoxic T cells are unable to kill by any other means.
(E) Apoptosis only requires the presence of C3b, which is usually available in abundance.

8. Schistosome worms are a good example of an infectious organism that evades the immune response by
(A) coating itself with host antigens
(B) decreasing the MHC I expression on the cells it infects
(C) frequently mutating its dominant antigens
(D) killing host T cells
(E) hiding within red blood cells

9. The "affinity maturation" of an immune response means that the
(A) response spreads from B cells to T cells
(B) response is caused by loss of suppressor T cells associated with advancing age
(C) response declines because of aging and death of the responding cells
(D) binding efficiency of the antibodies produced against a specific antigen decreases
(E) binding efficiency of the antibodies produced against a specific antigen increases

10. The immunoglobulin isotype most responsible for neutralization of infectious agents in the respiratory and gastrointestinal tract is
(A) monomeric (serum) IgA
(B) dimeric (secretory) IgA
(C) monomeric (serum) IgG
(D) dimeric (secretory) IgG
(E) pentameric IgM

11. Extracellular bacteria such as *Staphylococcus* and *Streptococcus* can be effectively cleared through
(A) antibody-mediated opsonization and complement activation
(B) apoptosis induced by cytotoxic T cells
(C) delayed (-type) hypersensitivity (DTH)
(D) histamine released by mast cells
(E) NK cells recognizing the absence on MHC I on bacterial surface

12. A 45-year-old man presented to the HIV clinic with symptoms of night sweats, fever, and cough. Pulmonary tuberculosis (*Mycobacterium tuberculosis*) was diagnosed. What element(s) of the immune system

would normally be primarily responsible for clearance of these intracellular bacteria?

(A) CD8$^+$ cytotoxic T cells

(B) Secretory IgA

(C) CD4$^+$ T cells and macrophages

(D) IgG and the components of the classical complement pathway

(E) IgG and eosinophils

13. A 30-year-old man presented with *Candida albicans* (fungus) growing widely over the mucosal surfaces of his oral cavity. Which of the following conditions should you suspect?

(A) Immune complex disease

(B) Hemophilia

(C) Deficiency of B cells/immunoglobulin

(D) Defective secretion of dimeric IgA

(E) Deficiency of cellular immune responses

14. A 65-year-old woman received pneumococcal vaccine, which contains capsular polysaccharides isolated from the 23 most prevalent types of *Streptococcus pneumoniae*. What type of vaccine is this?

(A) Live

(B) Attenuated

(C) Killed

(D) Extract

(E) Recombinant

Immune Deficiency

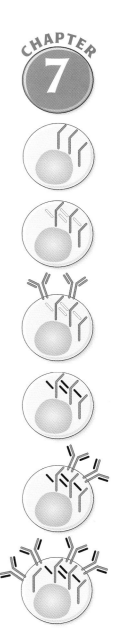

Chapter Outline

Introduction The complexity of diverse cells, specificities, molecules, and functions that must work in concert to make a functional immune system is truly remarkable. The vast numbers of cells and molecules that must migrate and interact precisely are so intricate that failure seems almost inevitable. Only rarely does the entire immune system fail and, when observed, it is far less frequent than one would expect. Dysfunction in one part of the immune system may be masked by the built-in redundancy in another part of the immune system. An example of such a fail-safe system occurs as part of the generation of B and T cell receptors. Because receptors are generated randomly (Chapter 4), it is not unusual for some of the epitopes on an infectious organism to go unrecognized by the TCR or by antibodies. However, recognition of other epitopes is normally sufficient to stimulate immune protection. Additional failsafe mechanisms are built into the immune system. For example, an antibody produced against a microbe may not activate the complement cascade or if complement is activated, the bacterial cell wall may resist complement-mediated lysis. All is not lost with the failure of antibody to neutralize or initiate complement-mediated lysis, because antibody and/or complement (C3b) binding to a microbe functions as an opsonin, targeting the infectious organism for lytic destruction by phagocytes. In addition, antibody may interfere with the binding of the infectious organism's binding to its obligate receptor molecule.

Yet, sometimes the system does fail. Defects in various components of the immune system—**immune deficiencies** or **immunodeficiencies**—are infrequent but not insignificant. They arise in two basic ways. **Primary immune deficiencies** are those that occur as intrinsic defects, usually genetic in nature but sometimes attributable to random developmental errors as well. Over 100 distinct human primary immune deficiency diseases and specific defective genes have been identified for many of them. The primary immunodeficiency diseases were originally thought to be quite rare. In fact, however, some of the primary immunodeficiency diseases are relatively common. For example, selective IgA deficiency occurs in as many as two individuals per thousand. Other primary immunodeficiency diseases are much less common and occur with a frequency of 1 to 10 per hundred thousand. However because there are so many primary immunodeficiency diseases, when taken together as a group of disorders, they become a significant health problem, occurring with a frequency comparable to leukemia and lymphoma in children and four times as frequently as cystic fibrosis.

Secondary immune deficiencies are characterized by reduced immune function attributable to environmental causes such as infection, therapeutic treatments, cancer, and malnutrition. Affected individuals are more susceptible to infectious disease than are normal individuals, and there may also be other side effects that accompany the immune deficiencies. Depending upon the nature of the defect, various therapies may be available to partially or fully restore normal immune function.

Immune deficiencies are recognized by a number of features. Some are common to most forms of immunodeficiency, while others are associated only with certain subsets of these diseases, and in some cases only with a single specific disease.

Characteristics common to most immune deficiency diseases are:

- Chronic infections
- Recurrent infections
- Incomplete clearance of infectious agents
- Infections with unusual agents (e.g., fungal infections)
- Incomplete response to standard antibiotic therapy

Characteristics common to several immune deficiency diseases include:

- Skin rashes [severe combined immune deficiency (SCID), Wiskott-Aldrich syndrome, X-linked agammaglobulinemia]
- Failure of infants to gain normal weight or "failure to thrive" (SCID, bare lymphocyte syndrome, interferon-γ receptor deficiency)
- Enlarged liver and spleen [common variable immune deficiency (CVID), Chediak-Higashi syndrome, interferon-γ receptor deficiency]
- Diarrhea [often due to gastrointestinal infection; CVID, Wiskott-Aldrich syndrome, X-linked agammaglobulinemia, bare lymphocyte syndrome, SCID, chronic granulomatous disease (CGD)]
- Recurrent abcesses (CGD, leukocyte adhesion molecule defects)

Nonimmunologic characteristics common to one or a few immune deficiency diseases include:

- Ataxia (loss of balance) and telangiectasia (widening of blood capillaries; immunodeficiency with ataxia-telangiectasia)

Patient Vignette 7.1

Daniel H., a 5-month-old boy, presents with bloody diarrhea and petechiae for several days. Since birth, he has had eczema and two episodes of pneumonia due to *Streptococcus pneumoniae*. Physical examination reveals an ill-appearing boy with eczema (scaling, itchy skin rashes) in the scalp, on the face, and in the diaper area. In addition, he has scattered petechiae on his body. Blood analyses are remarkable for low platelet counts and mild decreases in hemoglobin and white blood cell counts.

Q: What immunologic processes are likely to be involved in his problem?

A: This patient is likely to have Wiskott-Aldrich syndrome, an X-linked recessive disorder that includes thrombocytopenia (low platelet counts and small platelet size), eczema and recurrent infections that usually appear during the first year of life. In addition, individuals may have bloody diarrhea and excessive bruising. Immediate medical treatment for this patient includes platelet transfusion. Bone marrow transplantation may correct platelet and immunological disorders.

- Albinism (Chediak-Higashi syndrome)
- Platelet abnormalities (thrombocytopenias; Wiskott-Aldrich syndrome)

PRIMARY (CONGENITAL) IMMUNE DEFICIENCIES

Primary immune deficiencies can be categorized according to the tissue, cell, or molecule in which the defect occurs. Defects may involve the lymphoid cell lineage (T and B cells combined), the separate T and B cell lineages, and the lineages producing phagocytic cells and natural killer (NK) cells. In addition, dysfunctions of the thymus may affect the development and function of T cells that are intrinsically normal. Different immune cell lineages may interact in generating particular types of humoral and cell-mediated responses; therefore, defects in a single lineage may affect multiple types of responses. We will look more closely at defects in each of these categories and at a selected group of diseases that illustrate each.

Defects in autosomal genes, whether recessive or (less commonly) dominant, affect both

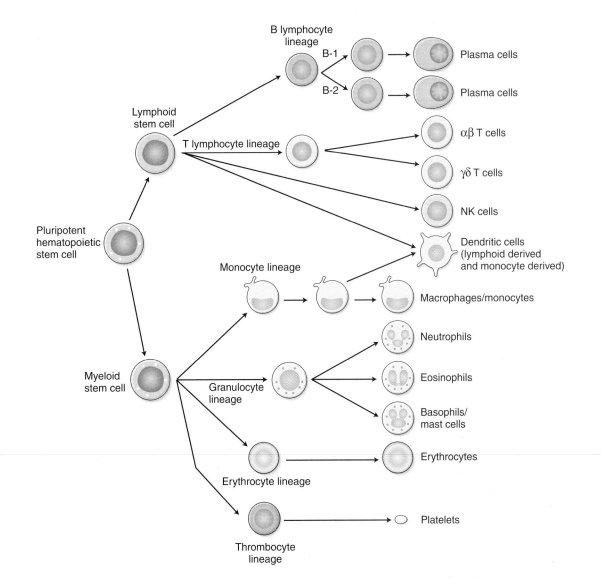

FIGURE 7-1. Hematopoeitic stem cells and their subsequent lineages. Pluripotent stem cells in the bone marrow are the source of lymphoid cells (T cells, B cells, natural killer cells, dendritic cells), thrombocytes (producing platelets), monocytic cells (monocytes, macrophages, dendritic cells), granulocytes (neutrophils, basophils, mast cells, eosinophils), and erythrocytes. Note that some dendritic cells are of lymphoid lineage, while others are derived from the monocytic series.

sexes equally. However, disorders caused by defective genes on the X chromosome are typically transmitted as X-linked recessive traits and occur far more often in males than in females. Females carry these defective genes, but their presence is usually masked by the presence of a normal counterpart on the other X chromosome. Males, however, receiving only a single X chromosome from their mothers, express the traits associated with every defective X-linked gene they inherit.

Defects in stem cells

The initial stem cell that ultimately generates the granulocytic, erythrocytic, monocytic, thrombocytic, and lymphocytic cell lineages is identifiable initially in the aorta-gonad-mesonephros (AGM), migrates during embryonic/fetal development to the liver, and then (by the time of birth) migrates to the bone marrow. Because it has the capacity to produce all of the hematopoietic cellular lineages, it is called a **pluripotent** stem cell. The pluripotent stem cell, in turn, gives rise to five sets of slightly more restricted stem cells, each capable of giving rise to one of the five hematopoietic lineages (Fig. 7-1). The lymphoid stem cells give rise to both B and T cell lineages. As described in Chapter 5, the B-2 cell lineage remains within the bone marrow for development, while the B-1 lineage is self-replicating within the peritoneal cavity and the T cell lineage migrates to the thymus.

Defects in the lymphoid stem cells giving rise to T and B cells cause malfunctions in both types of lymphocytes (Fig. 7-2). Numerous human diseases are attributed to defects in the lymphoid stem cells, and may be reflected in altered T and B cell numbers, in functions, or both. Cellular functions such as cell-mediated lysis and delayed hypersensitivity are usually reduced, as is production of immunoglobulins. However, the relative impact of the defects can vary between the two types of lymphocytes. In some immune deficiencies, the severity of the malfunctions may vary among affected individuals.

The classic example of lymphoid stem cell diseases is **severe combined immunodeficiency disease** (SCID). SCID is not a single disease but a group of diseases caused by different individual initial defects, but with similar consequences (Table 7-1). SCID may be caused by inherited genetic defects in several X-linked or autosomal genes. These include genes encoding enzymes (recombination activating gene, RAG-1, RAG-2) needed for the chromosomal rearrangement required to construct immunoglobulins and T cell receptors. Other defects are found in critical cytokine receptors and in molecules required for the intracellular signals necessary for the activation of lymphocytes following contact of their receptors with antigen. In some cases, these defects can have broad effects, as some gene products are components of receptors for several different cytokines (e.g., the γc chain that is part of the receptors for IL-2, IL-4, IL-7, IL-9, and IL-15).

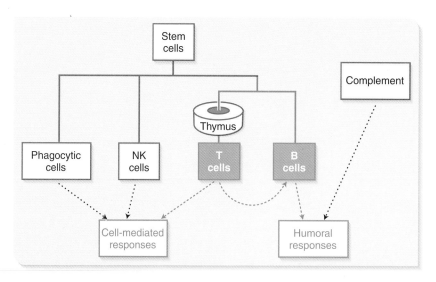

FIGURE 7-2. Deficiencies of the T and B cell lineage affect cell-mediated and humoral responses. Defects in the lineage producing T and B lymphocytes impair the cells' development and, consequently, their functions.

TABLE 7-1. **PRIMARY IMMUNE DEFICIENCY DISEASES OF STEM CELLS**

Disease	Inheritance	Molecular Basis	Consequences
Severe combined immunodeficiency disease (SCID)	Autosomal recessive	Defect in recombination-activating gene-1 (RAG-1) and/or RAG-2 genes (chromosome 11)	Inability to rearrange DNA to form variable regions of immunoglobulin and T cell receptor chains; reduced or absent numbers of T or B lymphocytes and functions; reduced or absent immunoglobulin levels; high susceptibility to infection
	X-linked recessive	Defect in common receptor γ chain (γc) gene (X chromosome)	Defective receptors for interleukin-2 (IL-2), IL-4, IL-7, IL-9, and IL-15; reduced immunoglobulin levels and T cell numbers; normal or elevated B cell numbers; increased susceptibility to infection
	Autosomal recessive	Defect in Jak 3 gene (chromosome 19)	Defective intracellular signaling; reduced immunoglobulin levels and T cell numbers but normal or elevated B cell numbers; increased susceptibility to infection
Adenosine deaminase (ADA) deficiency	Autosomal recessive	Defect in adenosine deaminase gene (chromosome 20)	Impaired purine metabolism; reduced numbers of T and B cells due to accumulation of toxic metabolites; reduced T and B cell functions; reduced immunoglobulin levels; high susceptibility to infection
Purine nucleoside phosphorylase (PNP) deficiency	Autosomal recessive	Defect in PNP gene (chromosome 14)	Impaired purine metabolism; decline in T cell numbers over time (they are more susceptible than B cells to the accumulated toxic metabolites); decrease in immunoglobulin levels due to decreased T cell help; increased susceptibility to infection
Immunodeficiency with ataxia-telangiectasia	Autosomal recessive	Protein kinase gene defect affecting DNA repair (chromosome 11)	Variable signs and symptoms, including problems with balance (ataxia) and areas of widened small capillaries (telangiectasia); immune deficiency signs (may at varying ages and in varying functions); may include reduced T cell number and function and reduced immunoglobulin levels (particularly IgG, IgA and IgE); B cell numbers may be normal, but autoantibodies often develop; frequent chromosomal abnormalities involving immunoglobulin and T cell receptor genes; increased susceptibility to infection; frequent sinus and pulmonary infections
Wiskott-Aldrich syndrome	X-linked recessive	Defect in Wiskott-Aldrich syndrome protein (WASP) (X chromosome)	Appears during infancy or early childhood; reduced T and B cell numbers and functions; reduced immunoglobulin; platelets abnormal and reduced in number; increased susceptibility to infection, especially by *S. aureus*

Patient Vignette 7.2

Stephen M., a 2-month-old infant, presents with persistent diarrhea and signs and symptoms of *Pneumocystis carinii* pneumonia and oral thrush (fungal infection by *Candida albicans*). His weight is well below average. The infant tests negative for HIV-DNA testing using polymerase chain reaction.

Q: What immunologic processes are likely to be involved in his problem?

A: This patient most likely has a form of SCID. Individuals with SCID usually develop symptoms during the first several months of life. They usually present with infections that are due to lack of T cell function, such as fungal infections or other opportunistic infections such as *Pneumocystis carinii* pneumonia.

While some defects are intrinsic to both B and T cells, they may have different effects in the two cell types. An excellent example of this is given by enzymatic defects in purine metabolism (Table 7-1). Defective production of **purine nucleoside phosphorylase** (PNP) results in accumulation of a different set of toxic metabolites that lead to defective function of T cells but have far less impact on B cells. Defective production of **adenosine deaminase** (ADA), on the other hand, results in accumulation of toxic purine metabolites that severely damage both T and B cells.

Defects in T cells

Primary immune deficiencies that are intrinsic to T cells result in abnormalities in T cell numbers and functions. However, because interactions with T cells are critical to the activation of B cells and to their subsequent ability to undergo isotype switching, these defects also cause abnormalities in B cell numbers and immunoglobulin levels (Fig. 7-3). Several diseases are listed in Table 7-2. Some are common to both CD4$^+$ and CD8$^+$ T cells (e.g., CD3 or XAP-70 deficiencies), while others affect only one cell type. Defects in the transporter associated with antigen presentation or the **TAP system** affect the ability to load cytoplasmically derived peptide fragments into MHC class I molecules for cell surface presentation. The reduced MHC I expression results in decreased CD8$^+$ T cell numbers and functions and will affect CTL responses against cytoplasmic pathogens and NK cell function. Defects in expression of MHC class II molecules have broader effects. While they directly affect immune responses mediated by CD4$^+$ T cells (e.g., delayed (-type) hypersensitivity), these defects also affect other functions that rely on interaction with CD4$^+$ T cells—B cell activation, isotype switching, and CD8$^+$ T cell activation.

A second category of T cell defects is illustrated by **DiGeorge syndrome** (Table 7-2). In this disease, there is no intrinsic defect in the T cells lineage. However, defective development of the thymus may result in an organ that is unable to carry out the necessary steps for development of the T cell precursors that migrate there. The defect arises from aberrant embryonic development of structures derived from the third pharyngeal pouch, which include the medullary and cortical regions of the thymus. While the extent of the deficiency varies, significant deficiencies in the number of functional T cells will result in diminished cell-mediated responses and B cell responses dependent upon interaction with T cells. Recently, the majority of individuals with DiGeorge syndrome have been shown to carry small deletions in chromosome 22, although the gene(s) have yet to be identified. Development associated with third pharyngeal pouch defects also lead to malformations of the aorta, the face and jaw, and the parathyroid glands (causing defective calcium metabolism). As a result, this disorder is often de-

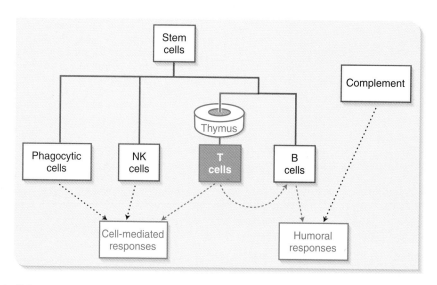

FIGURE 7-3. Deficiencies in the T lymphocyte lineage affect cell-mediated and humoral responses. Defects in T cells affect cell-mediated immune responses involving T cells as well as B-cell functions, due to the regulatory role that T cells play in B cell responses.

TABLE 7-2. **PRIMARY IMMUNE DEFICIENCY DISEASES CAUSED BY T CELL DEFECTS**

Disease	Inheritance	Molecular Basis	Consequences
Purine nucleoside phosphorylase (PNP) deficiency	Autosomal recessive	Defect in PNP gene (chromosome 14)	Impaired purine metabolism; decline in T cell numbers over time (more susceptible than B cells to the toxic metabolites that accumulate from this defect); low immunoglobulin levels due to decreased T cell help; increased susceptibility to infection
MHC class II deficiencies ("Bare lymphocyte syndrome")	Autosomal recessive	Defects in either the CIITA gene (chromosome 16) or the RFX-5 gene (chromosome 1)	Defective intracellular signaling; reduced $CD4^+$ T cell levels; decreased immunoglobulin levels due to defective T cell help; increased susceptibility to infection
CD3 deficiency	Autosomal recessive	Defects in the C3γ or C3ϵ genes (chromosome 11)	Variable effects on T cell function; increased susceptibility to infection
ZAP-70 deficiency	Autosomal recessive	Defect in ZAP-70 kinase gene (chromosome 2)	Defective signaling from TCR; $CD8^+$ from T cells absent; $CD4^+$ T cells present in normal numbers, but nonfunctional; recurrent severe infections
Transporter associated with antigen presentation-2 (TAP-2) deficiency	Autosomal recessive	Defect in TAP-2 gene (chromosome 6)	Reduced MHC I expression and associated antigen presentation; reduced numbers of CD8+ T cell numbers and functions; increased susceptibility to viral infections and to some intracellular bacteria
DiGeorge syndrome	Autosomal dominant or spontaneous	Impaired thymic development due to defects in embryonic development of structures derived from third and fourth brachial arches (when genetic, chromosome 22)	Intrinsically normal T cells; decreased T cell numbers and functions due to abnormal thymus; small deletions in the long arm of chromosome 22 frequently seen; accompanying defects in other systems (e.g., facial features, palate, aorta, and parathyroid glands and calcium metabolism) may be seen; variable severity of immune deficiency; variable immunoglobulin levels; increased susceptibility to infections

tected at birth, prior to the time (six months of age) when most immune deficiency symptoms become evident.

Defects in B cells

Many inherited genetic defects have been identified that are intrinsic to the B lymphocyte lineage or to immunoglobulin molecules themselves (Fig. 7-4). These defects comprise 80% or more of all immunodeficiency diseases. All affect immunoglobulin levels, but not necessarily B cell numbers. Some defects affect production of all immunoglobulin isotypes, while others affect only one or a few isotypes (Table 7-3). T cell functions are typically normal in these individuals.

Bruton's agammaglobulinemia, a recessive X-linked disorder, is often cited as the prototypical example of a B cell immunodeficiency. It stems from a defective Bruton tyrosine kinase (*btk*) gene whose product is crucial to the early development of B cells. As a result, few B cells are present and all immunoglobulin isotypes are diminished. Likewise, defects in several other autosomal genes can lead to aberrant B cell development, leading to a variety of agammaglobulinemias with similar features.

B cell activation is dependent in part on interaction with $CD4^+$ T cells. Some of this interaction occurs via CD40 on T cells binding to CD154 (CD40-ligand) on B cells. Defects in the gene encoding the CD40 ligand render the B cells unable to respond properly to signaling via this route and are unable to undergo isotype switching. As a result, individuals with this defect are able to produce IgM but are deficient in B cells capable of producing IgG, IgA or IgE.

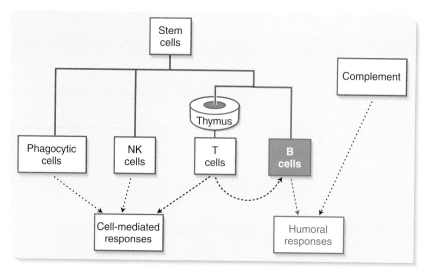

FIGURE 7-4. Deficiencies in the B lymphocyte lineage affect humoral responses. Defects in B cells affect humoral responses through alterations in the numbers and/or functions of B cells, including abnormal production of immunoglobulins. T cell numbers and functions are usually normal.

In addition to genetic defects that disrupt the normal development or activation of B cells, some immunodeficiencies result from defects in the genes that encode the light and heavy immunoglobulin chains (Table 7-3). In the case of those involving heavy chains, the constant genes affected determine the spectrum of isotypes that can be produced.

One disease involving a single isotype, **selective IgA deficiency**, is the single most common immune deficiency disease, with a frequency estimated as 1 to 2 per thousand individuals. Multiple gene defects produce it, and there is reason to believe that some forms of the disease may involve defective isotype switch signaling from T cells. Those with selective IgA deficiency often have other immunologic disorders such as allergy or autoimmunity.

Defects in phagocytes and natural killer cells

Immune deficiency diseases may also arise from defects in the so-called "accessory" cells such as phagocytes, neutrophils, NK cells, and others (Fig. 7-5, Table 7-4). Defects in phagocytic cells are pertinent because of their effects on both the innate and adaptive immune responses. These defects fall into two general categories. The first is an inability to kill microbes. In **chronic granulomatous disease** (CGD), defects in several different genes result in defective enzymes and other microcidal molecules (e.g., toxic oxygen metabolites) that prevent effective destruction of ingested microbes. In contrast, individuals with **Chediak-Higashi syndrome** are normal with respect to these destructive agents but are unable to deliver them to the microbes. Instead, a defect in the organelle membranes prevents the normal fusion of the lysosomes (carrying the enzymes and microcides) with phagosomes (containing the ingested microbes). Consequently, the cells fail to destroy their ingested microbial load. The organelle defect affects other functions as well, such as the formation of melanin granules necessary for normal pigmentation of the eyes and skin. Finally, some individuals cannot express receptors necessary for responding to critical signals that activate their phagocytic cells. Activation of phagocytic cells is critical to the ability of these cells to act against infectious microbes (Chapter 4) both via binding of pattern recognition receptors (innate) and IFN-γ produced by CD4$^+$ T cells (adaptive). Deficiencies in the receptor for IFN-γ render individuals susceptible to bacterial infections by inhibiting the ability to mount a delayed-type hypersensitivity response, a response crucial to combating infectious organisms such as *Mycobacterium*.

Other diseases arise from an inability of several types of leukocytes to interact with vascular endothelium and migrate from the vasculature

TABLE 7-3. **PRIMARY IMMUNE DEFICIENCY DISEASES CAUSED BY B CELL AND IMMUNOGLOBULIN DEFECTS**

Disease	Inheritance	Molecular Basis	Consequences
Bruton's agamma-globulinemia	X-linked recessive	Defect in Bruton's tyrosine kinase (*btk*) gene (X chromosome)	Drastic decrease in immunoglobulin levels and in numbers of B cells; increased susceptibility to infection; increased susceptibility to encapsulated bacteria (e.g., *H. influenzae*, *staphylococci*, and *streptococci*)
Ig heavy chain gene deletions	Autosomal recessive	Deletions in heavy chain constant genes (chromosome 14)	Various immunoglobulin isotypes absent (dependent upon the affected heavy chain gene); IgG most frequently affected; reduced B cell numbers frequent; increased susceptibility to infection; patients with IgG1 deficiency have increased susceptibility to pyogenic infections
Immunodeficiency with hyper-IgM	X-linked recessive Autosomal recessive	Defect in the CD154 (CD40 ligand) gene (X chromosome)	B cells unable to undergo isotype switches or somatic hypermutation; elevated IgM and reduced or absent IgG, IgA and IgE; 70% of cases due to X-linked defect; increased susceptibility to pyogenic infection
Kappa (κ) greek kappa chain deficiency	Autosomal recessive	Mutations in genes encoding the κ chain (chromosome 2)	Reduced or absent immunoglobulin containing κ chains
Common variable immuno-deficiency (CVI or CVID)	Multiple forms	Unknown	Variable symptoms; varying isotypes (or combinations of isotypes) reduced or absent; increased susceptibility to pyogenic infection
Selective IgA deficiency	Multiple forms	Multiple defects	Reduced or absent IgA-expressing B cells; reduced serum IgA, often accompanied by IgG subclass deficiency and allergic or autoimmune disorders; has a frequency of 1–2 per thousand individuals, making it one of the most common immune deficiency diseases; recurrent pyogenic bacterial infections in individuals with IgG2 deficiency
Autosomal recessive agamma-globulinemia	Autosomal recessive	Mutations in various genes involved in early differentiation	Failure in early differentiation of B cells; increased susceptibility to infection

into the tissues. This ability is necessary for the movement of lymphocytes, neutrophils, and phagocytes to the sites of infection where they can make contact with the microbe and/or the infected cells and tissues. They are thus unable to efficiently migrate to the organs in which lymphocyte activation occurs and to sites of infections where they are needed for clearance. These types of deficiencies are illustrated by the *leukocyte adhesion defect 1* (LAD-1) and LAD-2 deficiencies, in which molecules used for recognition and binding of leukocytes to endothelium are defective or lacking.

Defects in the complement system

Deficiencies in the complement system can impact humoral immune responses, both innate and adaptive (Fig. 7-6). The complement system consists of a series of soluble molecules capable of: (1) directly killing microbes; (2) increasing the killing of microbes by phagocytic cells; and (3) attracting and activating cells involved in inflammation (Chapters 3 and 4; Figs. 3-4, 3-5, 3-7, and 4-7). Defects in the complement system increase susceptibility to infection and sometimes also increase the risk of certain autoimmune disorders).

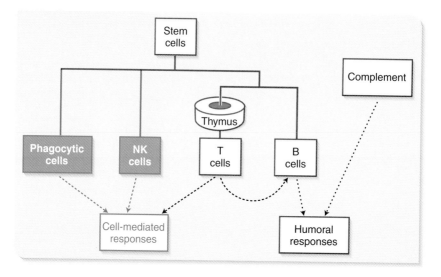

FIGURE 7-5. Deficiencies in phagocytic cells and natural killer cells affect cell-mediated responses. Defects in phagocytic cells impact both the innate and adaptive immune response by altering their ability to ingest infectious organisms, degrade them, and engage in antigen presentation to T cells. Defective NK cells are unable to assist in initial clearance of infections and development of adaptive Th1 immune responses.

TABLE 7-4. PRIMARY IMMUNE DEFICIENCY DISEASES OF LEUKOCYTES OTHER THAN T AND B CELLS

Disease	Inheritance	Molecular Basis	Consequences
Chronic granulomatous disease (CGD)	X-linked recessive	Defect in 91 kDa chain of cytochrome b (X chromosome)	Inability to produce superoxide metabolites for killing of ingested microbes, macrophages, and neutrophils affected; increased susceptibility to infection, especially *Staphylococcus aureus*, *Salmonella enterica* serovar, *Typhimurium*, *Serratia marcescens*
	Autosomal recessive	Multiple defects in 22 kDa chain of cytochrome b or of P47 or of p67 cytosolic factors (chromosomes 1, 7, 16, 21, and others)	Inability to produce superoxide metabolites for killing of ingested microbes; macrophages and neutrophils affected; increased susceptibility to infection
Chediak-Higashi syndromei	Autosomal recessive	Defective fusion of lysosomes and phagosomes due to defect in organelle membranes (chromosome 1)	Inability to kill ingested microbes; albinism of eyes and skin and other defects of organelle membranes; giant granules in neutrophils and other cells; decreased NK and T cell functions; increased susceptibility to infection by pyogenic bacteria
Leukocyte adhesion defect 1 (LAD-1)	Autosomal recessive	Defect in CD18, a component of several adhesion molecules (chromosome 21)	Defective chemotaxis and adherence to endothelial surfaces by macrophages, neutrophils and NK cells; increased susceptibility to recurrent infection by bacteria and nonresolving abscesses
Leukocyte adhesion defect 2 (LAD-2)	Autosomal recessive	Defect in gene (chromosome 11) encoding GDP-fucose transporter1, an enzyme responsible for synthesis of $CD15_\mu$, a carbohydrate adhesion molecule	Defects in ability of leukocytes to adhere to endothelial surfaces; reduced ability of leukocytes to move from vasculature into tissues; increased susceptibility to recurrent infection by bacteria and non-resolving abscesses; also causes Bombay blood group phenotype
IFN-γ receptor deficiency	Autosomal recessive	Defect in receptor for IFN-γ (chromosome 6)	High susceptibility to mycobacterial infections; macrophages, neutrophils and NK cells affected; defective Th1 cells

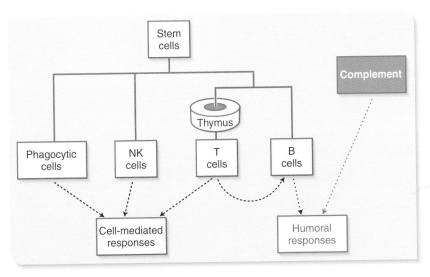

FIGURE 7-6. Deficiencies in the complement system affect humoral responses. Defective components in the complement system can impair complement-mediated responses, even in the presence of appropriate antibodies. Defects in some of the regulatory molecules of the immune system can lead to uncontrolled episodes of inflammation.

TABLE 7-5. PRIMARY IMMUNE DEFICIENCY DISEASES OF COMPLEMENT

Disease	Inheritance	Molecular Basis	Consequences
C1q, C1r deficiency	Autosomal recessive	Defects in C1q (chromosome 1) or C1r gene (chromosome 12)	Increased incidence of infections; systemic lupus erythematosus (SLE)-like syndromes (type III hypersensitivities; Chapter 8); impaired removal of immune complexes
C2 deficiency	Autosomal recessive	Defects in C2 gene (chromosome 6)	SLE-like syndromes; vasculitis; impaired removal of immune complexes
C3 deficiency	Autosomal recessive	Defects in C3 gene (chromosome 19)	Impaired opsonization; recurrent pyogenic infections
C4 deficiency	Autosomal recessive	Defects in C4 gene (chromosome 6)	Increased incidence of infections; SLE-like syndromes; impaired removal of immune complexes
C5, C6, C7 deficiency	Autosomal recessive	Defects in C5, C6 or C7 gene (chromsomes 9, 5, and 5, respectively)	Inability to form membrane attack complex; SLE-like syndromes; increased susceptibility to *Neisseria*
C8 deficiency	Autosomal recessive	Defects in C8α or C8β gene (chromosome 1)	Inability to form membrane attack complex; SLE-like syndromes; increased susceptibility to *Neisseria*
C9 deficiency	Autosomal recessive	Defects in C9 gene (chromosome 5)	Inability to form membrane attack complex; increased susceptibility to *Neisseria*
Factor H deficiency	Autosomal recessive	Defect in Factor H gene (chromosome 1)	Recurrent pyogenic infections; increased activation of alternative pathway
Factor P (Properdin) deficiency	X-linked recessive	Defect in properdin gene (X chromosome)	Reduced stability of C3bBb convertase on microbial surfaces; impaired alternative pathway; increased susceptibility to infection, particularly by *Neisseria*
Hereditary angioedema	Autosomal dominant	Defect in C1 inhibitor gene (chromosome 4)	Excessive spontaneous activation of classical complement pathway (especially C2) causing local inflammation; swelling of tracheal and bronchial passages that can be life-threatening
Paroxysmal nocturnal hemoglobinuria	X-linked recessive	Defect in gene (X chromosome) encoding enzyme responsible for synthesis of phosphinositol glycolipid (PIG)	Absence of PIG prevents fixation of DAF and CD59 to the host cell membrane; resulting inability to break down complement complexes on the host cell leads to excessive lysis of erythrocytes

Defects in genes encoding most of the complement components and regulatory molecules have been identified (Table 7-5). In general, defects in the components of the mannan-binding lectin (MBL) and alternative pathways lead to increased susceptibility to infection, particularly by pyogenic bacteria such as *Staphylococcus aureus* and *Streptococcus pneumoniae*. The importance of these activities is evident from the observation that defects in the classical pathway are not associated with significantly increased susceptibility to infection, except for those involving encapsulated bacteria, where the triad of antibody, complement, and neutrophils is required to bind, opsonize, phagocytose, and kill these bacteria. However, in individuals with deficiencies of C1, C2, and C4, clearance of immune complexes is inefficient, leading to renal damage, joint problems, and rashes that are characteristic of immune complex diseases (type III hypersensitivity), such as **systemic lupus erythematosus** (SLE) (Chapter 8).

Severity of disease susceptibility varies widely for individuals with complement deficiencies. A small number of individuals with complement deficiencies do not appear to experience any disease. In the absence of the classical pathway, the lectin-binding and alternative pathways are capable of generating sufficient complement-mediated protection against infection. Deficiencies in the components of the alternative pathway are associated with increased susceptibility to infection, but not with other immunologic abnormalities. Deficiencies of C3 result in severe problems with recurrent infection and with immune complex-mediated disease because of the central position of C3 in all three of the complement activation pathways.

Some complement-related diseases stem from deficiencies in factors that regulate complement activation. When absent, unregulated episodes of inflammation resulting from complement activation can create severe problems. Individuals with **paroxysmal nocturnal hemoglobinuria** experience periodic episodes of erythrocyte destruction because they lack *CD59* and **decay accelerating factor** (DAF) that prevent the accumulation of complement complexes, including C3b and the membrane attack complex, on the surface of host cells. Similarly, individuals deficient in the C1 inhibitor are unable to control the activation of the classical pathway, resulting in **hereditary angioedema** (or **hereditary angioneurotic edema**).

CLINICAL APPLICATION
HEREDITARY ANGIOEDEMA

Hereditary angioedema is a life-threatening condition caused by C1 esterase inhibitor deficiency (C1-INH). People with this condition exhibit nausea, cramping, and throat tightness due to the swelling of the submucosal and subcutaneous tissue of the gastrointestinal tract and larynx. The disease is caused by low levels of C1-INH. A deficiency of C1-INH permits autoactivation of the complement system and release of substances, causing angioedema. People can also exhibit C1-INH deficiency from acquired causes. Those with the acquired form may also have cancers or autoimmune disease.

SECONDARY (ACQUIRED) IMMUNE DEFICIENCIES

Not all immunodeficiency diseases arise from intrinsic defects. Secondary immune deficiencies result from environmental factors and may arise at any time of life (Table 7-6).

Therapeutic causes

Clinical situations often occur in which an individual's immune system is suppressed, either intentionally or as a consequence of treatment (iatrogenic). Both therapeutic and iatrogenic immunosuppression are discussed in Chapter 11. The immune systems of patients receiving transplanted organs from genetically nonidentical donors usually attack and destroy the transplanted tissue (Chapter 10). As a result, the organ recipient must undergo treatment to inhibit their immune responsiveness for at least a period of time. During this time, transplant recipients are very susceptible to *opportunistic infection* (occurring primarily in individuals with compromised immune systems) and must be constantly monitored and treated to prevent the rapid onset of overwhelming infection.

Similarly, those with autoimmune diseases (Chapter 9) must often be treated with agents that diminish immune responsiveness, again rendering them susceptible to infection. Finally, thera-

TABLE 7-6. CAUSES OF SECONDARY IMMUNE DEFICIENCY

Cause	Examples	Mechanisms
Therapeutic treatment	Ionizing radiation	Damages replicating cells; induces oxidative stress
	Cytotoxic drugs (including many used for cancer treatment)	Damage or kill replicating cells
	Antiinflammatory drugs (e.g., corticosteroids) Immunosuppressive drugs (e.g., cyclosporine A, tacrolimus, rapamycin)	Interfere with production of some cytokines
Infection	Human immunodeficiency virus (HIV)	Multiple effects; kills CD4$^+$ T cells, CD8$^+$ T cells and monocytes; in addition, the viral *nef* gene product redirects MHC I from surface and into lysosomes
	Epstein–Barr virus	Produces analog of interleukin-10
	Schistosoma	Secretes enzymes capable of cleaving immunoglobulins
	Herpesvirus	Interferes with MHC I maturation in ER
	Human cytomegalovirus (HCMV)	Interferes with transport of peptides into ER through TAP; redirects MHC I molecules into cytoplasm rather than to cell surface
	Adenovirus	Interferes with movement of MHC I out of ER
	Chlamydia	Interferes with phagocytic function by preventing fusion of phagosomes and lysosomes
	Staphylococcus	Produces toxin that kills phagocytic cells; produces protein that interferes with FcR-driven opsonization
	Yersinia	Produces toxin that kills phagocytes
	Streptococcus	Produces toxin that kills phagocytes
	Mycobacterium	Produces toxin that kills phagocytes; inhibits acidification within phagosomes by preventing fusion with lysosomes; inhibits oxidative degradation within phagosomes
	Salmonella	Inhibits oxidative degradation within phagosomes
	Leischmania	Inhibits oxidative degradation within phagosomes
Cancer	Multiple myeloma	Immune response becomes increasingly oligoclonal
	Burkitts's lymphoma	Causative agent (EBV) produces analog of interleukin-10
	Waldenstrom's macroglobulinemia	Excessive production of immunoglobulins
	Chronic lymphocytic leukemia (CLL), Small lymphocytic lymphoma (SLL)	Reduced production of immunoglobulins Reduced production of immunoglobulins
	Other forms of leukemia/lymphoma	Various
Physiological	General malnutrition	Has greatest impact on functions requiring highest energy metabolism
	Protein-energy malnutrition	Deficiency of amino acids crucial for energy metabolism
	Deficiencies of trace metals	Deficiencies in zinc, iron, selenium that are co-factors, etc.
	Vitamin deficiencies	Deficiencies in vitamins (e.g., A, B6, C, E) that are co-factors, etc.

peutic treatment directed against other medical problems may affect the immune system. For example, many of the physical (e.g., irradiation) and chemical (e.g., drugs) agents used in cancer therapy can profoundly damage the immune system. Again, these patients must be monitored to protect them against potential infection, and deliberate efforts must often be made to restore immune function following treatment.

Infectious causes

As discussed in greater detail in Chapter 6, many infectious organisms actively circumvent the immune responses generated against them. Several bacteria can impede processes within host cells that are aimed at their destruction. These include inhibiting fusion of phagosomes with enzyme-loaded lysosomes, altering intra-organelle pH, and inhibiting generation of microcidal molecules. Other pathogens can cleave immunoglobulins and complement components. Others secrete factors that inhibit the movement or function of phagocytes or lymphocytes in their vicinity. Many viruses are able to subvert the MHC class I peptide presentation by affecting different steps in the process. As a result, microbial and viral antigens are not effectively presented on the surface of the infected cell and evade detection by CD8$^+$ T cells. Finally, some infectious organisms can induce the immune system into the Th1 or Th2 pathway that is least effective for clearance of the microbe in question.

HIV, the virus that causes AIDS, illustrates the severe consequences that can result from the destruction of CD4$^+$ T cells, the so-called "conductors of the immune response." The progressive loss of CD4$^+$ T cells leads to gradual diminishment of humoral and cellular responses that should keep the virus in check. The eventual destruction and depletion of CD4$^+$ T cells leads to increasing susceptibility to opportunistic infections that are often fatal.

HIV utilizes the CD4 molecule expressed on subsets of T cells and macrophages as its major ligand for binding and entry into the cells. HIV also uses two chemokine receptor molecules as coreceptors: CCR5 on macrophages and dendritic cells and CXCR4 on lymphocytes. In the absence of these coreceptors, HIV is unable to successfully enter the cells. About 1% of Caucasians are homozygous for a "null" form of the gene encoding CCR5 and appear to be resistant to infection by HIV. Initial infections by HIV (e.g., through sexual contact) appear to preferentially involve macrophages and dendritic cells. These infected phagocytes remain largely sequestered in secondary lymphoid organs such as the spleen and lymph nodes with minimal destruction, and serve as a reservoir for subsequent spread of the virus to other sites in the body. Later, a "lymphotropic" form of the virus emerges and the infection spreads to CD4$^+$ T cells. HIV replicates most rapidly in activated T cells, and the increased infection of CD4$^+$ T cells is associated with a decline in the number of CD4$^+$ T cells, progressing to AIDS and an increasing susceptibility to infection.

Patient Vignette 7.3

George L, a 35-year-old man with a history of intravenous drug use, presents with signs and symptoms of *Pneumocystis* pneumonia.

Q: What immunologic processes are likely to be involved?

A: This patient likely has AIDS. The most common risk factors for HIV infection and AIDS include intravenous drug use and unprotected sexual activity (homosexual, bisexual, and heterosexual). The most common opportunistic infections in persons infected by HIV include *Pneumocystis carinii* pneumonia, *Mycobacterium avium* complex, Candida esophagitis, cytomegalovirus infection, toxoplasmosis, cryptococcal meningitis, and *M. tuberculosis*.

Cancer

Cancers of the hematopoietic tissues can have negative effects on immune function. Malignant lymphocytes can overtake the immune system, reducing the immune repertoire as the lymphocyte compartment is dominated by fewer and fewer clones. In addition, malignant cells can exhibit aberrant production of cytokines and aberrant expression of surface molecules. As a result, their interactions with other components of the immune system may become abnormal. Secreted immunoglobulins derived from malignant cells may flood the body fluids with partial or abnormal immunoglobulin molecules, or produce immunoglobulins in such excess that it can (as in Waldenstrom's macroglobulinemia) measurably increase the viscosity of the blood.

Physiological causes

Factors that affect the overall health of the body can also affect the immune system, such as fatigue and poor diet. One of the most general is nutrition. Malnourishment can significantly diminish the ability of the immune system to cope with infection. Shortages of specific dietary components can also have an effect. Insufficient amino acids such as glutamine can affect energy metabolism, and shortages of certain minerals (e.g., zinc, iron, and selenium) and vitamins (A, B6, C, and E) have been associated with reduced immune function.

THERAPEUTIC APPROACHES

A number of methods can be used to try to restore immune functions in immunodeficient individuals. Some of these provide only temporary benefits and must be repeated on a regular basis. Others have the possibility of providing a permanent benefit.

Passive supplementation

In some types of immune deficiencies, the defective or missing component can be supplied by passive administration. Injection of exogenous antibodies [**intravenous immunoglobulin (IVIG)**] is a straightforward method to augment insufficient immunoglobulin levels. Injections must be repeated at regular intervals, as the injected immunoglobulins have finite half-lives.

Foreign sources of immunoglobulin have been replaced by use of human immunoglobulin that has largely eliminated the danger of serum sickness. Other soluble products, such as cytokines or enzymes [e.g, adenosine deaminase (ADA)], can also be administered passively.

Bone marrow transplantation

Passive administration therapy can be effective but must be constantly repeated. A longer-term, potentially permanent solution is to replace the defective cells or tissues of the immune-deficient individual. With the exception of immune deficiencies due to defects of the thymus (e.g., DiGeorge syndrome), cell and tissue replacement can be approached by replacement of the patient's bone marrow with bone marrow from a normal donor. Because the bone marrow contains the stem cells that ultimately give rise to all the components of the immune system—lymphocytes, phagocytes, neutrophils, eosinophils, mast cells, and basophils—a normal and functioning immune system can be established in the recipient.

Transplantation of bone marrow poses special problems. Because it involves the placement of immunocompetent tissues into immunoincompetent recipients, the possibility exists that mature, immunocompetent T cells present in the transplanted marrow can recognize the recipient as nonself and attack the host tissues [**graft-versus-host disease (GVHD)**] unless certain precautions are taken (Chapter 10). This therapeutic method has been successfully used for several years, and its efficiency has increased as the techniques for bone marrow transplantation have been refined.

Genetic engineering

In recent years, the emerging technologies of genetic engineering have been applied to immune deficiencies. An individual's defective cells can be isolated, the normal gene inserted into them, and the new "repaired" cells put back into the patient. As with bone marrow transplantation, a number of technical problems must be solved before the approach can be applied more extensively. Unless the repaired cells are stem cells, the procedure must be periodically repeated as the injected cells die and require replacement. Even if stem cells are successfully engineered, additional problems may arise. Are the injected cells homing to sites where they can grow and develop properly? Is there a risk of malignancy developing within the engineered cell population? Will the expression of the repaired genes be properly regulated? Will the engineered cells respond appropriately to signals inducing expression and secretion of the required protein? These problems have not, at this point, been universally solved.

At least some partially successful attempts at genetic engineering of immune deficiencies have been carried out at the National Institutes of Health. A child with ADA deficiency underwent genetic therapy in 1990. A portion of her T cells appear to function normally, but the engineered cells were not stem cells, so replacement of the engineered cells must be periodically repeated and exogenous ADA is also required. Subsequent attempts to engineer hematopoietic stem cells have provided some degree of permanent relief for several other individuals with ADA deficiency. However, only a minor fraction of the T cells produced from the engineered bone marrow function normally, and the patients continue to require passive ADA administration. More recently, therapy of a patient with X-linked SCID has been reported in which a different method was used for insertion of the normal γc gene into the defective stem cells, but the long term results are not yet known.

Summary

- *Primary immune deficiencies* occur as a result of intrinsic defects, usually genetic in nature. *Secondary immune deficiencies* are characterized by reduced immune function attributable to environmental causes such as infection, therapeutic treatments, cancer, and malnutrition.
- Primary immune deficiencies can be subdivided according to the tissue, cell, or molecule in which the defect is expressed.
- Defects in autosomal genes affect both sexes equally. Disorders caused by defective genes on the X chromosome are typically transmitted as X-linked recessive traits and are expressed far more often in males than in females.
- Defects in the lymphoid stem cells giving rise to the both T and B cells cause malfunctions in both types of lymphocytes. The defects may be reflected in altered T and B cell numbers, T and B cell functions, or both.
- The classic example of lymphoid stem cell diseases is *severe combined immunodeficiency disease* (SCID), which occurs in several forms.
- Primary immune deficiencies that are intrinsic to T cells affect T cell numbers and functions, and may also affect B cell numbers and immunoglobulins because of diminished T cell help for B cell activation. A second category of T cell defects is illustrated by *DiGeorge syndrome,* in which the thymus does not develop normally.
- Many inherited genetic defects are intrinsic to the B lymphocyte lineage or to immunoglobulin molecules. *Bruton's agammaglobulinemia* is a recessive X-linked disorder. Defects in the gene encoding the CD40 ligand (CD154) renders the B cells unable to respond properly to defective communication between B and T cells. *Selective IgA deficiency* is the single most common immune deficiency disease, with a frequency estimated as 1/500 to 1/1000.
- In *chronic granulomatous disease*, defects in several different genes result in defective enzymes and other microcidal molecules (e.g., toxic oxygen metabolites), which affect the ability of phagocytic cells and natural killer cells to destroy ingested microbes.
- In the *complement* system, defects in the components of the lectin-binding and alternative pathways lead to increased susceptibility to infection, particularly by pyogenic bacteria. Defects in the classical pathway can usually be compensated for by the other two pathways.
- *HIV* destroys CD4$^+$ T cells and subsequently diminishes most T and B cell functions.
- Cancers of the hematopoietic tissues can have negative effects on immune function.
- Factors that affect the overall health of the body, such as fatigue and poor diet, can also affect the immune system.
- In some types of immune deficiencies, it is possible to supply the defective or missing component by passive administration. A longer-term, potentially permanent solution is to replace the defective cells or tissues of the immune-deficient individual by replacement of the patient's bone marrow with bone marrow from a normal donor.

Suggested readings

Buckley RH. Advances in immunology: Primary immunodeficiency diseases due to defects in lymphocytes. *N Engl J Med* 2000;343:1313.

Buckley RH. Primary immunodeficiency diseases: Dissectors of the immune system. *Immunol Rev* 2002;185:206.

Buckley RH. Molecular defects in human severe combined immunodeficiency and approaches to immune reconstitution. *Annu Rev Immunol* 2004;22:625.

Janeway CA Jr., Travers P, Walport M, Shlomchik P. Failures of host defenses. In *Immunobiology: The immune system in health and disease*, 6th ed. Philadephia: Garland Publishing, 2004.

Letvin NL, Barouch DH, Montefiori DC. Prospects for vaccine protection against HIV-1 infection and AIDS. *Annu Rev Immunol* 2002;20:73.

Moore MAS. The role of cell migration in the ontogeny of the lymphoid system. *Stem Cells Dev* 2004;13:1.

Rambaut A, Posad D, Crandall KA, Holmes EC. The causes and consequences of HIV evolution. *Nature Rev Gen* 2004;5: 52.

Wagner DK. Human immunodeficiency virus and the acquired immune deficiency syndrome. In *Kochar's concise textbook of medicine*, 4th ed. Philadelphia: Lippincott Williams & Wilkins, 2003.

Review questions

DIRECTIONS: Each of the numbered items or incomplete statements in this section is followed by answers or by completions of the statement. Select the ONE lettered answer or completion that is BEST in each case.

1. A major form of severe combined immune deficiency (SCID) is caused by an X-linked defect in the gene encoding:
   (A) btk (Bruton's tyrosine kinase).
   (B) γc, a common subunit of the receptors for IL-2, IL-4, IL-7, IL-9, and IL-15.
   (C) HLA-DR2.
   (D) CD3.
   (E) CD40L (CD154).

2. A patient with DiGeorge syndrome (absence of the thymus) displays which of the following changes in immune function?
   (A) Increased incidence of autoimmunity
   (B) Frequent uncontrolled complement activation
   (C) Recurrent viral infections
   (D) Increasingly severe contact sensitivity
   (E) Elevated levels of IgG

3. A patient with Bruton's agammaglobulinemia lacks the ability to do which of the following immune functions?
   (A) Mount delayed (-type) hypersensitivity (DTH) responses
   (B) Initiate complement activation leading to formation of the membrane attack complex
   (C) Clear infections of intracellular bacteria (e.g., *Mycobacteria*)
   (D) Clear infection of extracellular bacteria (e.g., *Streptococci*)
   (E) Clear fungal infections

4. Patients with genetically inherited deficiencies of complement component C3 display which of the following characteristics?
   (A) Autoimmune disease
   (B) Recurrent infections
   (C) Frequent incidents of uncontrolled systemic inflammation
   (D) Asthma
   (E) Anemia

5. An individual lacking complement component C1 is unable to:
   (A) assemble the membrane attack complex.
   (B) cleave and accumulate C3b.
   (C) generate a C5 convertase.
   (D) utilize bound immunoglobulin for activation of complement.
   (E) utilize the alternative pathway for complement activation.

6. Deficiencies in lymphoid stem cells generally result in:
   (A) selective absence of immunoglobulin isotypes.
   (B) deficiencies in both T and B cell functions.
   (C) diminished B cell function but normal T cell function.
   (D) heightened NK cell activity.
   (E) elevated IgM, and decreased IgG, IgA, and IgE levels.

7. For severe immunodeficiencies in which T and/or B cell development is defective, the most common strategy for permanent or long-term therapy is:
   (A) regular administration of an antibiotic "cocktail."

(B) regular administration of exogenous immunoglobulins.

(C) isolation.

(D) administration of thymic hormones.

(E) bone marrow transplantation.

8. A baby boy is born with hypocalcemia and cardiac abnormalities. Which of the following immunodeficiencies should be suspected in this patient?

(A) Wiskott-Aldrich syndrome

(B) DiGeorge syndrome

(C) Severe combine immunodeficiency disease (SCID)

(D) Adenosine deaminase (ADA) deficiency

(E) Chronic granulomatous disease

9. A 21- year-old woman has a history since childhood of episodes of angioedema of the respiratory and gastrointestinal tracts. Her C1 inhibitor level is nearly zero. Which of the following conditions is most likely?

(A) Wiskott-Aldrich syndrome

(B) C3 deficiency

(C) Severe combined immune deficiency (SCID)

(D) Nutritionally based immune deficiency

(E) Hereditary angioedema

10. A 3-month-old boy with chronic granulomatous disease (CGD) has recurrent infections. What component of the immune response is defective in this condition?

(A) Secretory IgA

(B) CD3

(C) IL-2 production

(D) Lysosomal enzymes and microcidal molecules

(E) IFN-γ receptor

Hypersensitivity Reactions

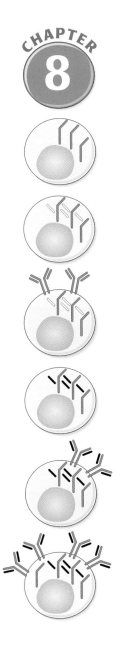

Chapter Outline

Introduction **Hypersensitivity** is the term applied to pathologies involving immune-mediated damage to host tissues (Fig. 8-1). There are four major categories of hypersensitivity reactions: Types I, II, III, and IV. In most cases, they involve an inflammatory process, although the mechanisms may vary from one type to another (Table 8-1). Most hypersensitivity reactions result in tissue injury mediated by the release of various chemical substances that attract and activate other cells and molecules responsible for inflammation (Chapters 3 and 5).

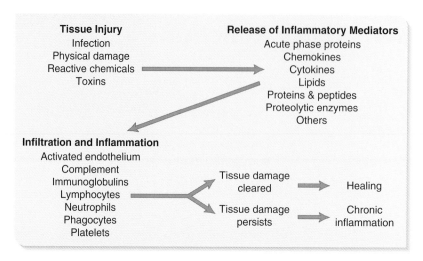

FIGURE 8-1. Generation of inflammatory responses. Tissue injury causes release of molecules that promote infiltration of the damaged tissue and initiation of inflammation. Upon destruction of the agent initiating injury, inflammation ceases and healing ensues. If the injury continues, inflammation becomes chronic and tissue damage accumulates.

Inflammation is a highly effective method for clearance of microbes or other intruding substances. However, in some cases, inflammation can become so intense or chronic that it inflicts permanent damage to body tissues. Hypersensitivity reactions also differ in the rate at which they can occur. Type I hypersensitivity reactions are the most rapid, sometimes occurring within minutes after exposure to an antigen, while Type IV hypersensitivity reactions generally require 2 to 4 days. Types II and III have even greater intervals. None of these occur during primary exposure; all are secondary (or subsequent) responses.

- **Type I hypersensitivity reactions** result from crosslinking of IgE molecules bound to the surfaces of mast cells, basophils, and eosinophils that causes the release of cytoplasmic granules from these cells. The cytoplasmic granules contain vasoactive amines and other substances that cause inflammation.
- **Type II hypersensitivity reactions** are those generated by the actions of antibodies (usually IgG, but sometimes also IgM) recognizing and binding antigens associated with host cell membranes or extracellular matrix. The antibodies may be directed against self (autoanti-

TABLE 8-1. HYPERSENSITIVITY RESPONSES

Type	Targets	Triggering response	Inflammatory mechanisms	Time course
Type I (Immediate)	Allergens	Ig-E mediated mast cell degranulation	Histamine and other inflammatory mediators (see Table 8-3)	Minutes to hours
Type II	Membrane autoantigens or neoantigens; intra-cellular matrix	IgG binding to membranes	Complement activation (classical pathway)	Hours to days
Type III (Immune complex disease)	Soluble antigens	Immune complex deposition in tissues	Complement activation (classical pathway)	Hours to days
Type IV (Delayed)	Infectious agents, reactive chemicals, neoantigens	CD4+ T cells and macrophages; less frequently, CD8+ T cells	Delayed type hypersensitivity; less frequently, cytotoxic T lymphocytes	Two to four days

bodies) or against neoantigens created by the binding of reactive substances to cell or matrix molecules. The damage occurs primarily through the activation of **complement** (via the classical pathway) or by **antibody-dependent cell-mediated cytotoxicity** (ADCC) mediated by NK cells or eosinophils. In some cases, the targeted surface molecules may be receptors whose function is interfered with by antibodies binding to them.

- **Type III hypersensitivity reactions** are those generated by the accumulation and sedimentation of large conglomerations of soluble antigen and antibodies called **immune complexes** (Chapter 4). The antibodies may sometimes be autoreactive antibodies, but the target self antigen is a soluble one. Either IgG or IgM may be involved and activate complement via the classical pathway.

- **Type IV hypersensitivity reactions** are those generated by cell-mediated immune processes. For the most part, these reactions are **delayed (-type) hypersensitivity** (DTH) **responses**, but under some circumstances, may also include damage inflicted by cytotoxic T cells.

TYPE I HYPERSENSITIVITY REACTIONS

Type I hypersensitivity reactions are also called **immediate hypersensitivity reactions** because they can literally occur within minutes to hours following exposure to an antigen. They are also termed **anaphylactic reactions** or, more commonly, **allergic reactions**. It is clear from the speed with which they can occur that they are secondary responses based on prior production of significant levels of IgE directed at specific antigens or *allergens* (Table 8-2). It is thought that type I hypersensitivity reactions evolved as a defense against parasitic infections. Unfortunately, many reactions also are directed at harmless molecules. Immediate hypersensitivity reactions are said to be *atopic*, meaning that responses against a given allergen occur only in a minority of individuals. For example, allergic responses to ragweed pollen (hay fever) or grass pollens occur in only about 15 to 20% of the U.S. population, despite widespread exposure to the allergen. Immediate hypersensitivity reactions are often directed at innocuous molecules. The likelihood that an individual might generate a strong IgE response to a particular antigen is determined by a combination of genetic and environmental factors. Allergies are often said to "run in families," although no individual genes have been identified as being primarily responsible. Genetic predispositions to allergies may also often be obscured by environmental factors. For example, hay fever is rare in Japan but far more common among those of Japanese descent living in the United States, because ragweed is more common in the U.S.

IgE is found at low levels in plasma because it is rapidly adsorbed onto the surfaces of mast cells and some basophils. These cells bear specialized receptors (FcRεs) that recognize and bind the Fc region of IgE that has not yet bound to antigen. In essence, mast cells and basophils adopt IgE for their own use as surface antigen receptors. Mast cells are found primarily in tissues that are at the body's frontiers with respect to contact with the environment, and basophils are found in the circulation. Mast cells accumulate in the respiratory passages, intestinal walls, and skin. In order to trigger a response, epitope-specific, surface-bound multiple IgE molecules must be crosslinked by binding to an antigen containing

TABLE 8-2. EXAMPLES OF TYPE I HYPERSENSITIVITY RESPONSES

Antigen (Allergen)	Entry	Location	Symptoms
Bee venom	Injected	Bloodstream (systemic)	Fluid loss from vasculature; potential vascular collapse
Pollen	Inhaled	Respiratory	Rhinitis, asthma
Food (various)	Ingested	Gastrointestinal	Gastrointestinal distress due to smooth muscle contraction
Animal dander/saliva	Contact Inhaled	Skin	Rashes; edema Rhinitis, asthma
House mites/dust mites	Inhaled	Respiratory	Rhinitis; asthma

multiple epitopes. The epitopes specifically recognized may be identical or different. Crosslinking of IgE generates an intracellular signal that prompts the mast cell or basophil to *degranulate* (Chapter 5, Fig. 5-17).

The cytoplasmic granules of mast cells and basophils contain a wide variety of mediators of inflammation, including *histamine* (Table 8-3). Histamine is one of the earliest-acting mediators in IgE-induced inflammation. Histamine and other mast cell products induce *vasodilation*, an increase in vascular permeability due to loosening of the junctions between the vascular endothelial cells of capillaries, which permits an increased flow of fluid out of the vasculature and into the tissues (Fig. 8-2). This added fluid produces a swelling of the tissues called *edema*. Histamine also causes constriction of the smooth muscle in walls of arteries and arterioles (*vasoconstriction*), an action that also accelerates fluid movement into the tissues. Other mast cell and basophil products [e.g., leukotrienes such as prostaglandin D2 (PGD2) and platelet activating factor (PAF)], also cause *bronchconstriction* and stimulate the secretion of mucus.

The symptoms of an allergic reaction are de-

TABLE 8-3. INFLAMMATORY MEDIATORS OF TYPE I HYPERSENSITIVITIES

Category	Molecule(s)	Effect	Produced By
Lipids	Prostaglandins	Elevate body temperature; stimulate pain receptors; increase vascular permeability	Mast cells; Eosinophils
	Leukotrienes	Attract and activate neutrophils; increase endothelial adhesion with leukocytes; constriction of vascular smooth muscle; increase vascular permeability; stimulate mucous production	Mast cells; Eosinophils
	Platelet-activating factor (PAF)	Increase adhesion between vascular endothelium and neutrophils	Mast cells; Eosinophils
Amines and other active peptides	Histamine	Increase vascular permeability and constriction of vascular smooth muscle	Mast cells; Basophils
	Heparin	Counters coagulation	Mast cells
Cytokines/chemokines	Interleukin-1 (IL-1); Interleukin-6 (IL-6)	Elevation of body temperature; release of acute phase proteins	Mast cells; Eosinophils
	Interleukin-5 (IL-5)	Chemotaxis of eosinophils	Mast cells
	Interleukin-8 (IL-8)	Attraction and adhesion of leukocytes to vascular endothelium	Mast cells; Eosinophils
	Macrophage chemotactic protein-1 (MCP-1)	Chemotaxis of monocytes	Mast cells; Eosinophils
	Macrophage inhibitory protein-1a (MIP-1a)	Chemotaxis of leukocytes	Mast cells; Eosinophils
	Interleukin-4 (IL-4); Interleukin-13 (IL-13)	Promote production of IgE	Mast cells;Eosinophils
	Interferon-γ (IFN-γ)	Activation of macrophages	Eosinophils
	Tumor necrosis factor (TNF)	Pro-inflammatory	Mast cells; Eosinophils Mast cells; Eosinophils
Cationic proteins of eosinophils	Major basic protein	Activation of platelets, mast cells and basophils	Eosinophils
	Eosinophil cationic protein (ECP)	Toxic to flatworms and roundworms	Eosinophils
	Eosinphil peroxidase (EPO)		
	Eosinophil-derived neurotoxin (EDN)		
Enzymes	Elastase Chymase Carboxypeptase Others	Breakdown/reconstruction of connective tissue	Mast cells; Eosinophils

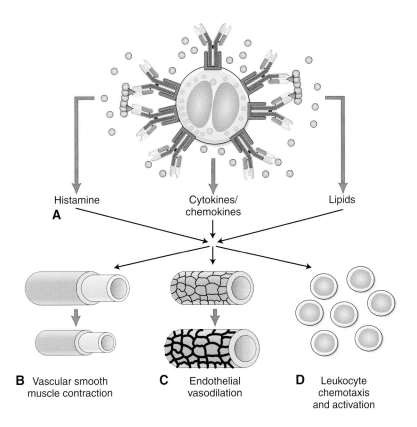

Histamine
A

Cytokines/
chemokines

Lipids

B Vascular smooth
muscle contraction

C Endothelial
vasodilation

D Leukocyte
chemotaxis
and activation

FIGURE 8-2. Mast cell inflammatory mediators affect vasculature and infiltration of tissues by leukocytes. Mast cell degranulation releases agents that contribute to inflammation **(A)** by affecting the ability of cells and fluids to leave the vasculature and enter the affected tissues. Among the effects are vasoconstriction due to contraction of smooth muscle of blood vessels **(B)**, vasodilation due to loosening of the junctions between vascular epithelial cells in capillaries **(C)**, and the attraction and activation of leukocytes that infiltrate the affected tissues **(D)**.

termined primarily by the location of the sensitizing antigen (Table 8-3). Antigens that enter the body by inhalation will be primarily localized to the nasopharyngeal and bronchial tissues where smooth muscle contraction and vasodilation will produce increased mucous production and constriction of the respiratory passages (Fig. 8-3). In combination, these responses can produce severe and potentially fatal respiratory difficulties such as *asthma*. Allergens that primarily contact the skin produce inflammatory responses resulting in rashes, often the classic "wheal and flare" appearance due to redness and edema. Those that are ingested can lead to food allergies that primarily affect the gastrointestinal (GI) tract. The most common food allergens are eggs, peanuts, milk, soy, tree nuts, crustaceans, and wheat. In the case of injected allergens (e.g., bee venom), the antigen may be disseminated via the bloodstream, and the resulting inflammation may be systemic. In these cases, the condition may become life-threatening as the vasoconstriction of the vascu-

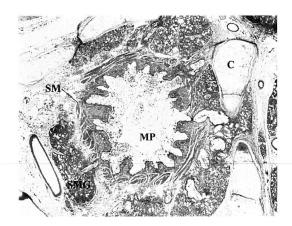

FIGURE 8-3. IgE-mediated hypersensitivity reactions—respiratory system and skin. Asthma results from contraction of smooth muscle of respiratory passages and excessive production of mucous by respiratory epithelium. The photomicrograph shows a section of lung from an asthmatic patient. Note the mucous plug (20×). (MP, mucous plug; SM, smooth muscle; SMG, submucosal gland; C, cartilage.)

lar smooth muscle, together with vasodilation of the vascular endothelium, can lead to severe fluid loss from the vasculature to produce shock. This condition is also called *anaphylactic shock*. In such cases, the prompt application of a systemic antagonist of histamine, such as epinephrine, is called for.

Patient Vignette 8.1

Wendy C., a 12-year-old girl with a suspected history of allergies to cats (Chapter 2, Question 7) goes camping regularly. When camping during late August and early fall, she sometimes had symptoms of sneezing, runny nose, nasal congestion, itchy eyes, and postnasal drip. She seldom has such problems when camping in the spring or early summer, but noticed that they tended to begin in late August and early fall.

Q: *What is causing these symptoms?*

A: Her symptoms are consistent with seasonal allergic rhinitis, an immediate hypersensitivity or allergy. Allergens that cause symptoms include pollens (trees, grasses, ragweeds), dust mites, animal danders, and molds. Patients with allergies often (but not always) show sensitivities to multiple allergens. Since Wendy has allergic rhinitis symptoms in the fall, this suggests that she may be sensitive to ragweed, which is prevalent in the early fall. Allergies to grass pollens, on the other hand, are usually seen in the spring. Diagnosis of allergic rhinitis includes a positive history of allergic symptoms, physical examination, and skin testing. A positive skin test to ragweed allergen correlating with her symptoms in the fall suggests that she has seasonal allergic rhinitis due to ragweed. Treatment for allergic rhinitis may include avoidance, antihistamines, sympathomimetic agents, topical nasal steroids and intranasal cromolyn, or immunotherapy.

Mast cells and basophils interact with eosinophils during inflammation. Mast cell products such as IL-5 and certain chemokines are chemoattractants for eosinophils. Eosinophils and basophils react to many of the same chemical signals as do mast cells, and eosinophils even ex-

press $FcR\varepsilon$ when activated, allowing them to bind free IgE. Eosinophils release a variety of enzymes, cytokines, chemokines, and other inflammatory mediators that contribute to inflammation in ways similar to those of mast cells (Table 8-3).

CLINICAL APPLICATION
ALLERGY TESTING

The precise allergen responsible for a particular patient's problems can sometimes be determined through allergy testing, if the allergen is one of the substances in the test panel. Such identification could help the patient to avoid contact in the future but, unfortunately, it is often impossible to pinpoint the culprit within the enormous number of potential allergens in the environment. Treatment with appropriate antiinflammatory agents can help minimize the effects of allergic responses but do not get at the root cause. Permanent alleviation of allergies is sometimes possible, but not guaranteed. In some cases, regular exposure to the allergen in an altered form or by an alternative route can provide benefit through a procedure called **allergen immunotherapy**. In older references, this is sometimes (inappropriately) called "desensitization." The rationale is that the intentional exposure might boost the production of IgG against the allergen and hasten its clearance. Rapid clearance of the allergen would reduce the likelihood of the allergen binding IgE on mast cells and triggering an inflammatory response.

Patient Vignette 8.2

Peter H., a 3-year-old boy with a history of allergies to peanuts (Chapter 1), presents to the emergency room with diffuse hives and pruritus of his skin, nose, and throat, a feeling of lightheadedness, and apparent difficulty breathing. According to his mother, he attended a birthday party and ate a cookie, and after a few minutes developed these symptoms. Because he has a history of peanut allergy, his mother immediately checked the ingredients listed on the

(continued)

cookie box and noted that the label stated "may contain peanuts." She immediately took an "Epi-pen" from her purse and administered a dose of epinephrine into Peter's thigh.

Q: What is Peter's condition, and why did his mother act as she did?

A: Peter's symptoms are consistent with anaphylaxis. Anaphylaxis is a potentially life-threatening condition caused by the release of histamines and other mediators. Symptoms and signs of anaphylaxis may include more than one organ system. Skin involvement may include pruritus (hives), flushing (erythema or redness of the skin), or angioedema (swelling of the skin). Respiratory symptoms may include shortness of breath, bronchospasms (contraction of the smooth muscles of the respiratory passages), or respiratory arrest. Gastrointestinal symptoms may include abdominal pain, nausea, vomiting, or diarrhea. Cardiovascular symptoms may include lightheadedness, syncope (loss of consciousness due to a sudden drop in blood pressure) or shock (vasodilatation—loosening of the endothelial junctions, leading to fluid loss from the vasculature), and cardiac arrest. Acute treatment for anaphylaxis includes basic life support, epinephrine (a histamine antagonist), and histamine-1 blockers. Peter's mother was correct in administering epinephrine immediately after checking the ingredients in the cookie. Individuals (or their caretakers) with severe allergies to foods or other environmental allergens (e.g., bee venom) are educated in avoidance and instructed to carry "Epi-pens" for rapid injection of epinephrine.

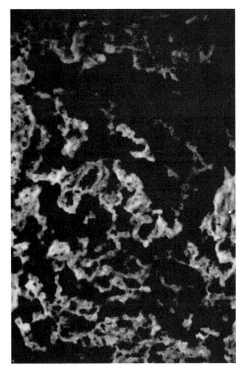

FIGURE 8-4. Type II hypersensitivity reactions—inflammation of basement membranes. Goodpasture's syndrome results from binding of autoantibodies to basement membranes in organs such as the lung (shown in photomicrograph) and kidney. The bright areas are sites of heavy binding of autoreactive IgG carrying a fluorescent marker. (Photo reprinted from Rubin E, Gorstein F, Rubin R, et al. *Rubin's pathology: Clincopathologic foundations of medicine,* 4th ed. Baltimore: Lippincott Williams & Wilkins, 2005.)

TYPE II HYPERSENSITIVITY REACTIONS

Type II hypersensitivity reactions are the result of antibodies (usually IgG) binding to epitopes associated with cell membranes or extracellular matrix. In this regard, these reactions differ from Type III hypersensitivity reactions that are directed at epitopes on soluble antigens. The epitopes targeted by immunoglobulin that can lead to Type II hypersensitivity reactions are of two broad types, self epitopes and exogenous epitopes. An example of a disease caused by reactions against self epitopes is Goodpasture's syndrome (Fig. 8-4). In this disease, antibodies, usually of the IgG isotype, are generated against epitopes of basement membranes in various tissues. These autoantibodies bind to these epitopes and subsequently activate complement via the classical pathway. The complement-induced inflammation is against the targeted tissues and can lead to significant damage. In other cases, the antibodies may be directed against externally derived molecules that have bound to host cell surfaces. An example of this mechanism is found in some hemolytic anemias, where exogenous drugs such as penicillin can bind to erythrocyte membranes (Fig. 8-5). If the individual produces antibodies against the penicillin, these antibodies can bind to penicillin on the erythrocyte surface, and

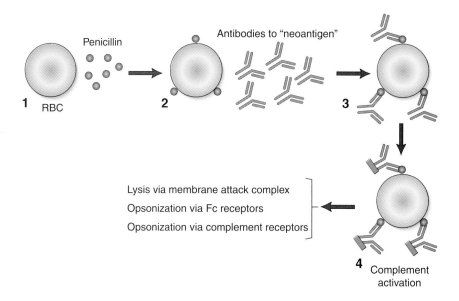

FIGURE 8-5. Drug-induced hemolytic anemia. (1) Erythrocytes are exposed to a reactive chemical such as penicillin; **(2)** Penicillin binds to molecules on the erythrocyte surface, forming neoantigens; **(3)** Antibodies are generated against the neoantigens and bind to the erythrocyte surfaces; **(4)** The bound IgG activates complement, leading to destruction of the erythrocyte.

activate complement. Complement activation can lead to lysis of the cell membrane and destruction of the cell.

Patient Vignette 8.3

Floyd E., a 50-year-old man, presents to the emergency room with symptoms of epistaxis (nose bleed), hematuria (blood in the urine), easy bruising and petechiae (hemorrhagic spots) with ecchymoses (purplish patches caused by extravasation of blood into skin). In addition, he complains of fatigue. Complete blood analyses reveal thrombocytopenia (low platelet count) and anemia. The patient states he was well until two weeks ago, when he was prescribed an antibiotic for symptoms of prostatitis.

Q: What is a likely explanation for his problems?

A: This patient may have a drug-induced thrombocytopenia. It is possible that the antibiotic acts as a hapten, binding to molecules on the platelets and causing the platelets to become immunogenic and induce antibody formation. The antibody response causes ly-

(continued)

Patient Vignette 8.3 (Continued)

sis (destruction) of the platelets, primarily by complement-mediated lysis. Treatment for this condition would be discontinuation of the antibiotic. Since this subject has significant ongoing bleeding and severe thrombocytopenia, platelet transfusion is indicated to deal with the immediate situation.

TYPE III HYPERSENSITIVITY REACTIONS

Like Type II hypersensitivity reactions, Type III hypersensitivity reactions are antibody-mediated, usually by the IgG isotype but sometimes by IgM as well. However, Type III hypersensitivity reactions are directed against soluble antigens. Under normal circumstances, antigen-antibody complexes are formed that include multiple antibodies and multiple antigens. The efficiency with which these complex are formed depends, to a large extent, on the size of the immune complex formed (Chapter 4 and Fig. 4-5). As long as these complexes are not extremely large and numerous, they are readily cleared by the **reticuloendothelial system** (RES). The RES consists of motile cells (e.g., some macrophages, dendritic cells, neutrophils) in the liver, spleen and bone marrow) that can ingest and degrade particles and debris—the "sanitation engineers" of the body. In large part, the antigen-antibody complexes are carried away by erythrocytes, via the FcR1 receptors on those cells, to the liver or spleen where the complexes are destroyed. However, in cases where high levels of both antigen and antibody are simultaneously present, the size and quantity of precipitated complexes may overwhelm the normal clearance mechanisms. As a result, the complexes accumulate in the tissues and the IgG and IgM antibodies within the antigen-antibody complexes can then bind complement component C1 and activate complement via the classical pathway (Chapter 5). The inflammation that ensues is targeted to the area of complex deposition.

It should be noted that the sites where immune complexes are deposited are not necessarily the

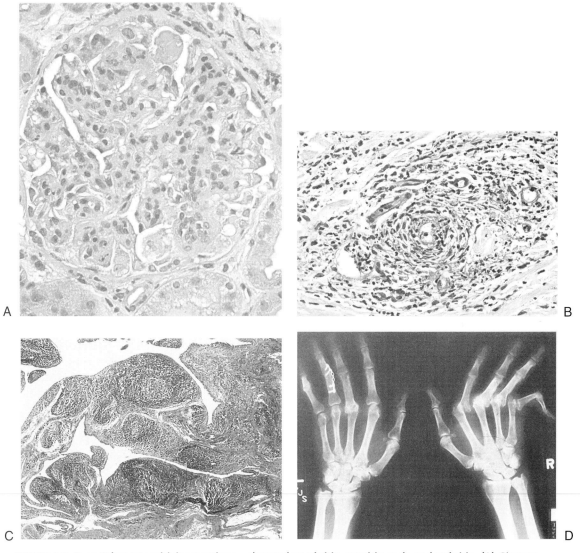

FIGURE 8-6. Type III hypersensitivity reactions—glomerulonephritis, arteritis, rash, and arthritis. (A) *Glomerulonephritis.* Note the monocytic infiltration and damage to the filtration structures. (Photo reprinted from Rubin E, Gorstein F, Rubin R, et al. *Rubin's pathology: Clincopathologic foundations of medicine*, 4th ed. Baltimore: Lippincott Williams & Wilkins, 2005.) **(B)** *Arteritis.* Inflammation results in heavy monocytic cell infiltration and damage to the vascular endothelium and surrounding structures. The blood vessel can become nonfunctional. (Photo reprinted from Rubin E, Gorstein F, Rubin R, et al. *Rubin's pathology: Clincopathologic foundations of medicine*, 4th ed. Baltimore: Lippincott Williams & Wilkins, 2005.) **(C)** *Rheumatoid arthritis.* Proliferative inflammation of the synovial membrane (40×). Note areas of mononuclear cell infiltration. **(D)** *Rheumatoid arthritis.* Damage to the synovial membrane and release of enzymes within the synovium lead to inflammation and destruction of joint bone and cartilage.

sites from which the antigen is derived. Thus, much of the damage that occurs may be of the "innocent bystander" variety. In essence, the adjacent tissues are damaged by "friendly fire." Several sites in the body seem to be particularly susceptible to these accumulations (Fig. 8-6A–D).

- **Glomeruli** of the kidney. The filtration of the blood that occurs in these structures makes them particularly susceptible to accumulation of precipitated immune complexes. The ensuing inflammation, driven by complement activation, can lead to permanent damage or destruction of the glomeruli (*glomerulonephritis*) and impaired kidney function.
- **Blood vessel walls.** Precipitated immune complexes can accumulate on the walls of veins and arteries, and the subsequent inflammation can damage the vasculature (**vasculitis**). This damage can sometimes be seen in skin lesions where the affected vasculature is close to the surface.
- **Synovial membranes** of joints. For unknown reasons, the membranes that line the synovial capsules that enclose articulating joints are common sites for deposition of precipitated immune complexes. Subsequent complement activation and inflammation can lead to considerable damage to the bone and cartilage of the

joint and sometimes cause total destruction and dysfunction of the joint (**rheumatoid arthritis**). Rheumatoid arthritis, like other rheumatoid diseases, presents an additional feature. The IgG in the immune complexes can become an antigen, stimulating the production of IgM against the bound IgG. The conformational changes in the Fc region of IgG molecules that occur when antigen is bound expose sites on the Fc region of those IgGs that become available for binding by IgM (Fig. 8-7). The anti-IgG IgM is also called "**rheumatoid factor.**"
- **Skin.** The skin is a common site for deposition of immune complexes, with the subsequent inflammation manifesting as rashes.

In addition to these four areas, some immune complex diseases are systemic in their distribution. Perhaps the best known example is **systemic lupus erythematosus** (SLE). Individuals with SLE have immune complex deposition and related inflammation in widespread regions of the body, often involving not only the kidney, joints, skin, and vasculature but also muscle tissue and other organs. SLE arises from autoantibodies formed against fragments of single- or double-stranded (ss or ds) DNA, RNA and some chromosomal proteins (e.g., histones). Because these molecules are widespread throughout the body, the inflammation is likewise broadly distributed.

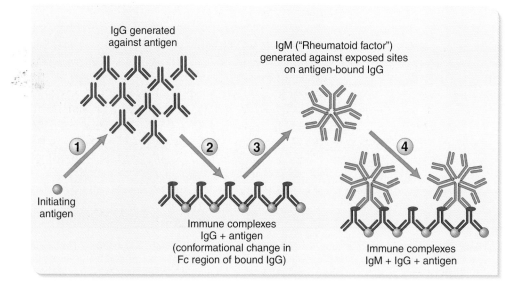

FIGURE 8-7. Formation of rheumatoid factor. (1) The first step in rheumatoid factor formation is the generation of a specific IgG against an antigen. **(2)** The antigen is bound by antibody, often as part of an antigen-antibody complex. Binding of the IgG causes conformational changes in the antibody's Fc region, exposing new sites on the IgG. **(3)** IgM is generated against the newly exposed sites on the antigen-bound IgG. The IgM generated against the IgG is the "rheumatoid factor." **(4)** IgM then binds to the exposed sites on the IgG molecules, augmenting the development of antigen-antibody complexes.

Type III hypersensitivity reactions are often diseases that occur secondarily to other conditions that increase the likelihood of high levels of immune complex formation. Successful treatment for these conditions may be helpful in treating type III hypersensitivities.

- *Autoimmune disease.* Because the stimulating antigen is never cleared from the body, disease caused by immune responses against self epitopes (autoimmune disease) presents a situation where constant stimulation can produce high levels of specific antibody in the simultaneous presence of high antigen levels.
- *Chronic or recurrent infections.* Chronic exposure to infectious organisms can cause sufficient antibody levels to facilitate high levels of immune complex deposition.
- *Cancer.* The steady presence of antigens that may be shed by tumors may stimulate simultaneous high levels of specific antibody, similar to that of autoimmune disease.
- *Repeated medications.* The recurrent presence of drugs or other medications in the body can, in some individuals, stimulate the presence of high levels of antibodies that can lead to immune complex deposition if the agent levels are high enough.

Patient Vignette 8.4

Wanda L., a 36-year-old woman, presents with symptoms of pain, pruritus, joint pain, weight loss, fever, and fatigue existing for several weeks. Blood analyses revealed the presence of antinuclear antibodies (ANA) with a specificity for dsDNA, anemia, and proteinuria (protein in her urine, a sign of damage to the filtration apparatus of the kidney). Physical examination was remarkable for a malar rash (a butterfly-shaped rash on the face) and bilateral swelling of the wrist and finger joints. The subject stated that she began taking isoniazid (INH) and pyridoxine several months ago because she had been exposed to a person with tuberculosis and had a positive PPD.

Q: *What is a likely explanation for her signs and symptoms?*

(continued)

Patient Vignette 8.4 (Continued)

A: This patient has symptoms and signs consistent with systemic lupus erythematosus (SLE). SLE is a chronic inflammatory multisystem autoimmune disease. SLE results from a Type III hypersensitivity response generated by tissue deposition of antigen-antibody complexes, and is typically associated with high levels of IgG against fragments of nucleic acids and chromosomal proteins. However, the diagnosis should not be rushed. In this patient, the underlying cause may be drug-induced (by the INH) and symptoms would usually resolve after discontinuing the drug, often within weeks after discontinuation. Blood tests for antihistone antibody may help to confirm the diagnosis.

TYPE IV HYPERSENSITIVITY REACTIONS

Unlike Type I, II, and III hypersensitivity responses that are based on antibody-mediated responses, type IV hypersensitivity reactions are entirely cell-mediated. Complement does not play a role in Type IV hypersensitivity reactions. The overwhelming majority of Type IV hypersensitivity reactions are actually CD4$^+$ T cell-mediated DTH responses. As noted in Chapter 5, macrophages that inflict the damage in this type of immune response are not specific; they kill both infected and uninfected tissues. The term "delayed" stems from the fact that it typically takes 2 to 4 days after exposure to an antigen for clinical signs to appear. In addition, it should be pointed out that these responses are secondary, resulting from the presence of already activated Th1 CD4$^+$ cells. In many cases, these cells are generated against infectious agents and result in levels of inflammation that may be intense or chronic enough to cause permanent damage. For example, DTH responses to bacteria such as *Listeria* or protozoa such as *Leishmania* can ultimately cause damage in infected tissues and organs. Likewise, much of the damage seen in the lungs of individuals with tuberculosis does not stem from the action of the infectious agent, *Mycobacterium tuberculosis*, but from the cellular inflammation generated against it within the delicate lung tissue. Similarly, *Mycobacterium leprae*, the causative agent of leprosy, is the stimulus for generation of DTH responses that lead to destruction of tissues, peripheral nerve damage, and disfigurement as they work to clear the bacteria. In addition to inflammation, delayed hypersensitivity responses attempt to prevent the spread of infectious organisms by walling them off, which is accomplished by forming **granulomas**. Granulomas are composed of lymphocytes and phagocytes that encase the infectious organisms while they are being destroyed (Fig. 8-8A,B). The remnants of these structures are the **tubercles** that are seen in the tissues of individuals with tuberculosis.

Contact sensitivities are a special category of DTH responses in which the stimulus is not an infectious agent, but is instead a reactive chemical

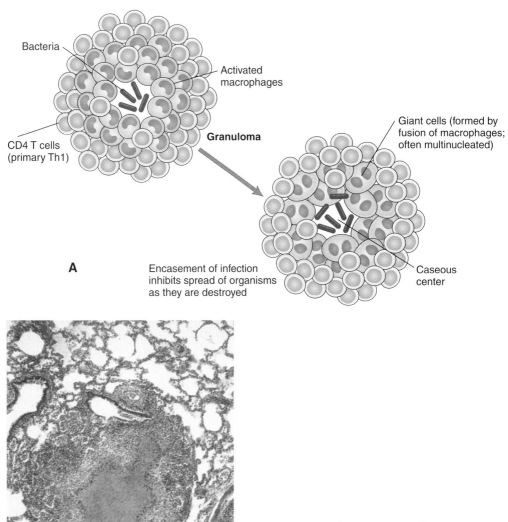

FIGURE 8-8. Granulomas in Type IV hypersensitivity reactions. (A) Granulomas are formed primarily by CD4[+] T cells and macrophages to isolate infectious agents and prevent their spread while they are destroyed. As the process proceeds, macrophages fuse to form multinucleated "giant cells." Caseous ("cheese-like") areas can develop as a result of the accumulated remains of destroyed microbes and host leukocytes. **(B)** Photomicrograph of granuloma. (Photo from Rubin E, Gorstein F, Rubin R, et al. *Rubin's pathology: Clincopathologic foundations of medicine*, 4th ed. Baltimore: Lippincott Williams & Wilkins, 2005.)

that attaches to cell surface proteins. In some cases, the reactive chemicals may alter the configurations of those proteins to create new forms called *neoantigens*. In other cases, the reactive chemicals are haptens that, once bound to cellular molecules, can provoke immune responses (see discussion of haptens in Chapter 1). These altered cellular molecules, neoantigens and haptenated molecules, are processed and presented by MHC class II molecules where they can trigger activation of Th1 CD4$^+$ T cells, which, in turn, activate macrophages and produce DTH responses. Many contact sensitivities occur in industrial settings where workers' skin may be exposed to reactive chemicals such as heavy metals. The best known examples, however, are the far more common afflictions known as **poison ivy**, **poison sumac**, or **poison oak**. These reactions result from exposure of the skin to **catechols**, reactive molecules produced in the leaves of the poison ivy, poison sumac, and poison oak plants.

> ### Patient Vignette 8.5
>
> Annabelle L., a 12-year-old girl, went camping. Two days after returning from camping Annabelle noticed itchy, red, indurated linear streaks on her left forearm.
>
> *Q: What is a likely explanation for Annabelle's signs and symptoms?*
>
> A: The timing, location, and type of the dermatitis suggest that she has poison ivy, a contact dermatitis. This is a Type IV hypersensitivity mediated by a delayed type hypersensitivity response. Other common causes of contact dermatitis include nickel, latex, and fragrances. Patch testing may help to confirm the diagnosis. The treatment includes application of topical steroids and antihistamines. Oral steroids may be indicated for severe cases.

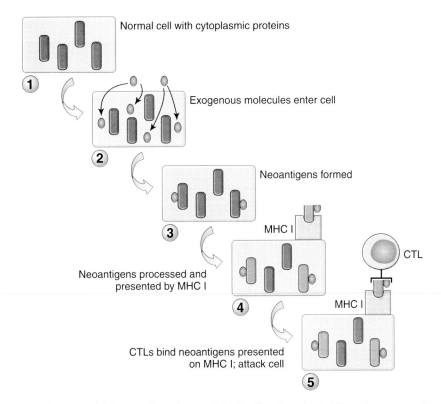

FIGURE 8-9. Type IV hypersensitivity reactions due to CD8$^+$ T cells. Normal cells **(1)** can be penetrated by some reactive agents **(2)** that bind directly to intracellular proteins, producing neoantigens **(3)**. As the cytoplasmic neoantigens are broken down and processed by proteasomes, the resulting fragments are presented by MHC class I molecules on the cell surfaces **(4),** where they can be recognized and bound by cytotoxic CD8$^+$ T cells **(5)** that can proceed to destroy the cells to which they bind.

Some specialized type IV hypersensitivity reactions are caused by CD8$^+$ cytotoxic T cell responses. Some active chemical agents can pass through the cell membrane and bind to internal cytoplasmic proteins, producing neoantigens. When these altered proteins are broken down for antigen processing and presentation via the MHC class I pathway, the affected cell becomes subject to destruction by CD8$^+$ T cells (Fig. 8-9).

Summary

- **Hypersensitivity** is the term applied to the pathologies involving immune-mediated damage to host tissues. There are four major categories of hypersensitivity reactions: types I, II, III, and IV.
- **Type I hypersensitivity reactions** are those generated by the actions of IgE and granulocytes, either mast cells or basophils. Type I hypersensitivity reactions are also known as **immediate hypersensitivities** because they can occur literally within minutes to hours following exposure to antigen. They are also termed **anaphylactic reactions**. Immediate hypersensitivities are often directed at totally harmless molecules. IgE can serve as passively acquired surface receptors for mast cells or basophils and can trigger release of inflammatory molecules stored as cytoplasmic granules. Crosslinking of IgE generates an intracellular signal for the mast cell or basophil to degranulate. The cytoplasmic granules of mast cells and basophils contain a wide variety of pharmacological mediators of inflammation, including **histamine**.
- **Type II hypersensitivity reactions** are those generated by the actions of antibodies (usually IgG, but sometimes also IgM) against antigens associated with cell membranes or extracellular matrix. Many of these diseases result from states of autoimmunity where the immune system has inappropriately begun to react against the body's own cells and molecules, as in the case of **Goodpasture's syndrome**. In other cases, the immunoglobulins may be directed against externally derived molecules that have bound to host cell surfaces. An example of this mechanism is found in some **hemolytic anemias.**
- **Type III hypersensitivity reactions** are those generated by the accumulation and precipitation of large conglomerations of soluble antigen and antibodies. Type III hypersensitivity reactions are antibody-mediated, usually by the IgG isotype but sometimes also involving IgM. Under normal circumstances, **antigen-antibody complexes** are formed that include multiple antibodies and multiple antigens. The antibodies within these complexes can activate **complement** via the classical pathway and initiate inflammation focused on the area of deposition. There are four sites in the body that seem to be particularly susceptible to the accumulation of precipitated immune complexes: glomeruli of the kidney, blood vessel walls, synovial membranes of joints, and the skin. In addition, some immune complex diseases are systemic in their distribution (e.g., systemic lupus erythematosus).
- **Type III hypersensitivity reactions** are diseases that often occur secondarily to other conditions that increase the likelihood of high levels of immune complex formation: autoimmune disease, chronic or recurrent infections, cancer, and repeated medications.
- **Type IV hypersensitivity reactions** are entirely cell-mediated. The majority of type IV hypersensitivities are actually CD4$^+$ T cell-mediated delayed type hypersensitivity (DTH) responses. Delayed (-type) hypersensitivity responses attempt to prevent the spread of infectious organisms by walling them off by forming **granulomas**, which are composed of lymphocytes and phagocytes that encase the infectious organisms while they are being destroyed. *Contact* **sensitivities** are a special category of DTH responses in which the stimulus is not an infectious agent, but is, instead, a reactive chemical that attaches to cell surface proteins.

Suggested readings

Dombrowicz D, Capron M. Eosinophils, allergy and parasites. *Curr Opin Immunol* 2001;12:728.

Gould HJ, Sutton BJ, Beavil AJ, et al. The biology of IgE and the basis of allergic disease. *Annu Rev Immunol* 2003;21:579.

Janeway CA Jr., Travers P, Walport M, Shlomchik P. Allergy and hypersensitivity. In *Immunobiology: The immune system in health and disease*, 5th ed. Philadephia: Garland Publishing, 2001.

Robbie-Ryan M, Brown M. The role of mast cells in allergy and autoimmunity. *Curr Opin Immunol* 2002;14:728.

Wills-Karp M, Khurana, Hershey GK. Immunological mechanisms of allergic disorders. In Paul WE, ed. *Fundamental immunology*, 5th ed. Philadelphia: Lippincott Williams & Wilkins, 2003.

Zeiss CR, Pruzansky JJ. Immunology of IgE-mediated and other hypersensitivity states. In Grammer LC, Greenberger PA, eds. *Patterson's allergic diseases*, 6th ed. Philadelphia: Lippincott Williams & Wilkins, 2002.

Review questions

DIRECTIONS: Each of the numbered items or incomplete statements in this section is followed by answers or by completions of the statement. Select the ONE lettered answer or completion that is BEST in each case.

1. When histamine is released during an acute inflammation, it _____ vascular permeability and _____ the movement of fluid out of the vasculature.
    (A) increases/inhibits
    (B) increases/promotes
    (C) decreases/promotes
    (D) decreases/inhibits
    (E) increases/does not affect

2. In systemic lupus erythematosus (SLE), kidney damage results primarily from:
    (A) cytotoxic T cells (CTLs) directed against kidney tubule cells.
    (B) type II hypersensitivity reaction directed against self antigens on the kidney cell surface.
    (C) precipitation of insoluble immune complexes in the glomeruli and complement activation.
    (D) IgE-mediated release of histamine.
    (E) delayed type hypersensitivity (DTH) responses against infectious agents in the kidney.

3. Exposure of industrial workers to heavy metals can lead to a contact sensitivity reaction, an inflammatory response mediated by which of the following?
    (A) IgG
    (B) IgE
    (C) NK cells
    (D) Th1 cells and macrophages
    (E) Immune complex deposition and complement activation

4. In type I (immediate) hypersensitivity reactions, one of the most important factors determining the nature of the symptoms is:
    (A) level of serum C4.
    (B) level of serum C3.
    (C) distribution/location of the antigen.
    (D) local concentration of NK cells.
    (E) levels of immune complex deposition.

5. Autoimmune diseases such as systemic lupus erythematosus (SLE) often predispose an individual toward subsequent development of which of the following types of diseases?
    (A) Immediate hypersensitivity
    (B) Delayed (-type) hypersensitivity (DTH)
    (C) Immunodeficiency
    (D) Contact sensitivity
    (E) Immune complex disease

6. Which of the following anatomical sites is a frequent target for deposition of precipitated antigen-antibody complex?
    (A) Brain
    (B) Liver
    (C) Eyes
    (D) Kidney
    (E) Bone

7. Rheumatoid arthritis is characterized by the presence of "rheumatoid factor," which actually consists of:
    (A) IgM antibodies directed against antigen-bound IgG molecules.
    (B) IL-4 and IL-10.
    (C) C5a.
    (D) secretory IgA bound to the synovial membrane and triggering the alternative pathway of complement.
    (E) antigen-IgE complexes.

8. A 6-year-old boy presents to the emergency room with a diffuse skin rash and difficulty breathing that began several minutes after eating a peanut butter cookie. His mother noted an episode with similar but milder symptoms several months ago after he ate a food containing peanuts. An allergy to peanuts is suspected. Which of the following treatments is the most appropriate to be used immediately?
    (A) Administration of epinephrine
    (B) Initiation of immunotherapy against peanut-associated allergens
    (C) Administration of antagonists against histamine receptors
    (D) Putting a moisturizing lotion on the rash
    (E) No treatment is called for.

9. A 50-year-old woman presents with symmetrical pain, swelling, and inflammation of the joints in her hands and in her wrists

and knees. She says this condition has been getting gradually worse over the past couple of years. You suspect rheumatoid arthritis. Which of the following tests would be most informative in your diagnosis?

(A) Increased anti-immunoglobulin levels
(B) CD4$^+$ T cell count
(C) CD8$^+$ T cell count
(D) Total immunoglobulin levels
(E) Histamine levels

10. A 25-year-old woman presents with a facial rash and pain and swelling in her joints. Blood tests reveal abnormal kidney function and anemia. Which of the following diseases would be most consistent with these symptoms?

(A) Immediate hypersensitivity reactions
(B) Delayed type hypersensitivity reactions
(C) Drug-induced hemolytic anemia
(D) Immune complex disease
(E) Contact sensitivity

Autoimmunity and Tolerance

Chapter Outline

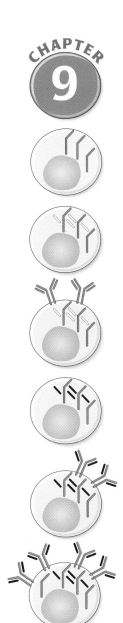

Introduction In this chapter, we consider how the immune system prevents responses against self and the consequences that ensue when that prevention is lost. The immune system has developed several mechanisms to prevent reactions against self antigens that provide overlapping layers of protection for the body. The loss of one or more of these preventive mechanisms can lead to **autoimmunity**, in which the immune system attacks the body's own normal cells and tissues that it is designed to protect.

THE THREAT OF RESPONSES AGAINST SELF

The role of the immune system is to attack "non-self," while leaving "self" relatively undisturbed. The innate immune system is able to make this distinction by expressing a relatively finite set of genetically programmed receptors that recognize molecules expressed by a wide variety of organisms. Some somatically generated receptors expressed by cells of the adaptive immune system, however, have the potential to recognize self. Some of the mechanisms that prevent damage to self, such as the negative selection process that occurs in the thymus to eliminate potentially self-reactive T cells, are discussed in Chapter 5. If these mechanisms fail to distinguish self from nonself, serious, even fatal, consequences may result. Once the self/nonself distinction is lost, damage can be inflicted on tissues and organs of the body. Autoimmunity is not rare or exotic. Autoimmune diseases and their sequelae occur with surprising frequency. Almost everyone knows someone with rheumatoid arthritis, psoriasis, multiple sclerosis, systemic lupus erythematosus (SLE), or other autoimmune disease (Table 9-1). Autoimmune diseases may also have effects beyond the specific immune responses involved. For example, they may lead to conditions that increase the risk of subsequent immune complex disease (type III hypersensitivity, Chapter 8).

The danger of autoimmunity was recognized by several pioneering immunologists, one of whom, Paul Ehrich, described it with the colorful term "**horror autotoxicus**" (the horror of self-toxicity). Since those early observations, it has been recognized that autoimmunity can sometimes be localized because of the limited distribution of the targeted self antigen(s) (Table 9-2). Other autoimmune diseases (e.g., rheumatoid arthritis, polymyositis, reactive arthritis, scleroderma, and

TABLE 9-1. AUTOIMMUNE DISEASES

Disease	Initial Target	Affected Tissue
Ankylosing spondylitis	Unknown	Lower spine
Autoimmune hemolytic anemia	Erythrocyte surface molecules	Erythrocytes
Crohn's disease	Unknown	Intestine
Goodpasture's syndrome	Type IV collagen of basement membranes	Kidneys, lungs
Graves' disease	TSH receptor	Thyroid
Hashimoto's thyroiditis	Thyroglobulin	Thyroid
Type I insulin-dependent diabetes mellitus	GAD; preproinsulin; other β-cell products	Pancreatic islet β-cells
Male sterility	Unknown	Seminiferous tubules, sperm
Multiple sclerosis	Myelin proteins (several)	Myelin
Myasthenia gravis	ACH receptor	Skeletal muscle
Rheumatic fever	Streptococcal M protein, cardiac muscle antigens	Heart valves
Rheumatoid arthritis	Unknown	Synovial membranes, joints
Pemphigus vulgaris	Desmoglein-3	Skin
Polymyositis	Jo-1; PM-Scl	Muscle
Psoriasis	Unknown, but there is some association with strep infections	Skin
Reiter's disease (reactive arthritis)	Possible association with infectious agents	Joints of lower extremities; eyes, genitals, urinary, or GI systems
Scleroderma	Scl-70; PM-Scl	Connective tissue
Sjögren's syndrome	Ro/SS-A	Tear ducts
Systemic lupus erythematosus (SLE)	Nucleic acids; chromosomal proteins	Skin, vasculature, muscle, joints, kidney
Thrombocytic purpura	Platelet integrin molecules	Platelets
Ulcerative colitis	Unknown	Intestine (small and large)
Uveitis (anterior)	Beta B1-crystallin and other proteins of the ciliary body epithelium	Eye

TABLE 9-2 EXAMPLES OF LOCALIZED AUTOIMMUNE DISEASES

Disease	Localization
Goodpasture's syndrome	Kidneys and lungs
Hashimoto's thyroiditis	Thyroid
Type I IDDM	Pancreatic β cells
Multiple sclerosis	Brain and spinal cord
Crohn's disease	Intestine
Sjögren's syndrome	Tear ducts

systemic lupus erythematosus) are systemically manifested because the antigens in question are found in many parts of the body. Infection may sometimes play a role in blurring the distinction between self and nonself as the development of autoimmunity is often associated with the occurrence of particular infectious diseases. Therefore, the genetic factors that provide variation in the immune capacity of different individuals can also make some individuals more susceptible to development of autoimmunity than others. Several specific genes have been identified that are associated with increased risk of certain autoimmune diseases. In humans, several genes within the HLA complex have been found to occur more frequently among patients with specific autoimmune diseases. In experimental animal systems, both MHC and non-MHC genes have been identified that appear to contribute to development of autoimmunity.

Autoimmunity is therefore a complex situation with multiple mechanisms, multiple causes, and multiple modifying factors. But what all of these factors have in common is that they contribute to a breakdown in the immune system's ability to refrain from attacking self antigens—in other words, a breakdown in self tolerance.

SELF TOLERANCE

A discussion of autoimmunity must begin with a discussion of **tolerance**, the normal and optimal state in which the immune system's offensive weaponry is reserved for use against external agents, such as infectious agents and toxins. This does not mean that the immune system cannot recognize self. It is clear that it can, for the ability to recognize what is nonself must be built upon a

knowledge of what is self. Tolerance requires that the immune system, when recognizing self, must adopt a nondestructive strategy. A variety of mechanisms is used for this purpose. Some eliminate potentially autoreactive cells, and others inactivate autoreactive cells that have slipped through the screening process and survived to circulate in the body. As we become increasingly aware of these natural mechanisms for maintaining tolerance, we may be able to duplicate them therapeutically in individuals in whom self tolerance has been lost.

Central tolerance

The initial attempt to prevent autoimmune responses occurs in the early developmental stages of T and B lymphocytes. During development, developing T and B cells are programmed to respond to binding of their antigen receptors (TCRs or antibodies). Once circulating in the body and in the secondary immune organs, B and T cells respond to this receptor binding by undergoing activation and proliferating in the presence of additional appropriate signals. However, as discussed in Chapter 5, potentially self-reactive are eliminated before they leave the primary immune organs in which they develop. This process is termed **central tolerance**.

During **negative selection** within the thymus, thymocytes that survive an earlier *positive selection* process are exposed to antigen-presenting cells (APCs) that display an array of self peptides (see Fig. 5-5 for review). Developing T cells with TCRs that can bind these self-peptides (whether presented by MHC class I or MHC class II on the APCs) receive a death signal as a result of that binding and undergo apoptotic death. T lymphocytes that fail to bind self antigens survive negative selection, leave the thymus, and adjust their physiology so that binding of their antigen receptors once again provides a positive signal for differentiation and proliferation. As a result of positive and negative selection, about 99% of the thymocytes that begin the developmental process within the thymus are eliminated. Among these are large numbers of self-reactive cells that will never enter the circulation and initiate autoimmune responses.

B lymphocytes also undergo a form of negative selection in the bone marrow. Once their initial surface antigen receptors (IgMs) are expressed, they have the potential to bind molecules in the local environment that might fit their receptors. Unless there are infectious agents in the bone marrow, any such binding must involve self antigens. At this point in their developmental program, such binding triggers apoptosis and self-reactive B cells are eliminated. Again, it must be remembered that not all self epitopes are necessarily present in the bone marrow during this process. B cells that survive this selection process, by not binding to antigen, subsequently alter their physiology so that future binding of surface immunoglobulin will trigger signals leading to activation and proliferation once they have successfully migrated to the lymph nodes.

Peripheral tolerance

While the process of central tolerance removes a large portion of potentially autoreactive lymphocytes from the primary immune organs, it is not foolproof. Many lymphocytes still enter the circulation with the potential for recognizing and binding self antigens. For example, it seems unlikely that all self antigens in the body are avail-

able in the thymus and bone marrow for presentation during negative selection. Several additional mechanisms, collectively called *peripheral tolerance*, operate to control or eliminate these cells. One such mechanism is the induction of *anergy*, a state of nonresponsiveness on the part of a lymphocyte, even after binding of its receptor to an appropriate peptide +MHC (pMHC; T cell) or antigen (B cell).

In the case of T cells, recall that that interaction with APCs is required for activation (Chapter 5). T cells require binding of their receptors to an appropriate combination of pMHC I (in the case of CD8$^+$ T cells) or of pMHC II (in the case of CD4$^+$ T cells) on the surface of APCs. They must also receive signals from the APCs, some transmitted through soluble molecules and others through interaction of surface molecules on the T cells and APCs.

Consider, in contrast, what might happen if an autoreactive CD8$^+$ T cell were to recognize and bind some self pMHC I on a cell other than an APC (Fig. 9-1). If the CD8$^+$ T cell was already activated, this binding would be sufficient for the T cell to proceed with killing its target

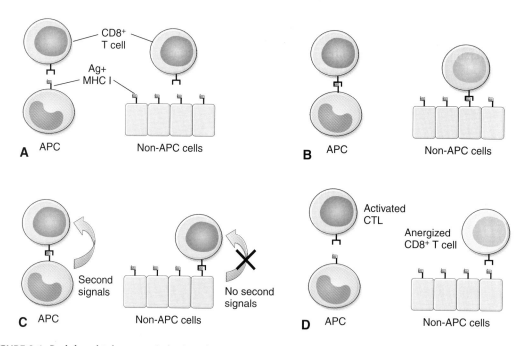

FIGURE 9-1. Peripheral tolerance—induction of anergy in naive CD8$^+$ T cells. Naive CD8$^+$ T cells can recognize **(A)** and bind **(B)** antigenic peptides presented by MHC class I molecules on both antigen-presenting cells (APCs) and non-APCs because all nucleated cells express MHC class I. Those binding to APCs receive second signals from the APCs that are necessary for activation and proliferation, while those binding to non-APCs do not **(C)**. Thus, those CD8$^+$ T cells that initially bind to APCs can be normally activated, but those that initially bind to non-APCs and fail to receive the second signals become permanently anergized **(D)**.

cell. This is the basis for some autoimmune diseases. The situation is different, however, for a "naïve" (never activated) CD8$^+$ T cell whose first act of recognition and binding is to a non-APC. If the mere act of TCR binding were sufficient for activation, such CD8$^+$ T cells could wreak havoc throughout the body because peptide-presenting MHC I molecules are expressed on all nucleated cells. However, the absence of APC-derived signals from the non-APC bound to the T cell prevents the normal activation process. Under experimental conditions, these APC signals can be supplied artificially, in which case activation proceeds.

Interaction of naive autoreactive T cells with non-APC targets is not without consequence, because in the absence of APC-derived second signals, the T cells become permanently anergized. The anergized cells are not killed but remain in circulation and, under most normal circumstances, cannot be activated by subsequent interaction with APCs. This state of anergy can be broken experimentally to activate these cells, and it may occur in the body under certain conditions (e.g., drug-induced autoimmune hepatitis). For example, a possible role for infection in breaking tolerance is described later in this chapter. In general, inducing anergy provides a major level of protection against autoreactive CD8$^+$ T cells that escape elimination through central tolerance.

Does this same method of inducing anergy also apply to naive CD4$^+$ T cells? Because APCs regularly ingest material from dead and dying cells, the regular presentation of self pMHC II to potentially self-reactive CD4$^+$ T cells must occur. CD4$^+$ T cells can be anergized in a way similar to CD8$^+$ cells. Under experimental conditions, the binding of naïve CD4$^+$ T cells to non-APCs renders them anergic because of the absence of necessary additional signals normally provided by APCs. Recall, however, that (with a few transient exceptions), MHC II molecules are expressed only by APCs, and so autoreactive CD4$^+$ T cells might not be expected to normally recognize and bind non-APC target cells because of the absence of a pMHC II combination on those target cell surfaces.

The need of naïve B cells for "help" from T cells through soluble signals and binding of surface molecules such as CD40 and CD154 (CD40 Ligand) (Chapter 5) provides a similar basis for inducing anergy in autoreactive B cells. Naïve B cells can be similarly anergized if their surface immunoglobulin binds to self antigens in the absence of the additional necessary T cell signals. Central and peripheral tolerance mechanisms should drastically reduce the chance that T cells specific for that same autoantigen will be available for interaction with the autoreactive B cells.

Suppression

Tolerance can also be maintained through the presence of regulatory cells that inhibit the activity of autoreactive lymphocytes. Numerous experimental systems have demonstrated that one subset of lymphocytes may inhibit the activity of other lymphocytes engaged in self-destructive responses. The molecular basis for these regulatory actions is still unclear but, in most cases, the regulatory cells are T cells. Among examples of this regulation are:

- CD4$^+$ T cells expressing CD25 may inhibit development of inflammatory bowel disease, an immune-mediated inflammatory disease.
- CD8$^+$ T cells may inhibit activation and proliferation of CD4$^+$ T cells, including some that mediate inflammatory delayed (-type) hypersensitivity (DTH) responses. Subpopulations of both CD8$^+$ and CD4$^+$ T cell subpopulations can inhibit the production of antibodies by specific B cells.

Alteration in the balance between Th1 and Th2 responses (Chapter 5) to a self antigen may sometimes result in autoimmune pathology. Consider a situation in which a Th2 response produces little or no pathology (because the relevant self-reactive B cells have been eliminated), but a Th1 response may produce a cell-mediated response such as DTH. If the response to that antigen in a particular individual becomes dominated by Th2 cells, then the Th1 cells are inhibited and the destructive processes leading to disease are diminished or eliminated. As discussed in Chapter 6, such a situation exists in the intestinal mucosal immune system of the gut-associated lymphoid tissues (GALT). The intestinal epithelial cells and the natural killer-like T cells (NKT cells) located within the intestinal epithelium produce IL-4, IL-10, and TGF-β, all antiinflammatory Th2 cytokines that create a microenvironment promoting production of antibodies, particularly IgA, and inhibiting inflammatory cellular responses.

Patient Vignette 9.1

Terence W., a 30-year-old man, presents with nonbloody diarrhea and right-sided abdominal pain. His laboratory tests reveal mild anemia and evidence of malabsorption. Imaging of the small intestine reveals evidence of mucosal swelling and ulceration.

Q: What is a likely explanation for this patient's problems?

A: The clinical signs and symptoms are consistent with Crohn's disease, a chronic inflammatory disorder involving the entire gastrointestinal tract. Crohn's disease is characterized by edema (swelling), fibrosis, and irregular ulcer formation in the gut wall. Fistulae may also form in the small intestine. For this patient, a biopsy of the intestinal mucosa may be helpful to support the diagnosis. Treatments for this disease include medications and, in cases unresponsive to medical therapy, surgery may be required. Therapy with antibodies against tumor necrosis factor-α may help to induce remission.

LOSS OF SELF TOLERANCE

Given all of the mechanisms that exist to maintain self tolerance, how does autoimmunity occur? What types of events can lead to a breakage of self tolerance? Several different situations have been found that create conditions under which this can occur.

Molecular mimicry and infectious agents

The antigenic molecules of some infectious agents bear structural similarities to molecules on host cells. This **molecular mimicry** provides an opportunity for autoimmunity triggered by cross-reactivity. If responses against the microbial antigen are sufficiently intense, they can also inflict injury on host cells and tissues that bear cross-reactive antigens (Fig. 9-2). The classic example of this mechanism is the heart damage that can follow **rheumatic fever**. Rheumatic fever is an inflammatory disease that can develop from pharyngeal infection with **Streptococcus pyogenes** ("strep"),

the causative agent of strep throat. Group A β-hemolytic strains of strep bacteria are rich in an antigen known as the M protein. IgM and IgG antibodies generated against M protein can cross-react with molecules on the sarcolemmal membranes and valves of the heart. If sufficiently intense, their binding can lead to valve damage that can impair cardiac function. Some of these antibodies are also able to cross-react with host molecules found in kidneys and joints. Over time, this damage may eventually lead to fatal complications. It is therefore important to identify the presence of strep when patients present with sore throats so that antibiotic treatment can be applied promptly to eliminate the infection before the patient's immune system generates high levels of antibody against strep antigens (Chapter 11).

Another example of molecular mimicry in autoimmune disease is type I diabetes mellitus, where the immune system attacks and destroys the pancreatic islet β cells that produce insulin. Cross-reactivity has been demonstrated between fragments of glutamate decarboxylase (GAD), a pancreatic islet β cell enzyme that is a major target of autoreactive T cells in individuals with type I diabetes, and peptide fragments from Cocksackie virus and cytomegalovirus. In addition, T cell cross-reactivity has been demonstrated between islet β cell tyrosine phosphatase IA-2 and peptides from several infectious agents (including cytomegalovirus, measles virus, hepatitis C virus, and *Hemophilus influenzae*).

Other autoimmune diseases may be attributable to molecular mimicry, although the mechanisms are not known as clearly as in the case of rheumatic fever. A group of diseases known as **reactive arthritis** are often associated with infectious organisms involved in food poisoning or diarrhea, and sometimes with other autoimmune diseases (e.g., psoriasis) as well. One of these, **ankylosing spondylitis** (an inflammatory disease usually involving the lower spine), occurs with elevated frequency in individuals carrying the HLA-B27 gene, as do several other forms of reactive arthritis. Some homology between the HLA-B27 molecules and a protein expressed by **Klebsiella** bacteria has been noted, and a similar homology between HLA-B27 and a *Klebsiella* protein occurs in **Reiter's disease** (a form of reactive arthritis affecting the joints of the lower limbs and the gastrointestinal/genital/urinary tracts). Protein sequence homologies have also been found between the acetylcholine receptor and poliovirus, and between papilloma virus and the insulin receptor. The acetylcholine receptor is the

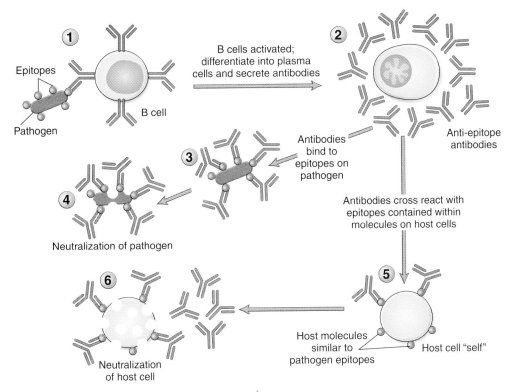

FIGURE 9-2. **Molecular mimicry as a source of autoimmunity.** Pathogen antigens are recognized by B cells **(1)**. With appropriate T cell help, activated B cells differentiate into plasma cells and secrete antibodies against the antigens of the pathogens **(2)**. The antibodies can bind to antigens on pathogens **(3)**, leading to their damage and death **(4)**. If host cells ("self") express molecules that are similar to the pathogen antigens, the antibodies can cross-react and bind to host cells **(5)**, a process that can lead to immune-mediated destruction of normal body cells **(6)**.

target antigen in **myasthenia gravis** (muscle weakness due to decreased ability to receive stimulation from motor nerves), and the insulin receptor in **hypoglycemia** (low blood sugar levels). Together, these types of homologies suggest that molecular mimicry is a strong possibility as a mechanism for generating some autoimmune diseases.

Infectious agents may play an additional role in facilitating the breakage of tolerance. It has been shown in experimental systems that the secondary signals produced by APCs for T cell activation can be mimicked by adding sufficient quantities of appropriate exogenous cytokines. Because of the innate and adaptive immune responses to microbes, areas of inflammation rich in proinflammatory cytokines can develop in vivo. An autoreactive T cell, binding to a self antigen within such an environment, could conceivably receive sufficient exogenous stimulation to undergo activation without direct interaction with an APC. Although demonstrated experimentally in vivo, activation of T cells in this way has yet to be clearly demonstrated in vitro because of

technical difficulties. However, the observation that autoimmune diseases often develop after infection is consistent with some research studies.

> ### Patient Vignette 9.2
>
> Tina W., a 13-year-old girl, presents with polyuria, polydipsia, and polyphagia over the past three days. In addition, she has noticed some weight loss despite eating a lot of food.
>
> Q: *What immunologic processes might be involved in her problems?*
>
> A: This patient probably has diabetes mellitus, most likely diabetes mellitus type I, an autoimmune disease in which the islet cells of the pancreas are destroyed. The onset of diabetes mellitus type I usually occurs in young individuals, such as this patient. Tina W.'s symptoms are due to high glucose levels causing glycosuria (urinary excretion of glucose).

Neoantigens

Responses to neoantigens are not truly autoimmune, because the neoantigens are altered self antigens rather than true self antigens. However, the consequences are similar and some diseases that are currently thought to be truly autoimmune might actually be caused by unidentified environmental agents creating neoantigens. Neoantigens are formed by modification of self antigens by, for example, the chemical binding of another reactive molecule (Chapter 8). The modified self antigen, however, may be sufficiently different from the native form to be perceived as foreign by the immune system. In general, responses against these neoantigens should resolve following the removal of the agent that is causing their formation. True autoantigens should be self-perpetuating, unless completely destroyed and eliminated.

An example of this mechanism occurs in some forms of **drug-induced hemolytic anemia** (Fig. 8-5). Penicillin is a small reactive molecule that can bind not only to microbial surfaces, but also to proteins on erythrocyte surfaces. Other drugs capable of similar actions include cephalosporins, levodopa, methyldopa, quinine, salicylic acid, sulfonimide, streptomycin, and others. The binding can create neoantigens on erythrocyte surfaces that, in some individuals, trigger antibodies that bind to the erythrocytes and lead to complement-mediated lysis.

Neoantigens can be formed by means other than chemical binding. If heat-denatured thyroglobulin is injected into an experimental animal, an experimental autoimmune thyroiditis develops. This disease can become self-perpetuating because the immune response against the denatured thyroglobulin could react with native thyroglobulin. In addition, the transformation of normal cells into cancer cells may include mutations of molecules into variant forms that may be recognized as foreign by the immune system. These could be viewed as another form of neoantigen, but one that is self-perpetuating.

Loss of suppression

As mentioned previously, some autoimmune responses are prevented by the action of suppressor cells. There is some evidence that the suppressor cells keeping self-reactive cells in check may be lost with age. Thus, as individuals get older, the opportunity increases for self-reactive lymphocytes to escape such regulation and begin to mount active autoimmune responses. This is one of the explanations postulated for some autoimmune diseases such as SLE, where the appearance of cells and antibodies reacting against fragments of nucleic acids and chromosomal proteins generally increases with age. It should be kept in mind that age-related increases in disease frequency may also simply reflect a longer time span over which the immune system has an opportunity for error.

Patient Vignette 9.3

Sharon T., a 30-year-old woman, presents with joint pain in the hands, malar rash (erythema on the nose and cheeks), fatigue, and weight loss. A blood test reveals a positive antinuclear antibody test and anemia.

Q: What immunologic processes might be involved in her problems?

A: This patient may have lupus erythematosus (SLE). The disease stems from the development of autoantibodies against fragments of nucleic acids and chromosomal proteins, and is conducive to secondary development of type III hypersensitivity reactions. In 1982, the American College of Rheumatology provided criteria for the diagnosis of SLE which requires the presence of four of the 11 following criteria: (1) malar ("butterfly") rash, (2) discoid skin lesion, (3) photosensitivity, (4) oral ulcers, (5) nonserosive arthritis, (6) serositis, (7) renal disorder, (8) neurological disorder, (9) hematologic disorder, (10) immunological disorder, (11) antinuclear antibody.

Sequestered antigens

The body contains some molecules that are seldom, if ever, available to the immune system for various reasons. In the seminiferous tubules, for example, the spermatogonia and developing sperm cells are not exposed to the immune system because the tubules are sealed off during fetal development by a sheath of tightly joined Sertoli cells prior to the development of the immune system. Thus, there is no opportunity for the immune system to "learn" that molecules unique to spermatogonia, and the subsequent multiple stages in development of sperm, are self antigens. If the immune system is exposed later to these molecules (e.g., through injury to the testicles), they will be viewed as foreign and may be attacked by the immune system (Fig. 9-3). Some cases of male sterility may be attributable to immune responses against an individual's own sperm.

Sheltered sites, such as the interior of the seminiferous tubules, are called **immunologically privileged sites**. Other examples include the anterior chamber and cornea of the eye, the brain, and the uterine environment surrounding the developing fetus. The anterior chamber and cornea of the eye are sequestered from the immune system because of minimal exposure to the vasculature, unless breached by injury or infection. With diminished access by the immune system, some molecules within these sites may not be recognized as self, and their subsequent release viewed by the immune system as an influx of foreign antigens. The blood-brain barrier limits passage of cells and molecules between the brain and the vasculature because the endothelial cells of capillaries in the central nervous system are denser and joined more tightly than in the rest of the body, allowing only small molecules such as oxygen, carbon dioxide, and sugars to pass without difficulty.

Mechanisms that are not yet clearly defined also prevent the maternal immune system from attacking paternally derived antigens of the fetus, with the exception of IgG crossing the placental barrier. Women frequently display antibodies and cellular responses against the foreign tissue antigens (histocompatibility antigens, Chapter 10) of their sexual partners. Yet these reactive cells and molecules are prevented from crossing the placenta to bind and attack antigens expressed by the fetus, and the uterine environment is considered by some to be an immunologically privileged site that protects the developing fetus.

A significant exception to this "placental protection" involves the Rh blood group antigen system. As described in Chapter 5, antibodies of the IgG isotype can cross the placenta to provide passive protection to the fetus. Thus, IgG antibodies generated against the Rh antigen by Rh^- mothers can cross the placenta and attack erythrocytes of Rh^+ fetuses. Sufficient destruction of fetal erythrocytes leads to **erythroblastosis fetalis**, a life threatening condition (see Chapters 10 and 11 for further discussion). That situation represents neither true autoimmunity nor tolerance, but reflects a natural breach in the ability of an immunologically privileged site to completely shelter internal elements from the immune system.

A molecular equivalent of privileged sites exists.

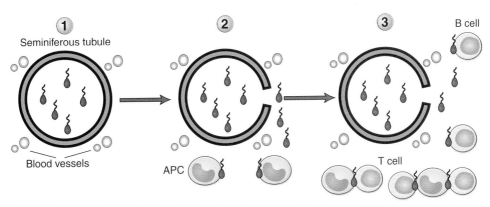

① Seminiferous tubule	②	③ B cell
Blood vessels	APC	T cell
Sperm-related cells and molecules are sequestered within seminiferous tubule	Breach of seminiferous tubules allows sperm-related cells and molecules to escape privileged site; peptides processed and presented by APCs	T and B lymphocytes specific for sperm-related antigens bind and become activated

FIGURE 9-3. Sequestered antigens—the seminiferous tubule. Cells and molecules related to formation of sperm are sequestered within the seminiferous tubules, which form prior to development of the immune system **(1)**, and tight gap junctions in the Sertoli cells surrounding the tubules seals the interior off from the rest of the body, including the immune system. Thus, the immune system does not learn to recognize them as "self." When a breach occurs in the seminiferous tubules, sperm-related cells and molecules can become available to the immune system **(2)**, which views them as "foreign" and may generate immune responses against them **(3)**. Autoimmune responses against sperm, etc. may account for 2–3% of male sterility cases.

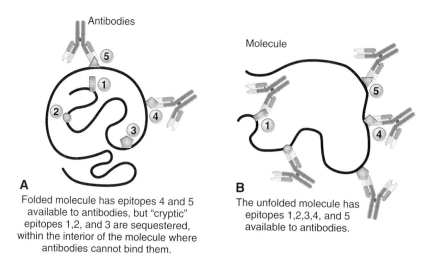

A
Folded molecule has epitopes 4 and 5 available to antibodies, but "cryptic" epitopes 1, 2, and 3 are sequestered, within the interior of the molecule where antibodies cannot bind them.

B
The unfolded molecule has epitopes 1, 2, 3, 4, and 5 available to antibodies.

FIGURE 9-4. Cryptic epitopes. (A) When molecules are in their normal folded and three-dimensional configurations, some epitopes may be "hidden" within the interior of the molecular scaffolding and unavailable for binding by antibodies. **(B)** When these molecules are unfolded (e.g., following denaturation), formerly cryptic or "hidden" epitopes may now be available to antibodies.

The three-dimensional configuration of molecules may conceal epitopes protected from the immune system by lying within folds or depressions (Fig. 9-4). However, if the molecule changes shape as the result of interaction with another molecule, or changes in pH or temperature, these **cryptic epitopes** may become exposed and available to binding by antibodies. **Rheumatoid factor** is an example of this process. When IgG antibodies bind to antigen, their Fc regions undergo conformational changes. These changes expose sites that are used for binding of complement component C1 and Fc receptors. They also expose sites that can serve as targets of IgM antibodies (see Fig. 8-7). These IgM anti-IgG antibodies are the rheumatoid factors and are characteristic of several inflammatory autoimmune diseases, including rheumatoid arthritis. Their ability to bind IgG molecules that are already bound to antigens can amplify the formation of immune complexes capable of generating type III hypersensitivity responses (immune complex disease, Chapter 8). Rheumatoid factors are found in other diseases as well and can sometimes be of the IgG or IgA isotype.

Epitope spreading

Multiple sclerosis results from immune-mediated destruction of myelin, the material that encloses and protects neuronal axons, like the insulation layer surrounding a telephone wire, to facilitate the transmission of electrochemical impulses from one neuron to another. Loss of myelin im-

pairs the conduction of nerve signals and subsequent motor responses. Experimental models suggest that anti-myelin immune responses are triggered in various ways, one involving infectious agents in areas that are rich in myelin. Immune responses to clear the infections can cause "innocent bystander" damage to the nearby myelin, and the debris generated as the myelin is destroyed can eventually trigger new immune responses directed at the myelin itself. Myelin is normally sequestered in the central nervous system because of the blood-brain barrier, but infection and other sources of inflammation can impair this barrier, permitting increased infiltration by cells and molecules of the immune system. Thus, responses originally directed at infectious agents can create conditions leading to subsequent autoimmune responses. This phenomenon, **epitope spreading**, provides another basis for the association seen between some autoimmune diseases and infectious agents. Epitope spreading has been suggested as contributing to SLE, inflammatory bowel disease, and some forms of diabetes.

HUMORAL AND CELL-MEDIATED PATHOLOGIES

Autoimmune diseases vary in the immune responses responsible for the pathological changes that occur (Table 9-3). Sometimes the inflammatory pathology is due to type II or type III hypersensitivity reactions triggered by autoantigen-spe-

TABLE 9-3. PATHOLOGICAL BASES OF AUTOIMMUNE DISEASES

Disease	Pathological Basis (Hypersensitivity Reactions)
Autoimmune hemolytic anemia	Type II
Goodpasture's syndrome	Type II
Hashimoto's thyroiditis	Type II
Type I insulin dependent diabetes mellitus	Type IV
Multiple sclerosis	Type IV
Reactive arthritis	Type IV
Rheumatoid arthritis	Type III; Type IV
Rheumatic fever	Type II
Systemic lupus erythematosus	Type II; Type III

cific antibodies. Autoreactive T cells are present in these diseases as well, and are required for activation of the autoreactive B cells, but do not contribute directly to the pathology. Other autoimmune diseases are based on pathology mediated by cytotoxic T cells or DTH (type IV hypersensitivity reactions). Some diseases involve both antibody-driven and cell-mediated pathologies. In some diseases, the determination of pathologies is determined from experimental models.

Patient Vignette 9.4

Bertha V., a 60-year-old woman, presents with atrial fibrillation (abnormal heart rhythm). The patient says that for the last several months she has experienced intermittent palpitation, has lost approximately ten pounds, and has mild heat intolerance and frequent bowel movements. Physical examination revealed an anxious female with slight exophthalmos (protrusion of the eyeball) and hand resting tremor (involuntary shaking). The patient also mentioned that her mother also had similar symptoms many years ago and died because there was no treatment.

Q: *What immunologic processes might be involved in her problems?*

A: This patient has the signs and symptoms of hyperthyroidism (increased thyroid hormone secretion) consistent with Grave's

(continued)

Patient Vignette 9.4 (Continued)

disease. The underlying mechanism of Grave's disease is the development of autoantibodies that bind to and activate the thyroid stimulating hormone receptor. This disease is more common in women than in men and there may be a positive family history. The diagnosis is confirmed by measuring thyroid hormone levels. In older patients, atrial fibrillation is a frequent presentation of Grave's disease.

HLA ASSOCIATION WITH AUTOIMMUNE DISEASES

We have previously discussed the fact that the frequency of the HLA-B27 gene is elevated in individuals with various forms of reactive arthritis, such as ankylosing spondylitis. An association is seen for many other autoimmune diseases, both organ-specific and systemic (Table 9-4). The precise molecular basis for these associations is still unclear, but the use of specific HLA genes for presentation of certain autoantigens must some-

TABLE 9-4. MHC ASSOCIATIONS WITH AUTOIMMUNE DISEASES

Disease	Associated HLA Gene[1]	Relative Risk[2]
Acute uveitis	B27	10
Ankylosing spondylitis	B27	100
Goodpasture's syndrome	DR2	15
Grave's disease	DR3	4
Hashimoto's thyroiditis	DR5	3
Type I insulin-dependent diabetes mellitus	DR3/DR4 heterozygote	2–25
Multiple sclerosis	DR2	5
	DR3	10
Myasthenia gravis	DR3	3
	B8	3
Pemphigus vulgaris	DR4	15
Psoriasis vulgaris	Cw6	5–13
Reiter's disease	B27	35
Rheumatoid arthritis	DR4	4
SLE	DR3	6

[1] Studies done with different populations may implicate different genes.
[2] Relative risks vary somewhat among different studies. Values given are typical.

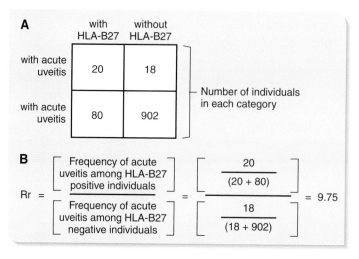

FIGURE 9-5. Relative risk. Relative risk (R_r) is a measure of the association between the development of a particular disease and the presence of some risk factor, such as a particular gene in the example presented. It represents the frequency of the disease (in this case, acute uveitis) among carriers of the gene in question (in this case, HLA-B27) compared to the frequency of the same disease among individuals without the gene in question. In the example presented, a survey found that 20/100 HLA-B27-positive individuals had acute uveitis. There were only 18 cases of acute uveitis among the 920 individuals in the study who were negative for HLA-B27. After determining the number of individuals (not the percentages!) in each possible category **(A)**, the R_r can be calculated as shown **(B)**. In this case, the risk of acute uveitis among HLA-B27 carriers is nearly ten-fold greater than among those who do not carry HLA-B27.

how preferentially trigger autoreactive T cells. Certain HLA genes (e.g., B27, DR2, DR3, DR4) appear to be implicated most frequently and are associated with multiple autoimmune diseases.

The strength of the association between the occurrence of an autoimmune disease and the presence of a particular HLA gene is expressed as *the relative risk*. Relative risk compares the frequency of the disease in question among individuals carrying a particular gene with the disease frequency among individuals who do not carry the gene (Fig. 9-5). For example, the risk of acute uveitis in carriers of HLA-B27 is approximately ten-fold greater than among those without HLA-B27 (see example in Fig. 9-5). While the relative risk may sometimes be very high, as in the case of ankylosing spondylitis and HLA-B27 (~100), it is more typically in the range of 2 to 5. A low relative risk is also a reminder that, while the gene in question may be involved, it is only one of several factors.

Summary

- **Autoimmune diseases** are common. Rheumatoid arthritis, psoriasis, multiple sclerosis, and some forms of diabetes are well known examples of such diseases. Autoimmunity is a complex situation with multiple mech-anisms, multiple causes, and multiple modifying factors.
- The process of eliminating potentially reactive lymphocytes before they leave the primary immune organs in which they develop is termed *central tolerance*.
- Several mechanisms, collectively called *peripheral tolerance*, have developed that can control or eliminate autoreactive cells. Tolerance can also be maintained through the presence of regulatory cells that inhibit the activity of autoreactive lymphocytes.
- The incidence of autoimmune diseases generally increases with age, possibly because suppressor T cells that inhibit some autoimmune responses are lost over time.
- *Molecular mimicry* provides an opportunity for autoimmunity triggered by cross-reactivity. The classic example of this mechanism involves rheumatic fever.
- A group of diseases known as *reactive arthritis* are often associated with infection by infectious organisms involved in food poisoning or diarrhea, and sometimes with other autoimmune diseases. *Ankylosing spondylitis* and other forms of reactive arthritis occur with elevated frequency in individuals carrying the HLA-B27 gene.

- Self antigens modified by reactions with externally derived agents may become sufficiently different from the native form to be recognized as foreign by the immune system. An example of this mechanism occurs in some forms of drug-induced hemolytic anemia.
- Molecules change shape as the result of interaction with another molecule, or because of changes in pH or temperature. In doing so, hidden or *cryptic epitopes* may become exposed and available to binding by other antibodies. *Rheumatoid factor* is an example of this process.
- *Epitope spreading*, in which immune responses against one epitope may facilitate the development of responses against other epitopes, provides a basis for the association seen between some infectious agents and autoimmune diseases.
- Autoimmune diseases vary in terms of the types of immune responses responsible for the pathological changes seen. In some cases, the inflammatory pathology is caused by type II or type III hypersensitivities triggered by binding

of autoantigen-specific antibodies. In other cases, the pathology may result from type IV cell-mediated hypersensitivities.
- Many autoimmune diseases, both local and systemic, are associated with certain HLA genes. The strength of the association between a particular HLA gene and an autoimmune disease is expressed as the *relative risk.*

Suggested readings

Cohen PL. Systemic autoimmunity. In Paul WE, ed. *Fundamental immunology*, 5th ed. Philadelphia: Lippincott Williams & Wilkins, 2003.

Eisenberg R. Mechanisms of autoimmunity. *Immunol Res* 2003;27:203.

Herrath MG, Homann D. Organ-specific autoimmunity. In Paul WE, ed. *Fundamental immunology*, 5th ed. Philadelphia: Lippincott Williams & Wilkins, 2003.

Janeway CA Jr., Travers P, Walport M, Shlomchik P. Autoimmunity and transplantation. In *Immunobiology: The immune system in health and disease*, 6th ed. Philadephia: Garland Publishing, 2004.

Pleister A, Eckels DD. Cryptic infection and autoimmunity. *Autoimmun Rev* 2003;2:126.

Shevach EM. Regulatory T cells in autoimmunity. *Annu Rev Immunol* 2002;18:423.

Review questions

DIRECTIONS: Each of the numbered items or incomplete statements in this section is followed by answers or by completions of the statement. Select the ONE lettered answer or completion that is BEST in each case.

1. An individual carrying which of the following HLA genes has an elevated risk of developing ankylosing spondylitis?
   (A) HLA-A8
   (B) HLA-DR3
   (C) HLA-B15
   (D) HLA-B27
   (E) HLA-DR2

2. Which of the following is a logical cause of autoimmunity?
   (A) Complete negative selection of T cells
   (B) Cross reactivity of self-antigens with antigens on infectious organisms
   (C) IgE-mediated inflammation
   (D) Ablation of the thymus
   (E) Increased numbers of suppressor cells

3. Individuals developing systemic lupus erythematosus (SLE) generate high levels of an-

tibodies against fragments of their own nucleic acids and chromosomal proteins. Many of the accompanying signs (skin rash, joint pain, kidney damage) are present because the individuals are predisposed toward what other types of diseases?
   (A) Immediate hypersensitivity
   (B) Delayed (-type) hypersensitivity
   (C) Immune complex disease
   (D) Contact sensitivity
   (E) Immunodeficiency

4. Individuals with rheumatoid arthritis usually display elevated levels of "rheumatoid factor." Rheumatoid factor in these patients consists of:
   (A) antigen-IgE complexes.
   (B) IL-4 and IL-10.
   (C) C5a.
   (D) IgM antibodies that are specific for exposed sites on Ag-bound IgG.
   (E) secretory IgA bound to the synovial membrane that triggers the alternative pathway of complement activation.

5. The binding of a naïve CD8+ T cell to an

antigenic peptide presented by an MHC class I molecule on the surface of a non-APC target cell results in what consequence for the T cell?

(A) Activation
(B) A lytic attack upon the target cell
(C) Proliferation
(D) Apoptosis
(E) Anergy

6. Drug-induced hemolytic anemias arise because of the development of neoantigens. Neoantigens can be formed by which of the following means?

(A) Binding of an antibody to its specific epitope
(B) Processing and presentation of epitopes derived from infectious agents
(C) Binding of a reactive chemical to a self molecule
(D) Mutation of a T cell receptor
(E) Release of sequestered antigens

7. Autoimmune responses against epitopes associated with development of sperm are thought most likely to arise through:

(A) the release of sequestered antigens from an immunologically privileged site.
(B) molecular mimicry following streptococcal infections.
(C) loss of immune suppression.
(D) action of the HLA-B27 gene.
(E) immune deficiency.

8. Individuals carrying HLA-B27 have a relative risk of 35 for developing Reiter's disease. This means that:

(A) the frequency of Reiter's disease in the population is 35 per 1000 individuals.
(B) they have a 35-fold greater risk of developing Reiter's disease than do individuals who do not carry HLA-B27.
(C) they have a 35% chance of having an affected blood relative with Reiter's disease.
(D) the likelihood is 35% that two individuals with Reiter's disease are related to each other by blood.
(E) 35% of families include an individual with Reiter's disease.

Transplantation

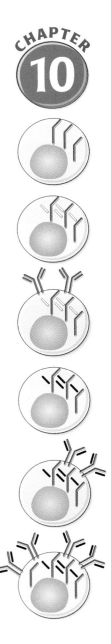

Chapter Outline

Introduction Organ and tissue transplantation has been a dream since ancient times. The possibility of removing body parts from the dead and using them to replace those of the living whose own had become diseased, injured, or lost seems a simple and logical idea. Indeed, as early as the first few centuries of the modern era, members of the potter's caste of India learned to shift skin on an individual's face in order to partially repair the mutilations (e.g., removal of the nose) that were used as a form of judicial punishment. This procedure did not reach Europe until 1597, when Gaspare Tagliacozzi used it on a patient in Bologna, Italy, transferring a piece of skin from the patient's arm to his face. Despite Fra Angelico's famous depiction of St. Cosmas and St. Damian performing a leg transplant in the third century, transplantation between different individuals was not realized until the mid-twentieth century.

The first systematic studies of transplantation were done in laboratory mice, often during studies on the role of the immune system in resisting cancer. If pieces of cancerous tissue were transplanted from one mouse to another, the cancerous graft would survive only occasionally. Shortly before 1930, Tyzzer and Little concluded that the deciding factor determining whether the transplanted tissue survived was the genetic relationship between the tissue donor and the recipient. The more closely related the host and donor, the more likely that the transplanted tissue would survive. Over the next two to three decades, pioneers in the field, such as Peter Gorer and George Snell, recognized that the immune system could recognize not only antigens from foreign sources (such as infectious microbes) but also molecules encoded within the body. The genes encoding these molecules were termed **histocompatibility genes** and their products were designated **histocompatibility antigens**. The first of these genes to be defined was the major histocompatibility complex (MHC) of the mouse, the H2 complex. The human equivalent, the human leukocyte antigen (HLA) complex, was discovered in the mid-1950s by Jean Daussett. It was later found that the MHC was not a single gene locus, but a tightly linked set of loci.

Histocompatibility antigens play a key role in the acceptance or rejection of transplanted tissue. When tissues are transplanted from one individual to another, the immune system of the recipient recognizes histocompatibility antigens on the cells of the donor tissue. If the donor tissue contains histocompatibility antigens that are not already present on host cells, the donor tissues are viewed as foreign and are destroyed.

While the initial experiments defining this phenomenon were done with transplanted tumor tissue, Dr. Peter Medawar demonstrated that the same principles applied to the transplantation of normal tissues. His immediate concern was the transplantation of tissue, particularly skin, to treat burn wounds suffered by pilots in World War II, but his discoveries held enormous implications for future clinical developments, such the therapeutic use of transplanted hearts, kidneys, bone marrow, and other organs. The next substantial advances toward successful transplantation were dependent upon the discovery of agents that could inhibit the immune system's ability to attack transplanted tissues without eradicating the entire immune response.

TYPES OF GRAFTS

Grafts, the transplanted pieces of tissue, are classified in a number of ways: by the genetic relationship between the donor and host; by the location; and, of course, by the type of tissue involved. Of these classifications, the most complex is the terminology used to define the genetic relationship. These terms arose with the development of specialized types of experimental animals, most commonly involving the mouse. In studying the genetic role in transplantation, researchers found it imperative to make the genetic component a controlled variable rather than an uncontrolled one. When tissues are exchanged between random members of a genetically diverse species (such as humans) it is difficult, if not impossible, to attribute the success or failure of a particular transplant to any gene or set of genes because the genetic combinations cannot be reliably repeated and confirmed in other individuals. In fact, it is usually not known which genes differ and which are the same between the host and donor. The solution to this problem lay with the development of specialized experimental organisms.

The development of specialized types of mice provided the key to understanding the role that genes play in transplantation. If mice are repeatedly bred by using brother × sister matings for 20 or more consecutive generations, the result is a set of mice that are more than 99% identical for all of their genes, with the obvious exception of those determining whether the mouse is male or female (Fig. 10-1). These sets, termed **inbred strains**, have been developed not only for mice, but for rats and rabbits and many experimental plants as well. With the availability of inbred strains, it is possible to repeat experimental transplants, for example between strain A and strain B, knowing that the genetics of the A and B mice are consistent from one experiment to another. Likewise, one can generate **hybrids** (offspring from genetically different parents) between inbred strains (e.g., AB hybrids from matings of type A mothers and type B fathers). Again, it is possible to utilize these hybrids with the assurance that the genetic combinations are consistent from experiment to experiment and that the genetic variation can be controlled by the appropriate selection of the animals to be used.

When tissues are transplanted between members of different inbred strains, they are typically rejected. While the results from one set of exper-

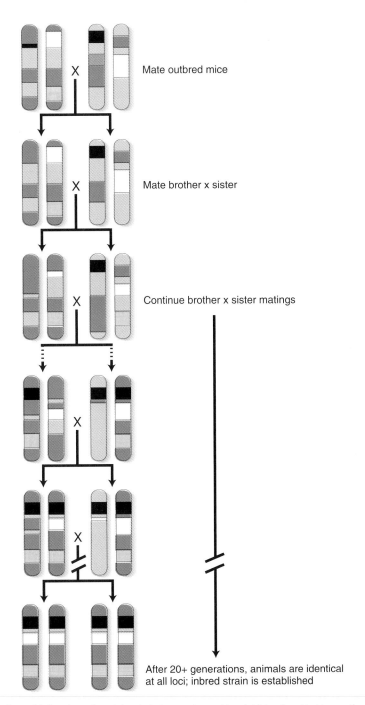

X — Mate outbred mice

X — Mate brother x sister

X — Continue brother x sister matings

X

X

After 20+ generations, animals are identical
at all loci; inbred strain is established

FIGURE 10-1. Formation of inbred strains. Inbred strains are formed by strict brother × sister matings for a minimum of 20 consecutive generations. The resulting animals are more than 99% homogenous, except for sex.

imental animals to the next may be consistent, inbred strains differ from one another at many genetic loci, and the role of any particular gene or set of genes can be determined only by developing additional types of experimental strains. With a careful program of breeding and selection, it is possible to "move" genes from one inbred strain into another to produce *congenic strains* (Fig. 10-2). Ten or more consecutive generations of such breeding and selection produces a set of animals that differs from one of its original parental types by only a small chromosomal segment. Thus, the influence of gene(s) lying within that segment on transplantation can be assessed (Fig. 10-3).

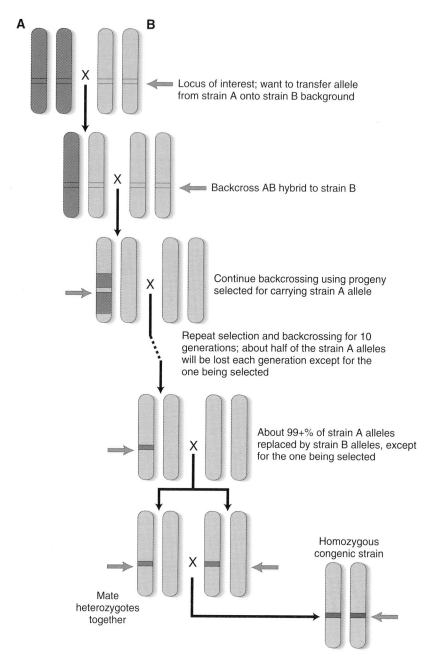

A

B

X

Locus of interest; want to transfer allele from strain A onto strain B background

X

Backcross AB hybrid to strain B

X

Continue backcrossing using progeny selected for carrying strain A allele

Repeat selection and backcrossing for 10 generations; about half of the strain A alleles will be lost each generation except for the one being selected

X

About 99+% of strain A alleles replaced by strain B alleles, except for the one being selected

Homozygous congenic strain

X

Mate heterozygotes together

FIGURE 10-2. Formation of congenic strains. Congenic strains result from the transfer of a particular gene from one inbred strain (A) to replace the equivalent gene in another inbred strain (B). They are formed by a systematic regiment in which animals are backcrossed to one of the parental inbred strains (B) for a minimum of ten generations. At each generation, only the animals carrying the desired A gene are selected to continue the breeding. After ten generations, almost all of the strain A genes (except the desired one that has been intentionally selected) have been replaced by strain B genes. By mating heterozygotes, homozygotes can be generated that differ from strain B only by the gene(s) derived from strain A.

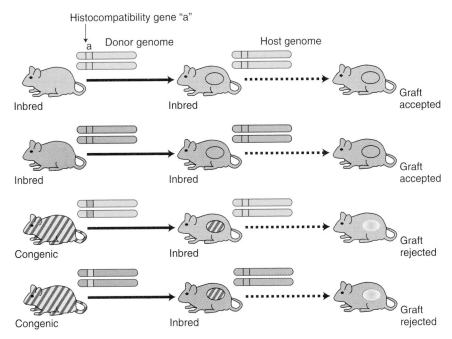

FIGURE 10-3. Association of gene (a) with transplant rejection using congenic strains. Transplants between experimental animals of different inbred strains are almost always rejected, but because they differ at so many histocompatibility genes, the effect is a composite one. Transplanting grafts between experimental animals differing at only one or a few histocompatibility genes allows assessment of the effects of individual gene differences on transplantation.

With these experiments in mind, the types of grafts based on the genetic relationship between the host and donor are:

- **Autograft**: a transplant from one part of an individual to another part of the same individual.
- **Syngeneic graft**: a transplant from one individual to a genetically identical individual, for example, an identical twin or another member of the same inbred strain. In older publications, these are sometimes also called **isografts**.
- **Allograft or allogeneic graft**: a transplant from one individual to a genetically different member of the same species. For example, a graft between a human parent and child would be an allograft. In older publications, these are sometimes also called **homografts**.
- **Xenograft**: a transplant between members of different species.

As stated previously, grafts are also sometimes classified by their locations:

- **Orthotopic graft**: a graft placed into its normal anatomical location.
- **Heterotopic graft**: a graft placed somewhere other than its normal anatomical location.

HISTOCOMPATIBILITY GENES AND ANTIGENS

All tissues express antigens consisting of genetically encoded molecules on the cell surfaces. These cell surface molecules identify the tissue genetically and are called **histocompatibility antigens**. The genes that encode the antigens are **histocompatibility genes**. Different allelic forms of these genes, carried by different inbred strains, account for the histocompatibility differences between different strains.

There are many histocompatibility loci (and antigens). Almost any surface or cytoplasmic protein that can exist in two different allelic forms can serve as a histocompatibility antigen. While the genetically outbred nature of humans makes it difficult to estimate the number of histocompatibility genes, experiments using inbred mice suggest that there are probably at least 100, about half of which have been individually identified.

Histocompatibility genes (and their antigenic products) are commonly divided into two broad groups: those encoded within the major histocompatibility complex and those encoded elsewhere (Table 10-1). The major histocompatibility genes are composed of the MHC I and MHC II

TABLE 10-1. HISTOCOMPATIBILITY GENES/ANTIGENS		
Location	Major MHC (Class I and II)	Minor All Chromosomes
Number of loci	5–10	100+
Rejection response	Typically rapid and vigorous	variable
Antibodies generated	++++	+/−
Cellular immunity	++++	++
Polymorphism	high	low
Function	Ag presentation	varied
Ease of tolerization	difficult	easier

loci. In experimental systems, where the effects of specific gene differences between hosts and donors can be studied with large sample sizes (in the absence of therapeutic intervention), differences at MHC class I and class II loci typically lead to strong, consistent destructive immune responses against the grafted tissues. At the other end of the spectrum, differences at the non-MHC histocompatibility genes (also called **minor histocompatibility genes**) generate, as a rule, weaker and less consistent rejections. The reasons for this disparity are unclear. However, m inor histocompatibility genes have a significant effect on graft survival because the large number of non-MHC molecules that can serve as minor histocompatibility antigens means that many such responses may be simultaneously generated.

T cells can be activated against histocompatibility antigens in two ways: by direct recognition or indirect recognition (Fig. 10-4). If at least some of the MHC class I or II molecules between the host and donor match, antigen-presenting cells (APCs) within the graft tissues may present antigen to host T cells and activate them. This constitutes **direct recognition** and can include presentation of foreign non-MHC molecules from the graft. In addition, if a graft bears MHC class I or II molecules that are "foreign" to the host, the MHC molecules themselves can serve as stimulating antigens. During their synthesis in the cytoplasm, some MHC molecules are degraded by proteasomes and the resulting fragments are presented, on the cell surface, by other intact MHC class I molecules. Foreign MHC (especially class I) molecules present a strong barrier to transplant survival, and it is estimated that 5% to 10% of an individual's T cells can recognize and bind fragments of foreign MHC I. **Indirect stimulation** occurs when a graft-borne MHC I that is not, in and of itself, foreign to the host presents a cytoplasmic peptide fragment that is foreign.

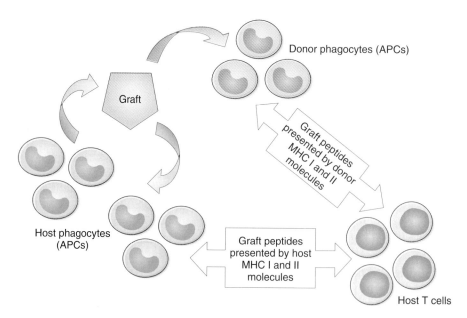

FIGURE 10-4. Direct and indirect recognition of graft antigens. Direct recognition occurs when donor antigen-presenting cells (APCs) within the graft present antigen directly to host T cells. Indirect recognition occurs when host APCs ingest material from the graft, process, and present the donor antigens to host T cells.

THE LAWS OF TRANSPLANTATION

With the discovery of a genetic influence on transplantation, researchers began to look intensively at the way in which these genes exerted their effects. Histocompatibility antigens are (with a very few rare and mysterious exceptions) codominantly expressed. That is, every functional allele encoded is expressed, whether homozygous or heterozygous. As a result, a general set of predictions can be made (Fig. 10-5), the basic "**laws of transplantation**." Hosts and donors that are identical (AA to AA, BB to BB, etc.) should be completely compatible. Hybrids (e.g., AB) should be able to accept grafts from either parental type (AA or BB), but their tissues should be rejected by those parents because they express histocompatibility antigens foreign to each parent. Simply put, *a host can recognize as foreign, and mount a response against, any histocompatibility antigen not encoded within its own cells.* The immune system can be exquisitely sensitive to the introduction of foreign tissue. In fact, it has been demonstrated in animal models that a difference of a single amino acid in a single histocompatibility antigen can be sufficient to trigger the destruction of transplanted tissue. This is not to say that such responses are always generated. As we have noted,

some histocompatibility antigens provoke only very weak responses, and sometimes only on rare occasions or only after the foreign graft has been in place for a very long time. But the potential is always there.

TRANSPLANT REJECTION

Initial rejections of transplanted grafts are typically mediated by T cells. This has been demonstrated by the transfer of cells or serum from individuals sensitized by prior rejection of grafts. Transferred T cells provide and augment the rejection of grafts by naïve recipients, while the transfer of serum does not. Both CD8$^+$ cytotoxic T cells and CD4$^+$ T cells mediating delayed (-type) hypersensitivity are involved in graft destruction. Antibodies, on the other hand, have only limited participation in graft destruction. Indeed, antibodies against histocompatibility antigens can be reliably generated only against MHC Class I and class II molecules. It is typically quite difficult to generate antibodies against minor histocompatibility antigens, for reasons that are unclear.

Types of rejection

Graft rejections fall into three general patterns:

- *Chronic rejection* is T cell-mediated. The grafts heal into place, establish vascular connections with the host, and function normally for a period of several weeks to years. Once the first signs of deterioration appear, the destruction proceeds slowly and gradually, and scar tissue slowly infiltrates and replaces the graft tissue. Chronic rejections are often associated with differences at minor histocompatibility genes.
- *Acute rejection* is T cell-mediated. The grafts heal into place, establish vascular connections with the host, and function normally for a relatively brief period, perhaps 7 to 12 days. Once the first signs of deterioration appear, the destruction then proceeds rapidly with an accumulation of blood and a strong infiltration of graft tissue by host monocytes and lymphocytes. The grafts may be totally destroyed in about two weeks. Acute rejection is often associated with differences at major histocompatibility genes.
- *Hyperacute rejection* is antibody-mediated. Hyperacute rejections occur in individuals with

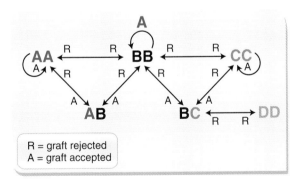

FIGURE 10-5. The laws of transplantation. Graft exchanges between different inbred strains (e.g., homozygous AA, BB, CC individuals) are normally rejected because of numerous differences in the histocompatibility genes carried by the different strains. Hybrids (e.g., AB or BC) are able to accept grafts from either parent because, although they carry only a single copy of each parental gene, none of the parental histocompatibility antigens are foreign to them. However, grafts from the hybrids to the parental strains fail, because some of the histocompatibility antigens of the hybrid are foreign to the parental strains (e.g., the "A" of the AB hybrid is foreign to the BB parent and the "B" of the AB hybrid is foreign to the AA parent).

preexisting high levels of antibodies specific for graft antigens. The antibodies attack the graft vasculature, preventing establishment of a connection to the host vasculature. Without a blood supply, the graft is lost rapidly, sometimes within a day or two.

Risk factors

Given that most grafts in humans are allogeneic, several factors contribute to the risk of rejection.

- **Prior exposure.** As a rule, individuals previously exposed to the foreign graft antigens are more likely to mount rejection responses on subsequent occasions. While this situation occurs primarily in experimental settings, it could present difficulties in rare clinical cases where repeated donations of cells from a limited number of donors may be necessary.
- **Degree of genetic difference between host and donor.** In general, the fewer genetic mismatches, the less likely that rejection will occur. Identical twins are identical at 100% of their genes. First-degree relatives are identical (on average) at 50% of their genes, and second-degree relatives (grandparents, grandchildren, aunts, uncles, nieces, and nephews) are identical at 25% of their genes. For MHC class I and II histocompatibility genes, the availability of antibodies and recently developed molecular techniques make it possible to determine the HLA genotypes of host and donors (HLA typing) and select the combination that matches most closely. For minor histocompatibility genes, there are no typing reagents available and the only means for minimizing genetic differences is to match the recipient with closely related donors.
- **Type of tissue transplanted.** The expression of histocompatibility antigens varies among tissues and organs. For example, MHC class I molecules are expressed heavily on lymphocytes and antigen-presenting cells, but less densely on other tissues such as the kidney and CNS. Mismatched tissues with low expression of histocompatibility antigens may have a better chance of survival within a recipient than those with high expression. In addition, some tissues—particularly the liver—appear to survive transplantation across histocompatibility differences that would doom other organs. In fact, some argue that typing and matching of host and donor for liver transplants are unnec-

essary. The reasons for these unusual properties of transplanted livers are unclear.

- *Functional status of the recipient immune system.* Patients whose immune systems are naturally or artificially suppressed are better able to accept mismatched grafts. However, this deficiency in immune function can have other serious consequences, such as an increased risk of opportunistic infection.

Patient Vignette 10.1

Lucinda Y., a 45-year-old woman with end-stage renal disease due to diabetes mellitus, underwent renal transplantation. She received a kidney from a living, unrelated donor. Approximately one month after transplantation, the patient's urine output and kidney function decreased. She developed tenderness, pain, and swelling at the graft site. In addition, she had nonspecific symptoms that included fever, decreased appetite, and myalgia (muscle pain).

Q: What immunologic processes might be involved in her problems?

A: The patient has signs and symptoms of acute rejection. To confirm the diagnosis, a renal biopsy must be performed. Acute rejection may be treated with intensive immunosuppressive drugs.

Avoiding transplant rejection

The key to survival of imperfectly matched grafts is to minimize immune responses against the graft antigens. This is approached in two general ways:

- **Immune suppression** (or **immunosuppression**) involves an inhibition of the immune response without regard to the specificity of the responses affected.
- **Specific immune tolerance** involves the selective inactivation or elimination of the response to a specific antigen or set of antigens.

While immune tolerance can be effectively induced in experimental systems, the complexity of the specific antigens involved and the need for sufficient lead time prior to the actual transplantation have prevented its use in humans to this

TABLE 10-2 IMMUNOSUPPRESSIVE AGENTS USED IN TRANSPLANTATION

Agent	Target	Action
Irradiation	Many cell types	DNA damage, especially in rapidly proliferating cells
Corticosteroids (e.g., prednisone)	Many cell types	Inhibits gene transcription of numerous cytokines and other products involved in inflammation
Cyclophosphamide	Many cell types	Inhibits nucleotide synthesis
Azathioprine	Many cell types	Inhibits nucleotide synthesis
Mycophenolate mofetil	Lymphocytes	Inhibits nucleotide synthesis and proliferation of lymphocytes
Cyclosporine	Lymphocytes	Inhibits gene transcription of several cytokines including IL-2 and IL-4
Tacrolimus (FK506)	T cells	Inhibits gene transcription in lymphocytes; inactivates calcineurin
Sirolimus (rapamycin)	T cells	Inhibits signal transduction induced by cytokines such as IL-2
Antilymphocyte serum;	Lymphocytes	Removal or inhibition of lymphocytes
Anti-CD3 antibodies	T Lymphocytes	Removal or blockade of T Lymphocytes
Anti-CD4 antibodies	CD4+ T cells	Blockade of CD4 molecules
Anti-CD8 antibodies	CD8+ types	Blockade of CD8 molecules
Anti-MHC I/II antibodies	APCs	Blockade of MHC molecules and inhibition of T cell activation

point. Therefore, immunosuppression remains the only viable option at present.

Originally, the immunosuppressive techniques used—whole body irradiation or toxic drugs—were highly effective at eliminating immune responses that could damage transplanted organs and tissues (Table 10-2). Unfortunately, these treatments are nonspecific and widespread ablation of immune responses left recipients susceptible to opportunistic infections that became the primary cause of death in transplant patients. Beginning in the 1960s, additional drugs became available that have more restricted effects on the immune system. These new agents could target their effects to only those cells responding to foreign graft antigens, while leaving the remainder of the immune system intact to deal with infectious organisms and other potential threats.

> **CLINICAL APPLICATION**
> **HEART TRANSPLANTATION**
>
> The first heart transplantation in the world was performed December 3, 1967 by Dr. Christiaan Barnard in Cape Town, South Africa. He transplanted the heart of a 25-year-old female accident victim into a 55-year-old South African grocer. The recipient died 18 days after surgery. The second heart transplantation patient lived for 18 months after surgery.
>
> *(continued)*

> **CLINICAL APPLICATION (Continued)**
>
> **The first adult heart transplant in the United States was performed by an American surgeon, Dr. Norman Shumway, in January, 1968. It was Dr. Shumway who began the practice of using cyclosporine to prevent organ rejection. In 1981, Dr. Shumway performed the first heart-lung transplant operation.**

One approach to a less global inhibition of the immune response has been the use of antibodies directed at molecules present on the surface of lymphocytes and antigen-presenting cells. For example, antibodies directed against MHC class I or class II molecules can interfere (at least temporarily) with T cell activation. Antibodies against CD4 or CD8 molecules, when administered during active rejection, can bind to and inhibit or destroy T cells and relieve the immediate crisis. However, applications of antibodies against broad categories of T lymphocytes (e.g., anti-CD3 antibodies) have many of the same problems as broadly reactive immunosuppressive drugs or irradiation in that their use, especially over an extended time span, can damage the immune system's ability to respond to infectious agents.

More recently, drugs have been developed that specifically target proliferating lymphocytes, the cells most likely to be involved in an active response against a newly placed graft. Judicious use of these agents can selectively inhibit or kill lymphocytes without extensive concomitant damage to the remainder of the immune system (Table 10-2). The drugs most frequently used for this purpose are cyclosporine, tacrolimus (also called FK506), and rapamycin. These drugs act to inhibit the proliferation and/or activation of T and B lymphocytes undergoing antigenic stimulation, but have little effect on quiescent lymphocytes. There is, however, some risk involved. Transplant patients must often receive the drugs over an extended period of time. If a significant infection occurs during this period, the patient's ability to recognize and respond to the infectious agent could be inhibited in the same way as are responses to graft alloantigens. In addition, the use of these drugs over extended periods of time has sometimes been associated with damage to organs, such as the liver. New drugs are being sought that provide the greatest benefit with the lowest risk of adverse side effects. Immunosuppressive agents are discussed further in Chapter 11.

Bone marrow transplantation

The transplantation of bone marrow has provided enormous benefits to patients with particular diseases, but carries with it certain unique risks. Because bone marrow contains the stem cells for the hematopoietic system—lymphocytic, monocytic, granulocytic, thrombocytic, and erythrocytic—its transplantation can be used to treat conditions in which these tissues are missing, defective, or damaged. In Chapter 7, we learned about a variety of diseases attributable to defects in hematopoietic cells participating in immune responses. In many cases, the preferred long-term solution to these diseases is to provide patients, through bone marrow transplantation, with a new supply of normal stem cells capable of generating the normal counterparts of the defective cells. For example, patients undergoing cancer therapy often must take drugs that are highly toxic to proliferating cells, including those of the immune system. The ability to replace cells damaged by these forms of therapy not only enhances recovery, but individuals with other conditions, such as some forms of anemia, can also benefit from bone marrow transplantation, which provides stem cells capable of generating normal populations of erythrocytes.

A risk in bone marrow transplantation lies in its placement of an immunocompetent tissue into a recipient who is usually immune deficient for natural or therapeutic reasons. Most recipients of bone marrow transplants are unable to mount effective *host-versus-graft* responses because they are immunodeficient or have undergone therapeutic treatment that damages the immune system. In addition, recipients (even those with intact immune systems) undergo procedures that deliberately damage their immune systems to enable the transplanted bone marrow to establish itself in its new environment, a process sometimes referred to as "*making space.*"

Under these circumstances, the cells in the transplanted bone marrow have the potential for recognizing histocompatibility antigens of the host, both MHC and non-MHC, as foreign and consequently attacking the host tissues. This is known as a **graft-versus-host** (GVH) response, and the resulting damage constitutes **graft-versus-host disease** (GVHD). GVHD can be fatal if not controlled. It can develop from two different sources within the transplanted bone marrow, the stem cells and mature T cells that may be present in the implanted bone marrow. Of these two sources, the most immediate and serious threat is the presence of mature T cells that can generate rapid and severe GVH responses. Careful removal of mature T cells from the bone marrow prior to implantation can usually minimize this danger. Lymphocytes generated from the implanted stem cells can also potentially become reactive against host antigens, but they can also often become tolerant as well, because in maturing within the new environment, they come to accept the "foreign" antigens they encounter as "self." GVH responses caused by lymphocytes generated from the new stem cells are usually more delayed, milder, and more transient than those resulting from mature T cells transferred in the bone marrow inoculum.

Patient Vignette 10.2

 Daniel H., a 5-month-old boy who was diagnosed with Wiskott-Aldrich syndrome (Chapter 7), received a bone marrow transplantation from a HLA-matched sibling donor. He was doing well until two weeks after transplantation, when he developed a rash. Subsequently, he developed diarrhea, an enlarged liver and spleen, and jaundice.

(continued)

Patient Vignette 10.2 (Continued)

Q: *What immunologic processes might be involved in his problems?*

A: Daniel has symptoms consistent with graft-versus-host disease. Other organs that may become involved in GVHD include the heart, lung, and central nervous system. The mortality for acute GVHD is high.

Some care must be taken in matching hosts and donors for bone marrow transplantation. T cells generated from the new stem cells must still undergo thymic education in the host thymus. Some degree of matching between the MHC class I and II genes of the host and donor is usually required for the generation of optimally functional T cell populations after undergoing positive and negative selection in the thymus. Once established and functioning within the new host, the transplanted hematopoietic stem cells can provide a normal or near-normal immune function to the recipient for life. Recipients are extremely vulnerable to infection until the engrafted marrow establishes itself and reconstitutes the immune system. During this time, patients must be carefully monitored for infection, and treated appropriately.

Xenotransplantation

With a shortage of donated organs and increasingly long waits for patients hoping to receive organs, research into use of nonhuman donors, at least as temporary measures, is currently ongoing. The first human xenogeneic transplantation of the modern era occurred in 1964, when a chimpanzee heart was placed into a human patient on an emergency basis because of the patient's rapid deterioration and the absence of an available human donor. This milestone, in fact, preceded the first human-to-human heart transplant by about three years. The transplanted chimpanzee heart failed shortly after the procedure, probably due to its small size. Since that time, attempts have been made to further utilize animal donors, primarily primates (chimpanzees and baboons) and swine. Primates are an obvious choice because of their close genetic relationship to humans. Pigs have many physiologic similarities to humans, and "miniswine" have been bred that weigh about 200 pounds, making their organs much more suitable than those of larger agricultural swine, in terms of

size, for human recipients. Pig skin has been used on occasion to provide temporary coverage of damaged areas in human burn victims.

However, xenotransplantation has not yielded great success thus far. Xenografts face numerous immunologic obstacles that often cause rapid rejection. Naturally existing antibodies in human serum, similar to those against the ABO antigens, can react with xenogeneic grafts and produce hyperacute rejection reactions. Natural killer (NK) cells readily detect the absence of human MHC class I molecules on xenogeneic cells and can kill them quite efficiently. Finally, xenogeneic cells lack enzymes that protect them against the attachment of human complement components and activation of the complement cascade leading to lysis. Pig cells, for example, bear enzymes that can protect them against pig complement, but they are ineffective against human complement. Together, these various mechanisms often destroy xenografts before the T cell-mediated responses typically associated with rejection can be generated.

Some attempts to resolve these immediate problems have been made by genetic engineering of the animal donors. Miniswine, for example, have been transfected with human HLA class I genes that can provide the signals that inhibit killing activity by NK cells. In addition, the transfection of human genes for complement regulatory factors such as DAF and CD59 can enable the pig cells to destroy human complement components that attach to them. One other major concern arises in xenotransplantation: the potential for introducing zoonotic infections (infections passed from one species to another) is heightened. There may well be many currently unknown infectious agents, including viruses integrated into the DNA of xenogeneic cells, that could have unforeseen adverse consequences when introduced into human recipients.

Organ procurement and distribution

Since its inception in the 1950s, organ transplantation has been increasingly used, and the total number of transplants performed since that time, on a worldwide basis, currently exceeds a half-million. The success of and increased reliance on transplantation has been possible because of constant improvements in surgical technique, in optimizing the matching of donors and recipients, and in the ability to manage the host immune system

TABLE 10-3. TRANSPLANT DATA FOR THE UNITED STATES[a]

Organ	Transplants Performed 7/1/2002–6/30/2003	Survival at One Year Post-transplant[b]	Patients Awaiting Transplants[c]
Kidney	14,981	96%	58,581
Liver	5,486	87%	17,001
Pancreas	548	96%	1,276
Kidney and pancreas	899	95%	2,356
Heart	2,143	8%	3,663
Heart and lung	30	71%	193
Lung	1,067	7%	3,841
Intestine	117	8%	169
Totals	25,271	—	87,080

[a]Data from 2003 OPTN/SRTR Annual Report: Transplant Data 1993–2002. HHS/HRSA/SPB/DOT; UNOS; URREA. www.ustransplant.org.
[b]Adult patients transplanted 7/1/2000–12/31/2002 (kidney, liver, kidney/pancreas, intestine) or 7/1/2000–6/30/2002 (heart, heart/lung, lung).
[c]As of 6/30/2003.

to permit graft survival without overwhelming sepsis (Table 10-3). With increased demand for donated organs, the problem of efficient and effective distribution of available organs has become increasingly complex. The ability of transplanted organs to cure or alleviate many diseases has resulted in a growing imbalance between the number of patients awaiting donated organs and the number of available organs. While organ donation has increased, it still falls far short of the need. In addition, numerous cultural and religious objections drastically inhibit the donation of organs. In the United States, organ distribution is currently managed through the United Network for Organ Sharing (UNOS). When an organ becomes available, UNOS utilizes various factors, including the degree of genetic matching, potential benefit to the recipient, and geographical priorities, to determine allocation of the organ. Detailed information is maintained and provided on the UNOS web site with respect to the type of organ, number of transplants performed, success rates, waiting lists, and other criteria. The information is frequently updated so that accurate and current information is available to the public.

Transfusion

There is another context in which antibodies play a major role in rejection of transplanted tissues—blood transfusion and erythrocytes, in particular. Blood transfusion has long been used in attempts to save lives and promote recovery. As early as 1492, Pope Innocent VIII received a transfusion that, alas, failed to save him. In the latter part of the seventeenth century, transfusion of blood from animals to humans was performed, but was subsequently banned because of the numbers of resulting deaths. Human-to-human and animal-to-human transfusions were attempted again during the 1800s with distinctly mixed results. The discovery of the ABO and other blood group antigens in the early 1900s led to donor-host matching which, together with continually improved methods for collection and storage, transfer techniques, and screening for infectious agents, have now made blood transfusion a routine and vital therapy. While hundreds of antigenic molecules are present on erythrocytes and other blood cells that can differ between blood donors and recipients, the overwhelming majority of them rarely trigger significant responses. Two systems of antigenic molecules, however, can trigger responses against transfused erythrocytes with severe clinical consequences, the ABO and Rh systems.

The ABO system

The **ABO antigen system** consists of a set of carbohydrate structures that are present on erythrocyte surfaces and on some endothelial and epithelial cells. They are determined by two loci, the H locus and the ABO locus (Fig. 10-6 and Table 10-4). The H locus has two alleles. A dominant H allele encodes a glycosyltransferase that adds a terminal fucose molecule to a precursor molecule normally present on erythrocyte surfaces. The resulting structure is known as the **H substance**. The recessive h allele encodes a nonfunctional enzyme. The H substance becomes the precursor for another set of glycosyltransferases encoded by the alleles of the ABO locus. The A and B alleles are codominantly expressed, while the O allele is recessive to both A and B. The glycosyltransferase

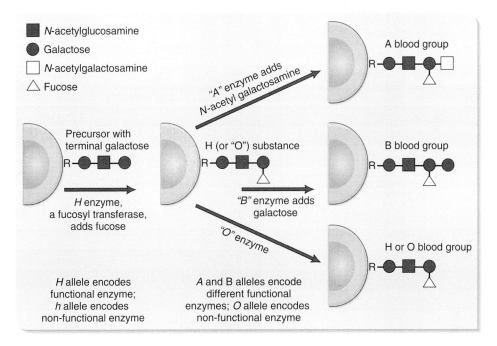

FIGURE 10-6. Genetic basis for ABO blood groups. The enzyme encoded by the H locus (functional H allele, nonfunctional h allele) adds a fucose to the terminal galactose of a precursor molecule normally present on erythrocyte surfaces. This creates a substrate (H substance) upon which the enzymes encoded by the ABO locus can act. The enzyme encoded by the A allele adds an N-acetylgalactosamine to the subterminal galactose, creating the A antigen. The enzyme encoded by the B allele adds a galactose to the subterminal galactose, creating the B antigen. Both enzymes can be active on different H substance precursors on the same cell surface, so that erythrocytes can carry both A and B antigens simultaneously. The enzyme encoded by the O allele is inactive, and does not modify the H substance to produce either A or B antigens.

encoded by the A allele attaches an N-acetyl galactosamine to the subterminal galactose, and the resulting structure (the A antigen) is recognized by anti-A antibodies. The glycosyltransferase encoded by the B allele attaches a galactose to the subterminal galactose (the B antigen) and the resulting structure is recognized by anti-B antibodies. AB individuals produce both types of enzymes and will modify some H to A and some to B. As a result, AB individuals express a mixture of A and B antigens on their erythrocytes. The nonfunctional enzyme produced by the O allele cannot be modified and the unaltered H substance (the O phenotype) is not recognized by either anti-A or anti-B antibodies.

A and B antigens are recognized and bound by IgM antibodies in the serum. They are called **naturally occurring antibodies** because they are present without any stimulation from prior transfusions or intentional immunizations. Antibodies against carbohydrate antigens are usually of the IgM isotype. These natural antibodies are thought to occur because the A and B antigens have some structural similarities to carbohydrates on normal

body flora and are produced by the stimulation provided by that flora. Individuals who have neither A nor B on their own erythrocytes generate IgM antibodies against both A and B. Individuals of blood type A, being tolerant to their own A antigens, will produce only anti-B antibodies. Type B individuals, for similar reasons, are tolerant to their own B antigens and generate only anti-A antibodies.

Mismatched transfusions (for example, when type A erythrocytes are given to a type B recipient) can have serious consequences. The preexisting IgM antibodies can react almost immediately with the transfused erythrocytes, leading to agglutination (clumping due to crosslinking by antibodies) and complement-mediated lysis. The massive destruction of red blood cells can produce a **transfusion reaction**. ABO mismatching can lead to a type of transfusion reaction known as an **acute hemolytic reaction** that may include fever, chills, shortness of breath, and urticaria, and eventually lead to disseminated intravascular coagulation (DIC), a potentially fatal condition. These signs often develop within 24 hours of transfusion and

TABLE 10-4. ABO AND RH BLOOD TYPES

Genotype			
H locus	ABO locus	Phenotype	Natural Antibodies Present Against A and B
HH	AA	A	Anti-B
HH	AO	A	Anti-B
HH	AB	AB	None
HH	BB	B	Anti-A
HH	BO	B	Anti-A
HH	OO	O	
Hh	AA	A	Anti-B
Hh	AO	A	Anti-B
Hh	AB	AB	
Hh	BB	B	Anti-A
Hh	BO	B	Anti-A
Hh	OO	O	Anti-A and Anti-B
hh	AA	O	Anti-A and Anti-B
hh	AO	O	Anti-A and Anti-B
hh	AB	O	Anti-A and Anti-B
hh	BB	O	Anti-A and Anti-B
hh	BO	O	Anti-A and Anti-B
hh	OO	O	Anti-A and Anti-B

Rh genotype		
D locus	CE loci	Rhphenotype
DD	CE, Ce, cE or ce	Rh+
Dd	CE, Ce, cE or ce	Rh+
dd	CE, Ce, cE or ce	Rh−

are caused by extensive hemolysis within the vasculature due to IgM and complement activation. Such mismatches can be avoided by typing of donors and recipients to determine their ABO phenotypes by simple methods such as agglutination (Appendix A). Type A individuals can safely be given blood of phenotypes A and O, while type B recipients can be given type B or O blood. Type O recipients should only be given erythrocytes from type O donors. AB individuals are "universal recipients," capable of safely accepting transfusions from type A, B, O, or AB donors.

Patient Vignette 10.3

Angelina S., a 55-year-old woman, requires a blood transfusion due to significant anemia associated with lower gastrointestinal bleeding. Several minutes after receiving the blood transfusion, the patient developed sudden fever, chills, flushing, nausea, and chest and back pain.

Q: *What immunologic processes might be involved in her problems?*

(continued)

Patient Vignette 10.3 (Continued)

A: This patient has symptoms of an acute transfusion reaction due to inadvertent administration of ABO-mismatched blood. The patient has an antibody against the transfused antigen of the red blood cell. The antibody is of the IgM isotype and, because it is a naturally occurring antibody, is present at a significant level. The immediate necessity is to stop the transfusion and evaluate the patient for other complications, including hypotension (reduced blood pressure) and renal failure. The mortality rate for transfusion reactions due to ABO-mismatched blood is 5% to 10%.

The Rh system

Rh antigens, unlike ABO antigens, are proteins. The antibodies recognizing Rh antigens are of the IgG isotype and are produced only when an Rh-negative individual is exposed to Rh-positive erythrocytes. IgG is the only immunoglobulin isotype that can cross the placenta. Because the Rh antigens can be typed prior to transfusion, the

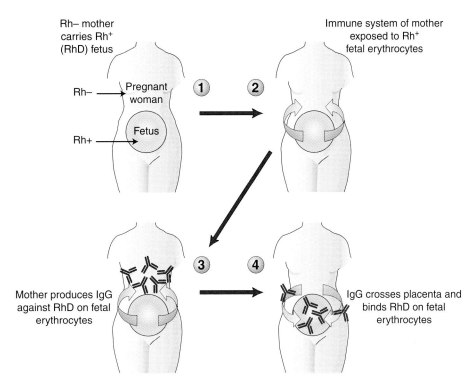

FIGURE 10-7. Hemolytic disease of the newborn. Rh^- mothers carrying an Rh^+ (RhD) fetus **(1)** can become exposed to the Rh^+ fetal erythrocytes during pregnancy and delivery **(2)**. The mother can generate IgG antibodies against RhD **(3)**. Because IgG can cross the placenta, the maternal antibodies can enter the fetal circulation and bind RhD on the fetal erythrocytes **(4)**. Antibody-induced damage to fetal erythrocytes can lead to anemia and other consequences.

avoidance of transfusing Rh-negative (Rh^-) recipients with Rh-positive (Rh^+) blood effectively prevents transfusion reactions. The primary danger from Rh mismatches occurs during pregnancy when an Rh^- mother carries an Rh^+ fetus.

Rh antigens are encoded by a series of closely linked loci (D and CE), each with dominant alleles (e.g., D) and recessive alleles (e.g., d). Of these, the critical locus is D. Individuals with DD or Dd genotypes are considered to be Rh^+, while those with dd are Rh^- (Table 10-4). When the father is Rh^+, an Rh^- mother may carry an Rh^+ fetus (Fig. 10-7). During labor and delivery, Rh^+ erythrocytes from the fetus may enter the maternal circulation. In addition, occasional leakage of fetal erythrocytes into the maternal blood may occur during pregnancy. This exposure can stimulate formation of anti-Rh IgG antibodies by the maternal immune system. Subsequent Rh^+ fetuses, are at risk because anti-Rh antibodies can pass from the maternal circulation into the fetus, and possibly causing anemia and damage to other organs as well. Preventive therapy is available for this situation and is described more fully in Chapter 11.

Summary

- Grafts are classified by the genetic relationship between the donor and host, by the location of the graft, and by the type of tissue involved.
- When tissues are transplanted between members of different inbred strains, they are typically rejected. It is possible, by a careful program of breeding and selection, to "move" genes from one inbred strain into another to produce congenic strains.
- Types of grafts that can thus be characterized by the genetic relationship between the host and donor are **autograft** (a transplant from one part of an individual to another part of the same individual); **syngeneic graft** (a transplant from one individual to a genetically identical individual, for example, an identical twin or another member of the same inbred strain); **allograft or allogeneic graft** (a transplant from one individual to a genetically different member of the same species); and **xenograft** (a transplant between members of different species).

- Target antigens on the donated tissue are genetically encoded molecules called *histocompatibility antigens*. The genes that encode them are *histocompatibility genes*.
- Histocompatibility genes (and their antigenic products) are commonly divided into two broad groups, those encoded within the major histocompatibility complex and those encoded elsewhere. The major histocompatibility genes are composed of the MHC I and MHC II loci. Differences at the non-MHC histocompatibility genes (also called minor histocompatibility genes) generate, as a rule, weaker and less consistent rejections.
- T cells can be activated against histocompatibility antigens in two ways, by *direct recognition* or *indirect recognition*.
- Grafts exchanged between hosts and donors that are genetically identical (AA to AA, BB to BB, etc.) should be completely compatible. *Hybrids* (e.g., AB) should be able to accept grafts from either parental type (AA or BB), but their tissues should be rejected by their parents because they express histocompatibility antigens foreign to each parent. Initial rejections of transplanted grafts are typically mediated by T cells. Both CD8$^+$ cytotoxic T cells and CD4$^+$ T cells mediating delayed type hypersensitivity have been demonstrated to be involved in graft destruction. Antibodies participate in graft destruction in a few situations.
- *Chronic rejection* is T cell-mediated. The grafts heal into place, establish vascular connections with the host, and functional normally for a period of several weeks to years. *Acute rejection* is T cell-mediated. The grafts may be totally destroyed in about two weeks, slowly infiltrating and replacing the graft tissue. *Hyperacute rejection* is antibody-mediated. Hyperacute rejections occur in individuals with preexisting high levels of antibodies specific for graft antigens.
- Patients whose immune systems are naturally or artificially suppressed are more likely to accept mismatched grafts.
- Improving the chance of survival for imperfectly matched grafts is approached in two general ways. Immune suppression involves a general inhibition of the immune response without regard to specificity. More recently, drugs and monoclonal antibodies have been developed that more specifically target the lymphocytes most likely to be involved in an active response against a newly placed graft.

- Transplantation of bone marrow can provide benefits to patients suffering from some types of immune deficiencies and anemias, and the side effects of some cancer therapies. The risk in bone marrow transplantation lies in the fact that it involves placement of an immuno-competent tissue into a recipient that is usually immune-deficient for natural or therapeutic reasons. Graft-versus-host disease can result when cells in the transplanted bone marrow recognize histocompatibility antigens of the host as foreign and attack host tissues.
- ABO blood group antigens are carbohydrate structures on erythrocyte surfaces and some other cell types. They are determined by the enzymatic products of two loci, the H locus and the ABO locus. Individuals who have neither A nor B on their own erythrocytes generate IgM antibodies against both A and B. Individuals of blood type A, being tolerant to their own A antigens, produce only anti-B antibodies. Type B individuals are tolerant of their own B antigens and generate only anti-A antibodies. ABO mismatching can lead to a type of transfusion reaction known as an acute hemolytic reaction. Antibodies against ABO antigens are preexisting and do not require deliberate immunization.
- *Erythroblastosis fetalis*, a condition that occurs when anti-Rh antibodies pass from the maternal circulation of an Rh$^-$ mother into the vasculature of an Rh$^+$ fetus, leading to destruction of fetal erythrocytes that can result in anemia and other potentially fatal damage to other organ systems.

Suggested readings

Appelbaum FR. The current status of hematopoietic cell transplantation. *Annu Rev Med* 2003;54:491.

Janeway CA Jr., Travers P, Walport M, Shlomchik P. Autoimmunity and Transplantation. In *Immunobiology: The immune system in health and disease*, 6th ed. Philadephia: Garland Publishing, 2004.

Masri MA. The mosaic of immunosuppressive drugs. *Mol Immunol* 2003;39:1073.

Sachs DH, Sykes M, Robson SC, Cooper DK. Xenotransplantation. *Adv Immunol* 2001;79:129.

Schroeder RA, Marroquin CE, Kuo PC. Tolerance and the "Holy Grail" of transplantation. *J Surg Res* 2003;111:109.

Strober S, Lowsky RJ, Shizuru JA, Scandling JD, Millan MT. Approaches to transplantation tolerance in humans. *Transplantation* 2004;77:932.

Sykes M, Auchincloss H Jr, Sachs DH. Transplantation immunology. In Paul WE, ed. *Fundamental immunology*, 5th ed. Philadelphia: Lippincott Williams & Wilkins, 2003.

Review questions

1. A 57-year-old man receives a heart transplant from an unrelated cadaver donor. As a precaution, he is administered a regimen including cyclosporine and tacrolimus. Immunosuppressive drugs such as cyclosporine and tacrolimus act primarily by:
   (A) lowering antibody levels by preventing expression of CD40 on B cells.
   (B) decreasing T-cell proliferation by preventing synthesis of IL-2.
   (C) interfering with antigen presentation by macrophages.
   (D) killing bone marrow stem cells.
   (E) causing involution of the thymus.

2. Which of the following treatments would be expected to result in the least severe (most targeted or limited) form of therapeutic immunosuppression?
   (A) Whole-body high dose irradiation
   (B) Administration of anti-CD3 antibodies
   (C) Administration of anti-CD4 antibodies
   (D) Administration of cyclosporine
   (E) Administration of corticosteroids (high dose)

3. Luiz P. requires a kidney graft. His HLA genotype is A3/A6, B27/B44, C1/C8 (the alleles for the A, B, and C loci are given, with the maternal allele listed first for each locus). Several potential donors are available. Which of the following potential donors is the best choice?
   (A) Donor of HLA type A3/A8, B7/B22, C4/C8
   (B) Donor of HLA type A6/A6, B27/B24, C12/C1
   (C) Donor of HLA type A27/A44, B1/B8, C3/C6
   (D) Donor of HLA type A3/A6, B24/B7, C2,C9
   (E) Donor of HLA type A3/A3, B27/B44, C6/C1

4. Yolanda R. required a bone marrow transplant following intensive chemotherapy for cancer. The donor was her mother. A primary concern in her recovery is the potential for:
   (A) host-versus-graft disease.
   (B) graft-versus-host disease.
   (C) type I (immediate) hypersensitivity.

   (D) type II hypersensitivity.
   (E) autoimmunity.

5. Grafts (excluding blood transfusion) exchanged between unrelated donors and recipients (without therapeutic intervention) who happen to be identical for HLA genes are:
   (A) impossible in humans.
   (B) likely to be rejected within 1–2 days.
   (C) likely to be rejected within 1–2 weeks.
   (D) likely to be rejected within months to years.
   (E) sure to succeed.

6. Several individuals have received heart transplants from primates, with only very short-term success at most. A major obstacle in the transplantation of organs from different species (xenografts) is:
   (A) strong graft-versus host disease.
   (B) strong binding of host T cells to MHC I antigens on the graft.
   (C) hyperacute rejection due to preexisting "natural" antibodies.
   (D) that they cannot be placed orthotopically.
   (E) xenografts trigger strong delayed (-type) hypersensitivity responses.

7. Which of the following organs can usually be successfully transplanted between fairly incompatible donors and hosts without requiring vigorous therapeutic intervention?
   (A) Bone marrow
   (B) Skin
   (C) Kidney
   (D) Liver
   (E) Heart

8. Among the following, the factor having the greatest effect on graft survival is:
   (A) the degree of genetic mismatch between host and donor.
   (B) graft size.
   (C) age of the donor.
   (D) sex of the donor.
   (E) whether the graft is orthotopic or heterotopic.

9. The ABO blood group is determined by a single autosomal locus with alleles A (codominant to B, but dominant to O), B

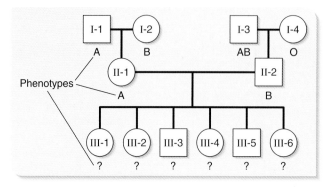

FIGURE 10-8.

(codominant to A, but dominant to O) and O (recessive to A and B). The pedigree shown (Fig. 10-8) gives the blood types (*phenotypes*) of the individuals in generations I and II. What are the possible phenotypes that should be found among the individuals in generation III?

(A) A, B, AB, and O
(B) B, AB
(C) A, AB
(D) A, B, AB
(E) AB and O

10. During Michelle T.'s fourth pregnancy, she saw an obstetrician because "she felt something was wrong." She had not sought regular prenatal care. The fetus she was carrying was found to be anemic in utero. Michelle was found to be Rh⁻ and the father was Rh⁺. Elevated levels of anti-Rh antibodies were found in Michelle's blood. Anti-Rh antibodies have the following characteristics:

(A) They are of the IgM isotype and can cross the placenta to attack Rh⁺ fetal erythrocytes.
(B) They are of the IgE isotype and can cross the placenta to cause type I hypersensitivity responses in the developing fetus.
(C) They are of the IgG isotype and can cross the placenta to attack Rh⁺ fetal erythrocytes.
(D) They are of fetal origin and can cross the placenta to attack maternal Rh⁺ erythrocytes.
(E) They are confined to the maternal circulation.

Immunotherapy and Immunosuppression

Chapter Outline

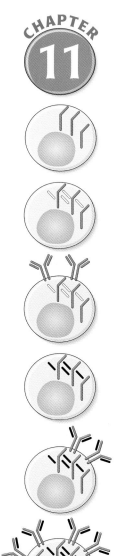

Introduction When the immune system is weakened by, for example, chemotherapy, or when it becomes overly aggressive, as in rejection of a transplanted organ or in an autoimmune response, it is possible to enhance, diminish, or alter the immune response. In this chapter, we describe several of the immunotherapeutic and immunosuppressive strategies to modify the immune response.

IMMUNOTHERAPY—STRATEGIES THAT ENHANCE THE IMMUNE RESPONSE

Immunotherapy is the use of different treatment strategies to enhance the immune system to fight a disease. For example, adjuvants nonspecifically stimulate the immune system either directly or indirectly; interferons have been used as immunotherapeutic agents; and human immune serum globulin may be used successfully to treat patients with generalized antibody deficiencies such as hypogammaglobulinemia or agammaglobulinemia.

Adjuvants

Adjuvants nonspecifically stimulate the immune system either directly or indirectly. In Chapter 6, we discuss the use of adjuvants with vaccines to stimulate development of an immune response. Adjuvants derived from microbial products may also be used to strengthen a weak immune response by increasing co-stimulatory molecule expression on antigen-presenting cells.

Bacillus Calmette-Guérin (BCG), commonly used as a tuberculosis vaccine, is also used to treat postsurgical superficial bladder cancer. A BCG solution is instilled into the bladder weekly for up to 6 weeks to stimulate inflammation and promote immune function. BCG has also been used in clinical trials to enhance immune function in the treatment of melanoma and certain other tumors, either by direct injection into a tumor nodule or by reintroducing tumor cells together with BCG into the patient. These studies have met with mixed results.

Levamisole is an antihelminthic drug used in veterinary medicine to treat parasitic infection. It is also an immunostimulant with low toxicity that has been used in conjunction with other therapies to restore cell-mediated immunity in certain chronic infections such as genital herpes or recurring infections such as viral respiratory infections.

Interleukin-12 (IL-12) is a cytokine produced by a variety of cells that promotes natural killer cell (NK) function and T cell activation, and is a B-cell growth factor. It may have therapeutic value as an adjuvant when co-administered with a vaccine. Immune responses to melanoma peptide vaccines appear to be enhanced when IL-12 is injected together with the vaccine.

Cytokine therapy

Cytokines, such as the interferons (IFNs), are involved in all aspects of the innate and adaptive immune response including cellular growth and differentiation, inflammation, and repair.

Both **type I (IFN-α/β)** and **type II (IFN-γ) interferons** have been used as immunotherapeutic agents. Recombinant IFN-α and IFN-β therapy has been shown to be effective in some patients with hepatitis B or hepatitis C viral infections. Like the naturally produced product, recombinant IFNs are rapidly cleared from the circulation. To prolong bioavailability and improve efficacy, polyethylene glycol (PEG) is conjugated to IFN-α to produce pegylated IFN-α. Chronic treatment with pegylated recombinant IFN-α decreases risk of subsequent hepatocarcinoma development in approximately 20% of individuals with chronic hepatitis C viral infection.

CLINICAL APPLICATION
HEPATITIS C VIRAL INFECTION

Approximately 4 million people in the United States (170 million worldwide) have **chronic hepatitis C** resulting from hepatitis C virus (HCV). HCV is transmitted by blood and body fluids. Risk factors associated with HCV infection include intravenous drug abuse, blood transfusions before 1992, frequent exposure to blood products, and high-risk sexual behavior. Approximately 80 % of the patients in whom HCV develops will progress to chronic infection that can cause cirrhosis, liver failure, and liver cancer.

Patients with chronic granulomatous disease (CGD) show diminished NADPH function, making them more susceptible to recurrent pyogenic (fever-causing) infections. The incidence of serious infection is greatly diminished in patients treated with recombinant IFN-γ. IFN-γ has also been used to treat patients with severe atopic (IgE-mediated) dermatitis. The rationale here is that of IFN-γ down-regulates IL-4 production and reduces the development of IgE responses.

The development of anti-tumor immunotherapy has proved elusive and certain treatment regimens have only recently become reliable. Systemic administration of type I IFN (IFN-α) has successfully increased some remissions of hairy-cell leukemia. Likewise, systemic IL-2 injection can prolong remission to some renal carcinomas and melanomas. Both IFN-γ and TNF-α administration have been used to treat ovarian tumors. IL-2 has also been shown to be an effective means of activating NK cells that subsequently attack and destroy tumor cells. These lymphokine-activated killer (LAK) cells (primarily NK) participate in the remission of melanoma.

Although tumors are often recognized by T cells, the growth rate of the tumor often outpaces the immune response. A novel immunotherapy has been developed in which T cells are isolated from excised tumors; the numbers of T cells are expanded in vitro using IL-2 and then are re-infused into the patient. The rationale for this approach is that CD8$^+$ tumor infiltrating lymphocytes (TILs) are more effective because they are specific for antigens of that tumor, and by expanding their numbers in vitro and returning these cells to the patient, these cytotoxic T lymphocytes (CTL) will efficiently kill tumor cells. In some instances, transfection of cytokine genes into TILs in vitro has increased their cytotoxicity in vivo. In another approach, tumor cells removed from the patient have been genetically engineered to constitutively express CD80/86 and IL-2. When returned to the patient, the engineered tumor cells function as antigen-presenting cells (APCs) to activate tumor-recognizing T cells, rather than causing them to become anergic. Additional clinical trials have used vaccines against tumor antigens. A major clinical trial involving uterine cancer has shown very promising results.

Antibody replacement therapy

Individuals with generalized antibody deficiency such as hypogammaglobulinemia or agammaglobulinemia may be successfully treated with human immune globulin (HIg). Administered intramuscularly, peak blood levels are achieved approximately 2 days after injection. Hig is composed primarily of IgG, with trace amounts of IgM and IgA. Because it is derived from pooled immune human sera, HIg provides a broad spectrum of antibody reactivity. The administered dose of HIg provides protection for approximately one month (recall that the serum half-life of IgG is approximately 23 days); therefore, injections must continue at monthly intervals.

People with selective antibody deficiencies, groups (elderly or infants) at high risk for certain infections, or those exposed to certain infectious diseases may benefit from intramuscular injection of either a broad-spectrum immune globulin or preparations of immune globulins containing specific antibodies. Among commercially available specific immune globulins are those for tetanus, hepatitis B, rabies, cytomegalovirus, and varicella zoster virus.

With the advent of monoclonal antibody technology, it is now possible to produce large quantities of antibodies against a specific epitope for certain cancers, such as anti-CD20 monoclonal antibody for the treatment of non-Hodgkin lymphoma. Monoclonal antibodies are used in approximately 20% of all immunotherapy patients.

Patient Vignette 11.1

Vera N., a 50-year-old woman (described in Chapter 4), has common variable immunodeficiency.

She has hypothyroidism, chronic diarrhea, and recurrent sinusitis and respiratory infections.

Q: What might be an appropriate type of immunotherapy for her?

A: This patient may benefit from receiving immune globulin therapy, which may reduce the incidence and severity of infection. The dose of the immune globulin is usually adjusted to achieve a good clinical response. No case of AIDS has been attributed to the use of immune globulin. Cases of hepatitis C were reported in Europe and Australia in the1980s and in the United States in 1993; these cases have been attributed to the use of immune globulin therapy. Currently, all immune globulin preparations are treated to eliminate viruses.

IMMUNOSUPPRESSION—STRATEGIES THAT DIMINISH THE IMMUNE RESPONSE

Sometimes the immune system responds too vigorously and needs to be calmed down. The term "immunosuppression" is used when an otherwise normal immune response is diminished. The immune response can be manipulated by using certain drugs to prevent the body from rejecting newly transplanted organs or to treat autoimmune diseases. Both specific and nonspecific strategies may be used.

Anti-inflammatory agents

Inflammation often results from the direct or indirect activation of the innate immune system and is characterized by leakage of plasma and blood components into the interstitial spaces and the migration of leukocytes into the inflamed site. Chemical mediators of inflammation such as histamine, serotonin, prostaglandins, bradykinin, chemokines, and leukotrienes are liberated from granulocytic cells such as mast cells, basophils, and eosinophils. Phagocytic cell activity may cause the release of lytic molecules. Anti-inflammatory drugs, such as corticosteroids (or, more specifically, adrenocorticosteroids), and nonsteroidal anti-inflammatory drugs (NSAIDs), such as aspirin, are used to control inflammation.

Corticosteroids

Since their first clinical application for the treatment of rheumatoid arthritis in 1949, the therapeutic role for **corticosteroids**, or glucocorticoids, has expanded. Corticosteroids are currently used to nonspecifically treat many diseases and conditions, including autoimmune disorders, allergic diseases, and bronchial asthma, and to prevent organ rejection. There are many ways to administer corticosteroids, including systemic therapy, inhalation, intranasal application, or topical application. Because adverse effects of the drug can be quite significant if high doses are used chronically, it is important to monitor the dosage and note any adverse reactions.

Although corticosteroids are effective anti-inflammatory agents, the mechanism of their anti-inflammatory effect is not completely understood. Some of the effects of corticosteroids include:

- Decreased size and lymphoid content of the spleen and lymph nodes
- Functional modification of certain T cell subsets
- Inhibition of inflammatory mediators, including histamine, prostaglandin, and leukotrienes
- Inhibition of monocyte and neutrophil chemotaxis
- Change in leukocyte distribution, causing lymphopenia (decreased numbers of lymphocyte) and neutrophilia (increased numbers of neutrophils)
- Inhibition of IL-1 production and decreased availability of IL-2 and decreased IgG blood concentration
- Decreased IgG blood levels

Corticosteroids can reduce the symptoms of certain autoimmune diseases such as inflammatory bowel diseases, systemic lupus erythematosus, autoimmune hemolytic anemia, idiopathic thrombocytopenic purpura, and rheumatoid arthritis. In the treatment of bronchial asthma, inhalation corticosteroids are the recommended first-line therapy. Because the key to the success of an imperfectly matched graft is to minimize immune responses against the graft antigens, corticosteroids are particularly useful in organ transplant rejection crises.

Many corticosteroid preparations are currently available. Systemic administration includes oral, intravenous, or intramuscular routes. Inhalation corticosteroids are used in the treatment of asthma, and intranasal corticosteroids are widely used in the treatment of rhinitis. Other preparations for topical administration are effective in the treatment of IgE-mediated atopic dermatitis and ocular allergy.

As with other medications, corticosteroids have risks and benefits. Complications and adverse effects of corticosteroids are related to the dose, duration, and route of administration. Adverse effects of high-dose and chronic high-dose systemic therapy can be significant. Potential adverse effects include suppression of the hypothalamic pituitary axis, infections, hypertension, cataracts, hyperglycemia, and osteoporosis.

Nonsteroidal anti-inflammatory agents

Nonsteroidal anti-inflammatory drugs (NSAIDs) have anti-inflammatory effects but are not corticosteroids. These agents include aspirin and similar drugs such as ibuprofen. The main effect of

NSAIDs is anti-inflammatory, but they also have antipyretic (fever-reducing) and analgesic effects. These drugs provide clinical benefit in the treatment of inflammatory diseases and other conditions requiring inhibition of platelet aggregation.

NSAIDs irreversibly block cyclooxygenase (prostaglandin synthase) and therefore inhibit prostaglandins and thromboxane synthesis. Inhibition of prostaglandins reduces the edema, leukocyte infiltration, and pain, and also helps to reduce fever. Inhibition of thromboxane production causes the inhibition of platelet aggregation. The anti-inflammatory effect of NSAIDs is usually observed at high doses, whereas the analgesic (pain-relieving) effect is dose-responsive.

NSAIDs are used clinically to reduce fever and to treat mild to moderate pain and inflammatory conditions, such as rheumatoid arthritis. One of the most beneficial uses of aspirin is the inhibition of platelet aggregation, including prevention of coronary artery thrombosis, and transient ischemic attack. Aspirin has demonstrated its clinical benefit in reducing the incidence of transient ischemic attack and unstable angina.

The main adverse effects of NSAIDs, such as aspirin, are gastrointestinal, which may include a range of effects from mild irritation to severe upper gastrointestinal bleeding caused by ulcers. Other adverse effects can include decreased glomerular filtration rate, acute renal failure, and interstitial nephritis. However, renal toxicity is unusual in patients with normal kidneys.

Immunosuppressive measures

Therapeutic intervention is often used to diminish autoimmune responses in diseases such as rheumatoid arthritis, inflammatory bowel disease, and systemic lupus erythematosus. Immune-suppressive measures are also used to diminish the overt and often catastrophic effects of bronchial asthma and graft rejection.

Rheumatoid arthritis therapy

Rheumatoid arthritis (RA) is a destructive inflammatory autoimmune disease that ultimately involves both cell-mediated and humoral immune responses. Initially, the synovia and cartilages of small joints are affected. The disease progresses to not only large joints but also other organ systems. Although the initiating mechanisms of RA are still unknown, it appears that CD4$^+$ T cell recognition of antigen(s) within the joint triggers the release of inflammatory cytokines that lead to the accumulation of neutrophils and macrophages that initiate cartilage damage. Also found within inflamed synovia are B cells, plasma cells, CD4$^+$ T cells, and a wide variety of cytokines, including tumor necrosis factor-α (TNF-α), IL-1, IL-8, and IFN-γ. Rheumatoid factors, IgM or IgG autoantibodies directed against the Fc region of circulating IgG molecules, are produced by CD4$^+$ T-cell-dependent B cells. The binding of rheumatoid factors to IgG augments the formation of immune complexes. The deposition and complement fixation of these complexes may contribute to joint destruction, as well as to the vasculitis and lung injury seen in advanced stages of RA.

Treatment of RA may include NSAIDs, disease-modifying antirheumatic drugs (DMARDs), corticosteroids, and biologic agents (TNF-α inhibitor and IL-1). As previously discussed, NSAIDs inhibit cyclooxygenase and block prostaglandin formation. Inhibition of prostaglandin helps to limit edema, leukocyte infiltration, and pain associated with RA. DMARDs include immunosuppressive agents, methotrexate, anti-malarial drugs, gold salt therapy, and sulfasalazine. These drugs can slow the disease process but usually do not lead to complete remission.

The mechanisms by which DMARDs work are not fully understood, but DMARDs appear to modify the immune system. It may take from many weeks up to 6 to 8 months to demonstrate a response to treatment. Studies have shown that DMARDs can be effective in treating RA and although their side effects are often significant and frequent, they can be minimized with frequent monitoring.

Methotrexate, an inhibitor of DNA synthesis, is the most widely used DMARD and is used as an immunosuppressive agent in the treatment of rheumatic disease. Methotrexate inhibits dihydrofolate reductase, an enzyme required for the conversion of folic acid into its active form, tetrahydrofolate, which is involved in the synthesis of thymidine. Adverse effects of methotrexate include hepatic fibrosis, hypersensitivity pneumonitis, mucositis, and bone marrow suppression. Because the treatment for RA requires only low doses of methotrexate, these adverse effects may not occur.

Other DMARDs agents used in the treatment of RA include alkylating agents and purine analogues that inhibit cell proliferation. Alkylating agents include cyclophosphamide and chlorambucil. Purine analogues include azathioprine and mercaptopurine. These immunosuppressive agents have significant adverse effects, including hepatic toxicity, and are associated with an increased risk of cancer and infection.

Because cytokines are involved in both the systemic inflammatory process and local joint destruction in RA, drugs that inhibit cytokine function can be useful RA therapies. Several approaches have been taken, including TNF-α neutralizing monoclonal antibodies, soluble recombinant TNF-α receptors, and IL-1 receptor-blocking proteins. Monoclonal antibodies effectively inactivate TNF-α, thus eliminating a cytokine that is crucial to the disease process. A second approach is to use a so-called **immunoadhesin** molecule, a fusion protein produced by recombinant DNA technology that combines the constant domain of an antibody molecule with the ligand-recognition domain of a cytokine receptor. In this approach, soluble immunoadhesin molecules successfully compete with cell-bound TNF-α receptors on cell surfaces and reduce the functional impact of TNF-α. The third approach uses a recombinant protein that mimics a naturally occurring IL-1 receptor antagonist. This protein effectively blocks the IL-1 binding site from occupancy by IL-1. Clinical trials have demonstrated that TNF-α can decrease the signs and symptoms of RA and reduce the progression of joint damage. In addition, their onset of action is faster than that of the traditional DMARDs. Adverse effects associated with cytokine inhibitors may include infections, such as the reactivation of latent tuberculosis infections.

Because an excess of IL-1 is found in individuals with RA, anti-IL-1 receptor antagonists are another new agent used in the treatment of RA. Because these drugs suppress the immune system, serious opportunistic infections may occur.

Patient Vignette 11.2

Chris B., a 52-year-old woman, presents with symptoms of joint pain and stiffness in hands, feet, and knees for the past 6 months. In addition, the patient also noted a 10-pound weight loss and a low-grade fever. She has been receiving an NSAID for 4 months and has not experienced much relief of her symptoms.

(continued)

Patient Vignette 11.2 (Continued)

Q: What immunological process is likely to be involved in her problems and what additional information would help you to confirm this?

A: This patient most likely has **rheumatoid arthritis**. In addition to a complete history and physical examination, radiographic evidence of joint erosions and a positive rheumatoid factor can confirm the diagnosis. Because this patient has tried an NSAID for 4 months without much relief, DMARDs and/or TNFα-inhibitors should be considered.

Bronchial asthma therapy

Bronchial asthma is a chronic inflammatory respiratory disorder. Inflammatory cells involved in the pathogenesis of bronchial asthma include mast cells, neutrophils, eosinophils, and CD4+ Th2 cells. This inflammation causes recurrent episodes of wheezing, restricted breathing, and cough in susceptible individuals. Episodes are most prevalent in the early morning and at night, and are accompanied by increased mucous production and bronchial obstruction. **Atopy** or the genetic predisposition to develop IgE-mediated responses to common allergens is a strong predisposing factor in the development of bronchial asthma. Airflow obstruction is often reversible, occurring either spontaneously or after treatment.

Current recommended drug therapies for asthma include β2-adrenergic receptor agonists, corticosteroids, theophylline (a bronchial smooth muscle relaxant closely related to caffeine), cromolyn (a blocker of mast cell degranulation), nedocromil (which prevents histamine release from mast cells), leukotriene antagonists, and anticholinergic agents. Because the underlying mechanism of asthma is inflammation, an inhaled corticosteroid is recommended and a β2-adrenergic receptor agonist should be used as needed.

Bronchial asthma is associated with increased IgE secretion. The Food and Drug Administration (FDA) recently approved a humanized monoclonal anti-IgE antibody for the treatment of moderate to persistent asthma. This neutralizing antibody prevents IgE from attaching to mast cells and other immune cells, and thus prevents IgE-mediated inflammatory changes.

Cytokines also play a role in asthma pathogenesis, especially IL-4, IL-5, and IL-13, and are potential targets for therapeutic intervention. Treatment with a recombinant IL-4 receptor has shown initial clinical benefits. Future therapies may rely on antagonists of cytokines or their receptors for effective asthma management.

Graft rejection

Most bone marrow allografts are imperfectly matched. Bone marrow transplantation is essentially the replacement of a defective or damaged immune system with a normal one and has been highly beneficial procedure for individuals with particular types of problems. The benefits and risks of this procedure have been discussed in Chapter 10. Bone marrow contains hematopoietic stem cells capable of establishing themselves and producing new monocytic, lymphocytic, granulocytic, thrombocytic, and erythrocytic cell populations (see Chapter 2). Individuals with primary immunodeficiencies, caused by defects in cells derived from the hematopoietic stem cells, are obvious candidates (see Chapter 7). In addition, the ability to replace bone marrow permits the use of much higher levels of therapeutic agents for treatment for other conditions (e.g., cancer) than was previously possible because of the toxic side effects of those agents on the immune system. The self-perpetuation of the transplanted stem cells in successful bone marrow transplantation offers the prospect for permanent cure rather than dependence on repeated applications of therapies with limited duration.

The risk involved in bone marrow transplantation arises from the placement of an immunocompetent tissue into a recipient (usually genetically disparate from the donor) that is often immunodeficient. Thus, whereas the immune system of the recipient is typically unable to react against foreign histocompatibility antigens that may be present on the cells of the inoculated bone marrow, the reverse is not true. Immunocompetent cells of the graft may recognize host antigens as foreign and react against them, leading to **graft-versus-host disease** (GVH or GVHD). Matching the histocompatibility antigens of the host and donor as closely as possible is important. GVHD is potentially fatal. Because the most severe and acute forms of GVHD are caused by mature T cells present in the bone marrow inoculate, careful removal of these cells can usually prevent acute GVHD. The hope is that newly arising lymphocytes derived from the en-

grafted marrow will adapt to their new surrounding and be tolerant of any "foreign" host histocompatibility antigens they may encounter. If GVHD does occur as a result of responses by newly arising lymphocytes, it is more likely to be mild and transient.

The key to graft survival is to minimize immune responses against alloantigens within the graft. Several approaches may be taken: global inhibition of the immune system, selective inhibition of a particular class of leukocytes, or the selective inhibition of graft-specific leukocytes.

- *Global approach.* Application of systemic immunosuppressive drugs such as corticosteroids or whole-body irradiation has met with limited success. Although effective at inhibiting host immune rejection of the engrafted tissue, these treatments also inhibit a normal immune response to environmental pathogens. Consequently, opportunistic infections often develop. Isolation of the patient from environmental flora is both difficult and costly. Graft-borne viral infections, such as cytomegalovirus, have been reported for patients who have undergone systemic immunosuppression.
- *Inhibition of a population of leukocytes.* A less drastic approach to inhibition of the immune response involves the use of antibodies directed at molecules present on the surface of lymphocytes and APCs. For example, antibodies directed against MHC class I or class II molecules can interfere (at least temporarily) with T cell activation. Antibodies against CD4 or CD8 molecules, when administered during active rejection, can bind to T cells to inhibit or destroy them and alleviate the immediate crisis.

Another approach involves inhibition of the immune response without regard to the specificity of the responses affected. However, applications of antibodies against broad categories of T lymphocytes (e.g., anti-CD3 antibodies) have many of the same problems as broadly reactive immunosuppressive drugs or irradiation in that their use, especially over an extended time span, can damage the ability to respond to infectious agents.

- *Inhibition of graft-specific leukocytes.* Beginning in the 1960s, additional drugs with more restricted effects on the immune system became available. These drugs target those immune cells responding to foreign graft antigens while leaving the remainder of the immune system intact to deal with infectious organisms and other potential threats. Among the drugs most frequently used for this purpose are **cyclosporine**, **tacrolimus** (also called FK506), and **rapamycin**. These drugs inhibit the proliferation and/or activation of T cells undergoing antigenic stimulation while having little effect on quiescent lymphocytes. However, some risk is involved.

Cyclosporine is an immunosuppressive agent with significant efficacy in the treatment of patients after transplantation of organs and tissues (including bone marrow), as well as selected autoimmune disorders. In vitro studies indicated that it selectively alters the immune regulation activities of helper T cells. Specifically, cyclosporine inhibits calcineurin, which is necessary for the activation of T cells. Therefore, it inhibits the gene transcription of IL-2, IL-3, IFN-γ, and other factors produced by antigen-stimulated T cells. Adverse effects include nephrotoxicity, neurotoxicity, hypertension, hyperbilirubinemia, reversible liver toxicity, and infections. It does not produce adverse effects on the bone marrow.

Tacrolimus is a macrolide antibiotic and is approximately 10 to 100 times more potent than cyclosporine. Its mechanism of action is similar to that of cyclosporine in that it also selectively alters the activities of helper T cells by inhibiting calcineurin and therefore inhibits IL-2 synthesis and secretion. The adverse effects of tacrolimus are similar to those for cyclosporine.

Rapamycin is also a macrolide antibiotic, structurally similar to tacrolimus. However, rapamycin blocks the response of T cells to cytokines and immunoglobulin production by B cells.

STRATEGIES TO ALTER THE IMMUNE RESPONSE

Sometimes the best strategy is to stop an immune response before it starts. Alternatively, an immune response that is annoying (such as allergy) or a life-threatening response (such as anaphylaxis) can be redirected in a less harmful direction.

Preemptive measures

Often an ongoing immune response cannot be fully suppressed. Although pathologies associated with adverse immune responses may be greatly diminished, it is difficult to obtain complete immunosuppression. A far more successful approach is to take therapeutic measures before an immune response develops, but this requires that a possible adverse immune response is imminent. Two such preemptive measures are Rh_0 (D) immune globulin and antibiotic therapy.

Rh_0 (D) immune globulin therapy

Pregnancy presents special problems to the immune system. Human fetuses derive nutrition *in utero* from the mother's circulation. Rh incompatibility can place the fetus at serious risk. Rh incompatibility between an Rh^- mother and an Rh^+ fetus can result in a hemolytic anemia affecting the fetus or neonate called **hemolytic disease of the newborn** (HDN) or sometimes **erythroblastosis fetalis**. The Rh antigen is a protein and elicits an IgG response. When maternal IgG crosses the placenta, a severe reaction can occur resulting in destruction of fetal tissues, most notably fetal erythrocytes. Complications from Rh disparity arise when Rh^+ fetal blood mixes with Rh^- maternal blood, causing maternal immunization and production of anti-Rh antibodies. The first pregnancy involving an Rh^+ fetus and an Rh^- mother often proceeds with little complication. Blood cells of fetal origin can be detected in the mother's bloodstream during the first trimester of pregnancy and these cells immunize the mother. It must be assumed that every conception between an Rh^+ male and Rh^- female will produce an Rh-incompatible fetus. Aborted (spontaneous or induced) conceptions can also lead to the development of an IgG antibody response to Rh_0 (D).

The severity of HDN varies widely. In the worst case, maternal IgG antibodies cross the placenta and bind to fetal erythrocytes. Fetal complement is activated, causing the erythrocytes to lyse. The resultant anemia may become so severe that the fetus sustains severe damage or dies in utero. To compensate for the anemia, the fetal bone marrow releases immature erythrocytes (or erythroblasts). The abnormal presence of these erythroblasts in the fetal circulation is the hallmark the disease (hence the term "erythroblastosis fetalis").

HDN can be prevented by the injection of a high-titer anti-Rh antibody preparation such as RhoGAM or MicoRhoGAM. These preparations consist of pooled anti-Rh antibodies, prepared from human serum obtained from mothers who have made antibodies to Rh antigens.

Anti-Rh antibodies must be given after every pregnancy (>12 weeks of gestation), even those that are terminated spontaneously or via induced abortion. Anti-Rh antibodies may also be indicated after a blood transfusion of an Rh⁻ female.

Antibiotic therapy

Sometimes antibiotics are administered to halt a bacterial infection and limit or prevent an adaptive immune response. Acute streptococcal pharyngitis or "strep throat" is generally a self-limiting illness of childhood and early adolescence in which symptoms spontaneously subside over a period of days in the majority of patients. Complications develop in a minority of patients, and these lead to the production of self-reactive antibodies. These antibodies are responsible for autoimmune acute rheumatic fever that can result

in rheumatic heart disease. Gram-positive group A streptococci (GAS), now classified as *Streptococcus pyogenes*, are characterized by the presence of a cell-wall carbohydrate (A carbohydrate) and cell-wall proteins termed M, T, and R. Penicillin is used to treat streptococcal pharyngitis, and no known penicillin resistance by GAS to penicillin has been shown. Penicillin accelerates bacterial clearance and in doing so limits immune involvement. Left untreated, an antibody response to the M protein of *S. pyogenes* develops in some patients. The anti-M antibodies cross-react with epitopes expressed by the lamella of the cardiac mitral valve.

Patient Vignette 11.3

Marilyn M., a 45-year-old woman, presents with increasing symptoms of shortness of breath when she walks up the stairs. In addition, she feels fatigue (tired) and has shortness of breath intermittently at night. Her physical examination was remarkable for a "heart murmur" and mild pedal edema (swelling of her feet).

Q: What immunologic processes might be involved in her problem?

A: This patient's symptoms suggest **mitral stenosis**. Mitral stenosis is a narrowing or constriction of the mitral valve opening. The underlying cause of mitral stenosis is rheumatic heart disease. Patients with mitral stenosis usually have a history of rheumatic fever, which can lead to rheumatic heart disease. Rheumatic heart disease is an inflammation of the heart that causes heart valve deformities, including stenosis. The suspected cause is the similarity of certain molecules on the streptococcal bacteria and human heart tissue.

The diagnosis of mitral stenosis includes medical history, physical examination, transthoracic echocardiography (ultrasound of the chest), and confirmation with cardiac catheterization. Patients with moderate to severe mitral stenosis with symptoms require surgical intervention.

Modification of ongoing disease

Often it is not possible to predict that an adverse immune response will occur. In such cases, therapeutic measures are applied to minimize the course of the disease.

Cytokines

Systemic administration of cytokines has been used clinically to alter the course of a number of diseases. One of the most successful applications has been the use of IFN-α to treat metastatic melanoma. Granulocyte-monocyte colony-stimulating factor (GM-CSF) treatment dramatically increased survival times in melanoma patients. Independent clinical trials have shown that intravenous IFN-α treatment of melanoma patients shows overall survival benefit. Certain renal carcinoma patients have benefited from IL-2 therapy.

With the advent of highly active antiretroviral therapy (HAART), deaths caused by HIV infection in developed countries have declined dramatically. Despite the success of HAART to decrease viral load, the virus is not eliminated. Chronic HIV infection causes the gradual depletion not only of CD4$^+$ T cells but also of monocytes/macrophages and CD8$^+$ T cells. A major clinical challenge is the restoration of functional immune cells. A number of cytokine therapies are currently being tested in clinical or preclinical trials. These include IL-2 to reverse CD4$^+$ T cell lymphopenia, IL-12 to enhance HIV-specific cell-mediated immunity, IL-15 to enhance CD8$^+$ T cell function, IFN-α/IFN-γ to enhance CTL responses, GM-CSF to enhance monocyte/ macrophage function, and G-CSF to increase myeloid cell precursors. The goal of all cytokine therapies is to preserve and enhance immunity to HIV and prevent opportunistic infections. Unfortunately, systemic cytokine therapy is accompanied by adverse side effects. For example, IL-2 supports the growth of T lymphocytes and NK cells, but it also increases apoptosis in T cell populations. IL-15 also simulates proliferation of both CD8$^+$ and CD4$^+$ T cell populations and appears to be anti-apoptotic.

Allergy desensitization

When it is not possible to avoid exposure to an allergen and when pharmacologic therapy does not prove to be effective in the treatment of allergic rhinitis or allergic asthma, allergen immunotherapy may be attempted. An aqueous extract of the allergen is repeatedly injected subcutaneously over a period of weeks to months in gradually increasing doses. The repeated immunization regimen is designed to increase the amount (titer) of IgG antibody produced to the allergen. In older sources, allergen immunotherapy is known as desensitization. The term "desensitization" is a misnomer. The goal of repeated immunization is to redirect antibody production from predominantly IgE to predominantly IgG. IgG antibodies bind and remove the allergen before it can interact with IgE antibodies bound to the surfaces of mast cells. Because anaphylactic reactions may develop in patients injected with an allergen, the patient undergo observation for at least 20 minutes after injection, and emergency treatments including antihistamine and epinephrine should be available if necessary.

Summary

- **Adjuvants** derived from microbial products may be used to strengthen a weak immune response by increasing co-stimulatory molecule expression on antigen-presenting cells. Examples of adjuvants are Bacillus Calmette-Guérin, Levamisole, and interleukin-12.
- **Cytokines** are soluble molecules produced by a variety of cells that affect immune function. Examples of cytokines that have been used as immunotherapeutic agents are type I (IFN α/β) and type II (IFN-γ) interferons.
- Individuals with generalized antibody deficiency such as hypogammaglobulinemia or agammaglobulinemia may be successfully treated with human immune globulin (HIg), which is composed primarily of IgG.
- Anti-inflammatory drugs, such as **corticosteroids** and **nonsteroidal anti-inflammatory drugs (NSAIDs)**, are used to control inflammation. Corticosteroids are currently used to treat many diseases and conditions, including autoimmune disorders, allergic diseases, and bronchial asthma, and to prevent organ rejection.
- **Rheumatoid arthritis (RA)** is a destructive inflammatory autoimmune disease that ultimately involves both cell-mediated and humoral immune responses. Treatment of RA may include NSAIDs, disease-modifying antirheumatic drugs (DMARDs), corticosteroids, and biologic agents (TNF-α inhibitor and IL-1).
- **Bronchial asthma** is a chronic inflammatory respiratory disorder. Drug therapies for

asthma include β_2-adrenergic receptor agonist, corticosteroids, theophylline, cromolyn, nedocromil, leukotriene antagonists, and anticholinergic agents.

- Several approaches to minimize immune responses against alloantigens within the graft include: global inhibition of the immune system, selective inhibition of a particular class of leukocytes, or the selective inhibition of graft-specific leukocytes. The global approach is to use systemic immunosuppressive drugs such as corticosteroids or whole-body irradiation. Another approach is the use of antibodies directed at molecules present on the surface of lymphocytes and antigen-presenting cells. Yet another is using drugs with more restricted effects on the immune system such as cyclosporine, tacrolimus, and rapamycin.

- A strategy to stop an immune response before it starts is using RhoGAM or MicoRhoGAM to prevent **hemolytic disease of the newborn (HDN)**. Rh incompatibility between an Rh$^-$ mother and an Rh$^+$ fetus can result in a hemolytic anemia affecting the fetus or neonate, causing HDN, sometimes also called erythroblastosis fetalis. HDN can be prevented by the injection of a high-titer anti-Rh antibody preparation such as RhoGAM or MicoRhoGAM.

- Systemic administration of cytokines has been used clinically to alter the course of a number of diseases. For examples, the successful uses of IFN-α to treat metastatic melanoma and granulocyte-monocyte colony-stimulating factor (GM-CSF) treatment in increasing the survival times in melanoma patients.

- In the treatment of allergic rhinitis or allergic asthma, allergen immunotherapy may be used. The main goal of treatment to redirect antibody production from predominantly IgE to predominantly IgG.

Suggested readings

Alexandre J, Barbuto M, Akporiaye ET, et al. Immunopharmacology. In Katzung BG, ed. *Basic & Clinical Pharmacology,* 7th ed. New York: Appleton and Lange, 1998.

Ashby B. Prostaglandins and Related Autocoids. In Brody TM, Larner J, Minneman KP, eds. *Human Pharmacology: Molecular to Clinical*, 3rd ed. St. Louis: Mosby, 1998.

Foegh ML, Hecker M, Ramwell PW. The Eicosanoids: Prostaglandins, Thromboxanes, Leukotrienes, and Related Compounds. In Katzung BG, ed. *Basic & Clinical Pharmacology*, 7th ed. New York: Appleton and Lange, 1998.

Greenberger PA. Asthma. In Grammer LC, Greenberger PA, eds. *Patterson's Allergic Diseases*. 6th ed. Philadelphia: Lippincott Williams & Wilkins, 2002.

National Institutes of Health, National Heart, Lung, and Blood Institute. Expert Panel Report: Guidelines for the Diagnosis and Management of Asthma. Bethesda, MD: U.S. Department of Health and Human Services, 2002. NIH publication no. 02-5074.

Nimmagadda SR. Corticosteroids. In Grammer LC, Greenberger PA, eds. *Patterson's Allergic Diseases*, 6th ed. Philadelphia: Lippincott Williams & Wilkins, 2002.

Van Everdinglen AA, Jacobs JWG, van Reseema DRS, et al. Low Dose Prednisone Therapy for Patients with Early Active Rheumatoid Arthritis: Clinical Efficacy, Disease Modifying Properties, and Side Effects. *Ann Intern Med* 2002;136:1–12.

Review questions

1. Which of the following has shown promise as an adjuvant in vaccine therapy?
   (A) IFN-α
   (B) IFN-γ
   (C) IL-2
   (D) IL-12
   (E) IL-15

2. Which of the following has shown promise as an adjuvant in the treatment of superficial bladder cancer?
   (A) BCG (Bacillus Calmette-Guérin)
   (B) Pegylated IFN-γ
   (C) Rheumatoid factor
   (D) FK506
   (E) NSAIDs

3. The antibody isotype most commonly used for antibody replacement therapy therapy is:
   (A) IgM
   (B) IgD
   (C) IgG
   (D) IgA
   (E) IgE

4. For the past several weeks, a 14-year-old boy has had daily bouts of coughing and intermittent wheezing. His symptoms worsen at night. His pediatrician suspects asthma. In

addition to albuterol (a β2-adrenergic) in-haler, which of the following may help the patient in long-term control of his symptoms?

(A) A course of antibiotic therapy
(B) NSAID
(C) Inhaled corticosteroid
(D) Monoclonal IgE
(E) No additional medication is needed

5. A 55-year-old woman with a 1-year history of severe rheumatoid arthritis has been treated with NSAIDs and methotrexate for many months without much relief of her symptoms. Which of the following medications is considered the next best option?

(A) Gold salt therapy
(B) Anti-malarial agent
(C) IL-1
(D) Theophylline
(E) TNF-α inhibitor

6. A 60-year-old man is brought to the emergency room for recurrent chest pain. He has hypertension, diabetes, and smokes cigarettes. In the emergency room, his electrocardiogram shows that he has myocardial ischemia (inadequate circulation of blood to the heart muscle). Immediate general treatment for this patient should include oxygen followed by:

(A) Corticosteroid
(B) Aspirin
(C) NSAID
(D) Epinephrine
(E) Cyclosporine

Tools and Assays of Immune Function

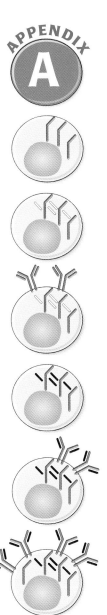

Appendix Outline

Introduction Clinical laboratories use antibodies as tools in a variety of assays to specifically detect antigens as soluble, particulate-bound, and cell-bound molecules. In routine tests (e.g., blood typing) antibodies agglutinate (causing to clump together) particles such as erythrocytes. In other tests [e.g., radial immunodiffusion (RID) and immunoelectrophoresis (IEP)], the binding of soluble antibody to soluble antigen forms precipitating antigen–antibody complexes (precipitin reaction, see Fig. 4-5) that are readily visualized. Antibodies labeled with either radioactive molecules or enzymes are used in assays [e.g., radioimmunoassay (RIA) and enzyme-linked immunosorbent assays (ELISA)]. Among the most sensitive biological tests known, RIA and ELISA use antibodies to detect picrogram (10^{-9} gram) quantities of antigen. Antibodies may also be labeled with fluorescent molecules to detect epitopes on single cells either by light microscopy or by flow cytometry.

Immune function can also be assayed in the laboratory. In vitro tests may be used to assess the function of the soluble molecules such as complement system components and to determine whether neutralizing antibodies have been produced against a bacterium, virus, or toxin. Leukocyte function is assessed by the ability of cells to respond to mitogens (substances that induce cells to proliferate) or to specific antigens. Chemoattractant stimuli are used to determine the leukocyte homing ability in leukocyte migration assays. The function of cytotoxic T lymphocytes (CTLs) and natural killer (NK) cells are determined in cytotoxicity assays. Leukocyte phagocytic activity can also be assessed. In vivo hypersensitivity function may be determined through allergy, delayed (-type) hypersensitivity (DTH), and contact skin testing.

ANTIBODIES AS EPITOPE-DETECTING TOOLS

Molecules recognized by the immune system are known as antigens. Some antigens are simple and others are large and complex. Antibodies, as antigen-recognizing structures, "see" only a limited portion of most antigens. The smallest part of an antigen recognized by the immune system is known as an antigenic determinant or **epitope** and is typically contained within a sequence of approximately 6 to 10 amino acids for protein antigens. Antibody-based assays are epitope-detecting tools.

Many diagnostic clinical tests are derived from the quantitative precipitin reaction (see Fig 4-5). These tests can be grouped according to whether antibodies bind to particulate antigens to cross-link (agglutination), interact with soluble molecules to form a precipitin reaction (RID, Ouchterlony, and IEP), or bind with a labeled ligand (RIA and ELISA).

Detection of particulate antigens

Not all antigens are soluble. The **agglutination reaction** measures the interaction of antibody with epitopes on the surface of a particulate antigen. Cross-linking of particulate antigen by antibody results in clumping or **agglutination** or, when erythrocytes are the particulate antigen, **hemagglutination** (Fig. A-1A). Hemagglutination is frequently used to determine blood type. IgM antibodies are large molecules with 10 antigen-binding sites that span a relatively large molecular distance, efficiently cross-link epitope-bearing particles, and are effective in the **direct agglutination test** (Fig. A-1B). Other immunoglobulin isotypes, because they are smaller and have fewer antigen-binding sites, are less efficient at direct agglutination.

The same rules that govern the quantitative precipitin reaction (see Fig. 4-5) apply to agglutination tests. Addition of too much antibody inhibits agglutination, similar to the zone of antibody excess in which too much antibody inhibits precipitation (Fig. A-1C). The inhibition of agglutination by antibody excess is known as the **prozone**. To circumvent prozone inhibition of agglutination, dilutions of antibody are added to identical samples of particulate antigen. Two-fold or serial dilutions of antibody are typically prepared. Each dilution is half as concentrated as the preceding one. The lowest concentration of antibody that causes agglutination is called the **titer**. Titers are relative measures of antibody activity and are typically expressed as the reciprocal of the dilution, e.g., 1:16; 1:32, 1:64, etc.

Sometimes IgM antibodies are present in concentrations too low to be detected by direct agglutination. Antibodies other than IgM may be present but are not detected by direct agglutination. The sensitivity of the agglutination test may be enhanced using anti-immunoglobulin antibodies in the so-called **indirect** or **passive agglutination technique**. When a small amount of human serum containing mostly IgG antibodies is incubated with antigen-bearing particles, agglutination may not be seen (Fig. A-1D). Addition of a rabbit anti-human IgG antibody causes agglutination of the particles to which human IgG is bound (Fig. A-1E). The use of anti-immunoglobulin antibody, sometimes called a **second-step antibody**, finds application in a number of diagnostic methods.

Detection of soluble antigens by precipitation

The classical quantitative precipitin reaction requires the preparation of a number of antigen/antibody samples. The preparation of these is often too cumbersome and time-consuming to find application in most clinical laboratories. Fortunately, the quantitative precipitin reaction has been adapted through several simple modifica-

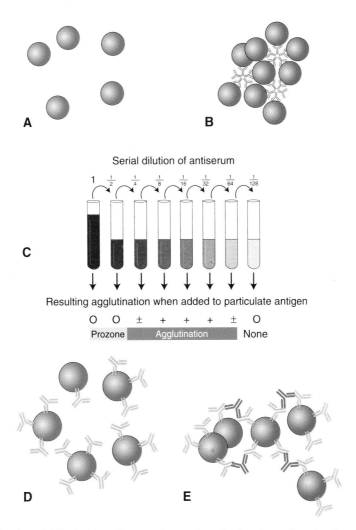

FIGURE A-1. Agglutination. (A) Particulate antigens such as erythrocytes (or other antigen-bearing particles such as bacteria or latex particles) are normally evenly dispersed in suspension. **(B)** Cross-linking of antigen-bearing particles by IgM antibodies causes them to clump, a process known as agglutination. **(C)** Agglutination reactions are governed by the same rules as the quantitative precipitin reaction; excessive antibody concentrations inhibit agglutination. Antibodies must be diluted to the "proper" concentration for maximum agglutination to occur. Serial dilutions of antibody are prepared and added to identical samples of particulate antigen. After a brief incubation period, the agglutination patterns are determined. Those dilutions in which antibody inhibits agglutination form the prozone (similar to the zone of antibody excess in the quantitative precipitin reaction). Dilutions that cause agglutination are similar to the equivalence zone in the quantitative precipitin reaction. The lowest concentration of antibody that causes agglutination is known as the titer (this occurs in at a 1/64 dilution in this example. **(D)** Non-IgM antibodies agglutinate poorly. **(E)** An anti-immunoglobulin or second-step antibody (blue) may be used to cross-link antibodies bound to a particle in indirect or passive agglutination.

tions for application in the clinical laboratory. Several of these reactions involve visualization of immune precipitates in a semi-solid medium, agar.

Radial immunodiffusion

Single or **radial immunodiffusion** (RID), originally called the **Mancini technique**, is based on the diffusion of soluble antigen through an agar gel that contains a uniform concentration of antibody. Antibody-containing molten agar is poured onto a glass slide or plastic dish, the agar is allowed to cool, wells are cut into the gel matrix, and soluble antigen is placed into the well cut (Fig. A-2). As the antigen diffuses radially through the antibody-containing gel, a precipitin ring forms around the well and moves outward,

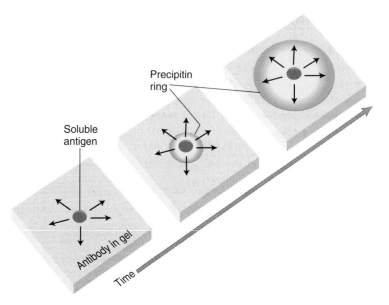

FIGURE A-2. Radial immunodiffusion (RID). The amount of antigen in a solution can be quantified using the radial immunodiffusion (RID) technique. A low concentration of antibody is added to molten agar and the uniform mixture is poured on a glass slide or plastic dish. Several minutes later, once the agar has gelled, wells are cut into the agar layer and antigen is placed in the well. The soluble antigen readily diffuses through the gel matrix. The initial antigen concentration around the well is great enough that soluble complexes are formed and precipitin formation is inhibited (zone of antigen excess). As the antigen continues to diffuse from the well and its concentration diminishes by the square of the radius, eventually an equivalence point is reached and a precipitin ring is formed. As more antigen enters the gel, the precipitated antigen–antibody complexes dissolve and the equivalence zone is re-established at a distance further from the well. When no additional antigen diffuses into the gel (approximately 24 hours), the diameter of the zone of equivalence stabilizes and is directly proportional to the concentration of the antigen loaded into the well. Concentrations of antigens (unknowns) are determined by comparing the diameters of their precipitin rings with a standard curve constructed from the precipitin ring diameters of different known concentrations.

eventually becoming stationary at equivalence. The diameter of the ring is directly proportional to the antigen concentration originally loaded into the well. By comparing the precipitin ring diameter of a test sample of unknown concentration with a standard calibration curve of known antigen concentration, the concentration of an antigen in a test sample can be accurately determined.

Double diffusion

In the **double diffusion** or **Ouchterlony technique,** both antigen and antibody are allowed to diffuse through the gel. An antigen–antibody precipitin line is formed at equivalence. Solubility, molecular size, and charge affect the local concentration of each reactant and their diffusion rates through the gel. This technique is qualitatively sensitive but not quantitative.

Multiple precipitin lines will be present if antigen and antibodies contain several molecular species. Multiple precipitin lines often form depending on the molecular size of the antibody

(IgM diffuses slower than IgG) and if the antibodies detect epitopes on different-sized antigens. This technique has the advantage that several antigens or antibodies can be compared around a single well and can distinguish **identity, partial identity,** and **nonidentity** between antigens and/or antibodies. To illustrate the power of this technique, we use three examples.

In the first example, three wells are cut into an agar layer. A mixture of insulin (a) and thyroglobulin (b) are loaded into the upper left well and insulin only is loaded into the upper right well (Fig. A-3A). Rabbit antisera to both proinsulin (anti-a′) and thyroglobulin (anti-b) are loaded into the bottom well. After several hours, precipitin lines form, bisecting the axis of the antigen–antibody wells. Two precipitin bands are formed (Fig. A-3A). One line results from reaction of thyroglobulin with anti-thyroglobulin (blue). A second line indicates that anti-proinsulin (anti-a′) reacts with insulin (a). The formation of an arc (a smooth joining of two lines; see example A in Fig. A-3) indicates antigenic **iden-**

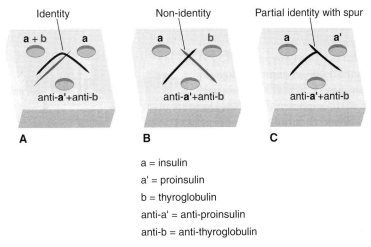

a = insulin
a' = proinsulin
b = thyroglobulin
anti-a' = anti-proinsulin
anti-b = anti-thyroglobulin

FIGURE A-3. Double diffusion or Ouchterlony technique. In the double diffusion or Ouchterlony technique, both antigens and antibodies diffuse through the gel. Molten agar is poured onto a glass slide or plastic plate and allowed to gel. Wells are punched into the gel and loaded with soluble antigen or antibody. In this example, the bottom well in each gel is loaded with rabbit antisera to proinsulin (anti-a') and thyroglobulin (anti-b). Proinsulin is a single chain precursor of the insulin A and B chains and a C peptide that is absent from mature insulin. **(A)** Insulin (a) and thyroglobulin (b) have been loaded into one antigen well and insulin only was loaded into the other antigen well. Anti-thyroglobulin reacts with thyroglobulin to form a precipitin line (blue). Anti-proinsulin reacts with insulin from both antigen wells (black precipitin arc). This shows that antibodies to proinsulin recognize insulin and, by forming a precipitin arc, indicate that the antigens loaded into the adjacent wells have identical epitopes in common. **(B)** A second gel is loaded with insulin (black a) in one antigen well and thyroglobulin (blue b) in the other. The crossed precipitin lines indicate nonidentity—that the antigens do not share any epitopes in common. **(C)** Insulin (a) and proinsulin (a') have been loaded in separate antigen wells. A precipitin arc is formed as in the first gel, but with a spur, indicating the recognition of additional epitopes on proinsulin that are not present on insulin.

tity (in this case insulin) for antigens loaded into the upper wells.

A second gel is prepared in which insulin (a) and thyroglobulin (b) are placed in the upper left and upper right wells (Fig. A-3B). Precipitin bands formed between insulin and thyroglobulin with their respective antibodies show a **nonidentity** pattern.

In a third gel (Fig. A-3C), one antigen well is loaded with insulin (a) and the other is loaded with proinsulin (a'). Anti-proinsulin antibodies react with both insulin and proinsulin. However, anti-proinsulin reacts with additional epitopes in proinsulin, represented as a **spur**, that are not present in insulin, demonstrating **partial identity**.

Immunoelectrophoresis

A modification of the double diffusion technique, **immunoelectrophoresis (IEP)** separates antigens according to charge and size before their reaction with antibody. Antigens are loaded into a well in an agar layer, an electrical current is passed through the agar, and the antigens migrate according to their size and charge (Fig. A-4). The

electrical current is removed, and a trough is cut into the gel, which is loaded with antiserum. The antigens and antibodies diffuse through and precipitin arcs are formed in the gel. More than 80 different serum molecules can be identified by this technique, although not all at once. The choice of antibody used in the trough determines which antigens will precipitate. The precipitin lines that are formed are not always symmetrical. This effect is often caused by the heterogeneous mobility of the antigen through the gel. Various factors can affect the electrophoretic mobility of serum molecules, including the presence of isomers (e.g., isozymes) and different degrees of glycosylation.

Monoclonal antibodies

For years, serum-derived antibodies produced by immunizing animals with multiple antigen injections were used in epitope-detecting assays. Because of animal-to-animal variability in antibody quality and relatively small batch size, each antiserum batch had to be extensively characterized before use in the clinical laboratory. This all changed in 1975 when Georges Kohler and Cesar

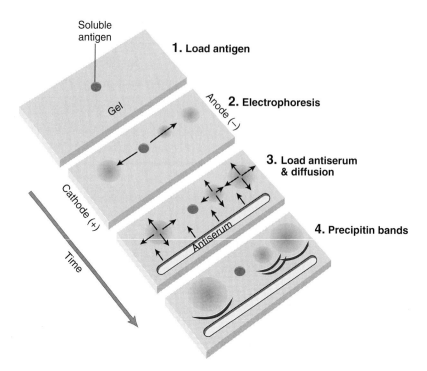

FIGURE A-4. Immunoelectrophoresis (IEP) is a variation of the double diffusion technique. Molten agar is poured onto a glass slide, allowed to cool, and a well is cut into the gel. **(1)** Soluble antigen is loaded into a well on a glass slide. **(2)** An electrical current is passed through the gel causing the antigen to migrate according to both their electric charge and size. **(3)** The electrical current is removed, a trough is cut into the gel, and antiserum is loaded into the trough. Similar to the double diffusion technique, both antigens and antibodies diffuse through the gel matrix. **(4)** After several hours, precipitin bands form. Sometimes the precipitin bands are asymmetrical, because of different forms (isomers) of the same antigen and glycosylation differences. IEP is a sensitive, qualitative, but not quantitative, technique.

Milstein developed a method to produce antibodies derived from the progeny of a single antibody-producing cell, or **monoclonal antibodies**.

The method for creating monoclonal antibodies begins by immunizing a mouse with antigen (Fig. A-5). Splenic B cells from an immunized mouse are fused with B-cell lineage tumor cells (myeloma) using polyethylene glycol to promote fusion of cell membranes.

Only a small proportion of the splenic B cells and myeloma cells successfully fuse to make a **hybridoma**, although several cell types are also present in the fusion mixture, including splenic B cells, myeloma cells, and homokaryons (fusion of two like cells).

The myeloma cells used as a fusion partner lack thymidine kinase (TK) required for the synthesis of purines by the *de novo* DNA synthetic pathway. Instead, these myeloma cells use hypoxanthine–guanine phosphoribosil transferase (HGPT) to synthesize purines from hypoxanthine via the salvage pathway. On exposure of these myeloma cells to aminopterin, a drug that selec-

tively blocks HGPT activity, all DNA synthetic activity is blocked and the cells die. Cells of the fusion mixture are cultured in a selective culture medium containing hypoxanthine, aminopterin, and thymidine (**HAT medium**). Splenic B cells and B-cell homokaryons naturally die in culture after several weeks. Myeloma cells and myeloma homokaryons, because they cannot synthesize purines by either the *de novo* or salvage pathways, cannot grow in HAT medium. Only hybridomas that have acquired both the TK gene from the B-cell parent and the transformed trait from the myeloma will grow in HAT medium. Not all hybridoma cells, however, produce antibody. Hybridoma cells are placed in wells in a tissue culture plate and ELISA or other immunoassay is used to identify those wells with antibody-producing cells. Cells from antibody-producing wells are cloned by placing a single cell in a single well. A clone of antibody-producing cells derived from a single progenitor cell is immortal and produces monoclonal antibody. Because the hybridoma cell line is immortal and produces antibody of a single

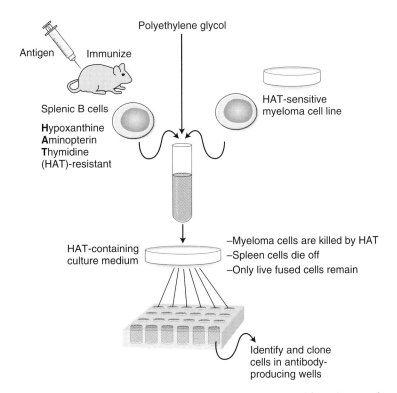

FIGURE A-5. Monoclonal antibody creation. Before 1975, antibodies were isolated from the sera of immunized animals, resulting in different isotypes, affinity, and specificity between animals and production lots of antisera. With the advent of hybridoma technology, antibodies derived a single antibody-producing progenitor (monoclonal antibody), allowing the production of unlimited amounts of antibody with the same isotype, affinity, and specificity. The creation of a monoclonal antibody begins by immunizing a mouse with antigen. Several days after the last immunization, spleen cells are harvested and placed in a test tube. Cells of a B-cell lineage tumor cell line (myeloma) that lack immunoglobulin genes and have a defective thymidine kinase (TK) gene are added to the test tube. Polyethylene glycol is added to the test tube to promote cell membrane fusion. Only a small percentage of heterokaryons (cells containing genetic material from two different genomes) are fused to form hybridomas. Two selective methods are used for nonhybridoma cells in the fusion mixture. Parental spleen cells and splenic homokaryons (fusion of two or more like cells) normally die in culture after several weeks. Myleoma cells, because they lack TK, cannot use the *de novo* DNA synthetic pathway for purine synthesis and must rely on hypoxanthine–guanine phosphoribosyl transferase (HGPT) for the synthesis of purines from hypoxanthine by the salvage pathway. The cells of the fusion mixture are cultured with a selective medium containing *hypoxanthine, aminopterin,* and *thymidine* (HAT). Aminopterin is an HGPT-specific toxin. TK-defective myeloma cells and myeloma homokaryons die, because they cannot synthesize purines via the *de novo* pathway (TK defect) and aminopterin poisons HGPT activity necessary for the salvage pathway. Only hybridoma cells survive, because the TK gene is supplied by the spleen cell partner and cell line immortality is supplied by the myeloma cell. Not all hybridomas produce antibody. The cells are cultured in individual wells of a tissue culture plate and antibody-containing wells are identified by immunoassay. Cells from antibody-containing wells are cloned by placing a single cell. This assures that antibody-producing daughter cells derive from a single progenitor cell or clone and that the antibodies are monoclonal. Unlimited amounts of antibody of a single specificity can be produced from this cell line.

known specificity, an unlimited amount of monoclonal antibody can be produced now and for years to come.

Quantitative methods using labeled antibodies

Antibodies or antigens may be labeled with radioactivity or with a wide variety of readily detectable molecules, such as enzymes, fluorescent molecules, or heavy metals. An extensive description of immunoassays and their application is beyond the scope of this book. Here we describe two types of immunoassay, radioimmunoassay using soluble antigen and antibodies, and enzyme-linked immunosorbent assay.

Radioimmunoassay

Radioimmunoassay (RIA) is widely used in clinical diagnostic laboratories and is a theme with many variations. In general, antibodies are directly radiolabeled if the antibodies are readily available and/or the epitopes to be detected are in relative abundance. If, however, an epitope is present in low frequency, a radiolabeled antibody to the detecting antibody (an anti-immunoglobulin) is used to amplify the sensitivity of the reaction. Figure A-6 shows direct RIA using radiolabeled primary antibody and indirect RIA in which an anti-immunoglobulin antibody is radiolabeled. Antigen–antibody complexes are separated from free-radiolabeled ligand by precipitation, centrifugation, or other means, and the radioactivity bound to the complex is measured. In competitive-binding RIA, a test sample containing an unlabeled ligand is allowed to react with the antibody, and then a known amount of radioactively labeled ligand is added. Inhibition of binding by the radiolabeled ligand may then be used to quantify the amount of unlabeled ligand in the test sample. RIAs, although very sensitive, generate radioactive waste and, because of radioactive decay, the reagents have a limited shelf life.

RIA can detect ligands in the range of nanograms to picograms per milliliter. A variation of this assay relies on the fluorescent properties of a class of rare earth elements, such as europium, and detection sensitivities in the attomole (10^{-18} M) range are possible.

Enzyme-linked immunosorbent assay

Enzyme-lined immunosorbent assay (ELISA) [sometimes called enzyme immunoassay (EIA)]

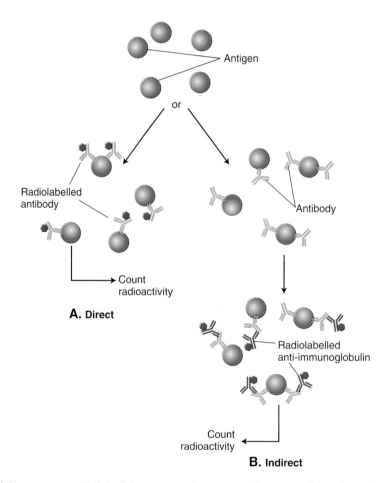

FIGURE A-6. Radioimmunoassay (RIA). Radioimmunoassay is a very sensitive means of detecting antigen. The presence of epitope-bearing antigens may be detected by either direct or indirect immunoassay. **(A)** In direct RIA, radiolabeled, epitope-specific antibodies directly bind directly to the antigen. The degree of radiolabel binding is determined by a radioactivity counter. **(B)** In indirect RIA, two antibodies are used. An unlabeled first or epitope-specific antibody is incubated with the antigen. A radiolabeled, second, or anti-immunoglobulin antibody with specificity for antigenic determinants on the first antibody is then added. The extent of radiolabeled antibody binding by the second antibody is used as a measure of the amount of epitope detected by the first antibody and is determined by a radioactivity counter.

has replaced RIA in a number of tests. ELISA offers the advantage of safety, rapidity, and reagent stability and has a sensitivity that equals or exceeds that of RIA. Enzyme-labeled antibody or enzyme-labeled antigen conjugates are used. The assay relies on nonspecific binding of antigen to a solid substrate, such as polystyrene, in a 96-well plate (Fig. A-7). After several hours, unbound antigen is washed away, and subsequent nonspecific binding is minimized by addition of a

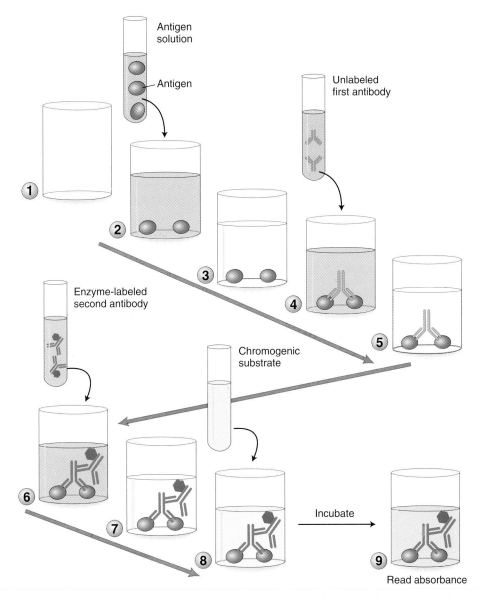

FIGURE A-7. Enzyme-linked immunosorbent assay (ELISA). The enzyme-linked immunosorbent assay (ELISA) uses enzyme-labeled antibody for epitope detection. Because of its safety, the long shelf life of the labeled antibody, and low cost, ELISA has replaced RIA for many laboratory assays. **(1)** The assay is generally performed in a 96-well plate constructed of a special protein-adsorbing polystyrene (a single well is shown here). **(2)** Antigen solution is added to the well and allowed to noncovalently bind to the plastic. **(3)** Unbound antigen is removed by washing the plastic with a saline (0.15 M NaCl) solution. A protein solution, generally an albumin, is added to the well to nonspecifically block any protein-binding sites on the plastic, followed by a saline wash (not shown). **(4)** Unlabeled, first antibody is added to the well and allowed to bind to specific epitopes. **(5)** Unbound first antibody is removed by washing the well with a saline solution. **(6)** An enzyme-labeled, anti-immunoglobulin solution is added to the well and allowed to bind to the first antibody. **(7)** Unbound anti-immunoglobulin is removed by a saline wash. **(8)** A chromogenic substrate is added to the well and allowed to incubate. **(9)** Change in the color of the substrate indicates the presence of enzyme-labeled antibody. Because the enzyme-labeled antibody only detects the first antibody, and the first antibody detects a specific epitope, the degree of color change indicates the amount of epitope detected.

substance such as albumin that will bind to the plastic but not interfere with the subsequent binding of antibody. The test sample containing putative antibodies to the substrate-bound antigen is then added, incubated, and the well is washed again. An enzyme-labeled second antibody is added, incubated, and the well is washed again. A chromogenic substrate that changes color on cleavage by the enzyme coupled to the second antibody is then added to the wells. Presence of enzyme-labeled antibody is visualized by a color change in the substrate. Enzyme activity is measured spectrophotometrically. The amount of primary antibody bound is determined by comparing the test serum to a control or reference serum containing known amounts of antigen.

Antigen detection in and on cells

Antibodies can be used to detect epitopes in and on cells in a wide variety of tissues. Both radioac-

tivity and enzymes are used to label antibodies for detection of epitopes in tissues. Another method for labeling antibodies is by covalently coupling a fluorescent molecule such as fluorescein as a marker for detection. Antibodies labeled with fluorescent molecules are used to detect epitopes on single cells either by light microscopy or by flow cytometry.

Immunofluorescence

Fluorescent dyes, such as fluorescein isothiocyanate (FITC), are covalently attached to an antibody. FITC will fluoresce green light (535 nm) when excited by light of a shorter wavelength (485 nm). In the example (Fig. A-8), a thin, frozen section of tissue is prepared and mounted on a glass slide. Epitopes may be detected by either **direct** or **indirect immunofluorescence**. In the direct technique (Fig. A-8A), the tissue section is bathed in a solution containing FITC-la-

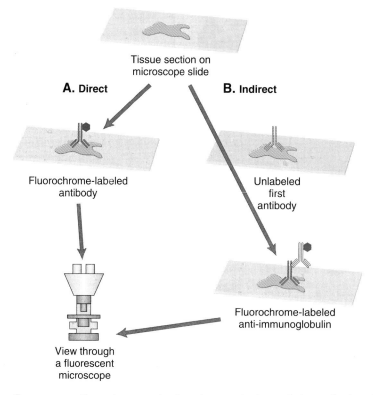

Tissue section on microscope slide

A. Direct

B. Indirect

Fluorochrome-labeled antibody

Unlabeled first antibody

Fluorochrome-labeled anti-immunoglobulin

View through a fluorescent microscope

FIGURE A-8. **Immunofluorescence.** Fluorochrome molecules, when covalently coupled to antibody molecules, can be used to identify epitopes within a tissue preparation. A thin tissue section is prepared and mounted on a glass microscope slide. **(A)** Fluorochrome-labeled antibody is incubated with the tissue section in the direct immunofluorescent technique. After an incubation period, unbound antibody is washed away with a mild (0.15 M) salt solution. Presence of epitopes can be visualized using a fluorescent microscope. **(B)** In the indirect immunofluorescent technique an unlabeled, epitope-specific antibody is allowed to bind to the tissue section, then the preparation is washed with a mild (0.15 M) salt solution. A fluorochrome-labeled anti-immunoglobulin is then incubated with the preparation and unbound labeled antibody is washed away. Presence of epitopes is visualized with a fluorescent microscope.

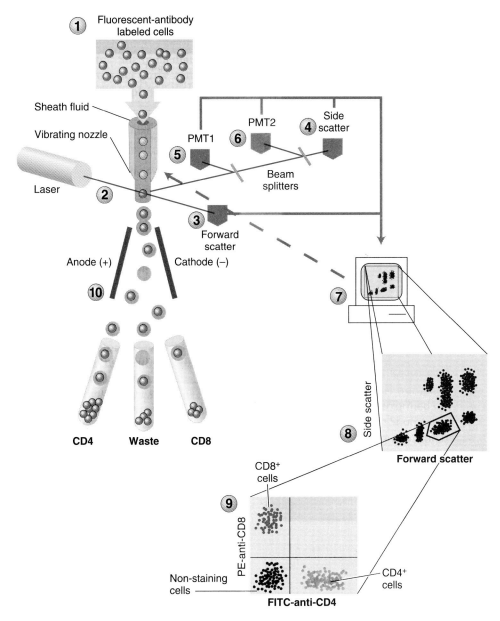

FIGURE A-9. Flow cytometry. The percentages of cells in a population bearing one or more epitopes of interest can be readily identified and isolated by flow cytometry. **(1)** A single-cell suspension of leukocytes is prepared and stained with fluorochrome-labeled antibodies. The labeled cells pass flow pass through a chamber (flow cell) as a single-cell stream contained within an aqueous sheath (sheath fluid). The sheath fluid passes through a vibrating nozzle as it exits the flow cell, causing stream to break into individual droplets. **(2)** A laser beam passes through the stream just before droplets are formed. The laser beam is refracted and reflected when a particle passes through the stream. **(3)** Refracted light is measured as forward scatter and is a measure of cellular volume. **(4)** Reflected light (measured at right angles to the laser beam) is a measure of cellular granularity. Beam splitters sample the reflected light beam using photomultiplier tubes (PMT) to measure **(5)** green and **(6)** red fluorescence. **(7)** A computer analyzes the sensor data and represents these graphically on a screen. **(8)** Data using two sensors, forward and side scatter, allow the flow cytometer operator to distinguish cells based on their morphology. In the example, a box has been drawn around the lymphocyte population. This electronically identified or "gated" population can be further analyzed. **(9)** Analysis of the lymphocyte-gated population shows a population of CD4+ staining cells (x axis) and a population of CD8+ staining cells (y axis). **(10)** Populations identified can then be isolated (sorted) by the flow cytometer. The computer signals the flow cytometer to apply a negative or positive charge to the aqueous sheath before droplet formation. Droplets that carry a negative charge will be attracted to the anode and those with a positive charge will be attracted to the cathode deflection plate and are collected in a test tube. Uncharged droplets are consigned to waste.

beled antibody and after an incubation period, unbound antibody is removed by washing the preparation with a mild (0.15 M) salt solution. Bound labeled antibody is visualized with a fluorescent microscope. In the indirect technique (Fig A-8B), the tissue section is bathed in a solution containing unlabeled, anti-epitope antibody and after an incubation period, unbound, anti-epitope antibody is washed away. The preparation is then bathed in a solution containing fluorochrome-labeled anti-immunoglobulin, incubated, and washed with a mild salt solution. Bound labeled antibody is visualized with a fluorescent microscope. By giving antibodies "tail-lights," antigens and the cells that express these molecules may be readily detected by fluorescent light microscopy or flow cytometry.

Flow cytometry

A powerful modification of the immunofluorescent technique is known as **flow cytometry**. Leukocytes or other cells are stained with fluorochrome-labeled antibodies. As an example, we outline the procedure used to detect and quantify $CD4^+$ and $CD8^+$ lymphocytes using FITC-labeled anti-CD4 and phycoerythrin (PE)-labeled anti-CD8 antibodies.

Single-cell suspensions containing both labeled and unlabeled cells (Fig. A-9.1) flow through a vibrating chamber (flow cell) in an aqueous stream (sheath fluid) so that they pass through a laser beam (Fig. A-9.2). Each cell is measured for the amount of light it refracts (forward scatter, a measure of cell volume; Fig. A-9.3) and the amount of light that is scattered at approximately right angles to the laser beam (a measure of cellular granularity; Fig. A-9.4). Additional filters and photomultiplier tubes (PMT) detect green (FITC, 535 nm; Fig. A-9.5) and red (PE, 570 nm; Fig A-9.6) fluorescence. Data signals from the PMTs feed into a computer (Fig. A-9.7) for real-time data analysis. Cellular morphology can be readily distinguished using forward and side scatter (Fig A-9.8). Signals from lymphocytes are electronically identified (gated) and data for FITC-anti-CD4 and PE-anti-CD8 labeled cells may be plotted (Fig. A-9.9) and the percentage of each population determined.

Four cell populations may be identified by this technique. $CD4^+$ cells are displayed in the lower right quadrant and $CD8^+$ cells in the upper left quadrant. Dual $CD4^+CD8^+$ immature T cells, if present, would be displayed in the upper right quadrant, and cells that are neither $CD4^+$ nor $CD8^+$, such as B cells and NK cells, are displayed in the lower left quadrant. Computer analysis of the signals allows immediate quantification of the different cell populations. In addition, the vibrating nozzle on the flow cell breaks the sample stream into droplets. Analysis by the computer allows an electrical charge to be placed on the stream such that each droplet may carry a positive, negative, or no charge (Fig. A-9.10). The individual droplets then pass between electrically charged deflection plates and into appropriate collection tubes so that different cell populations can be isolated for further analysis.

ASSESSMENT OF IMMUNE FUNCTION

The function of molecules and cells of the immune system can also be assessed.

In vitro assessment of molecular function

The functional activity of molecules generated by the immune system can be assessed in the laboratory. We give two examples here.

Complement

Complement fixation (CF) test detects the presence of antigen–antibody complexes in the serum (Fig. A-10). The test consists of two parts, the indicator system and the assay for complement fixation. The indicator system (Fig. A-10A) contains three components—complement, sheep erythrocytes, and complement-fixing antibody specific for sheep erythrocytes. Sheep erythrocytes are incubated with anti-erythrocyte antibodies to form antigen–antibody complexes. On the addition of limiting quantities of complement, the erythrocytes are lysed, the reaction tube is centrifuged, and the amount of hemoglobulin released from the erythrocyte may be determined spectrophotometrically. To assay serum for complement activity (Fig. A-10B) requires incubation of the serum with a known antigen (or the serum may have preformed antigen–antibody complexes) with complement. The presence of antigen and complement-fixing antibody complexes depletes the limited quantity of complement so that antibody-coated erythrocytes, when added to the reaction mixture, are not lysed and hemoglobulin is not released.

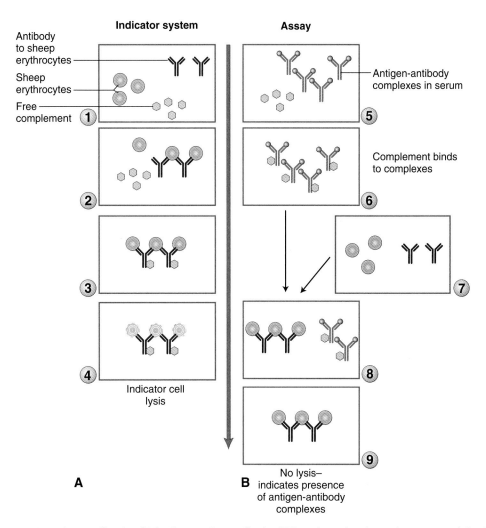

FIGURE A-10. Complement fixation (CF). The complement fixation (CF) test is used to detect the presence of circulating antigen–antibody complexes. This is a two-part test—an indicator system and the assay. **(A) Indicator system.** 1) Antibodies to sheep erythrocytes, sheep erythrocytes, and complement are combined in a test tube. 2) Anti-erythrocyte antibody combines with the sheep erythrocytes. 3) The resulting antigen–antibody complex activates the complement cascade, resulting in 4) the lysis of the sheep erythrocytes (indicator cells). **(B) Assay.** 5) Serum from an individual is collected, heated to 56°C for 30 minutes (to inactivate endogenous complement), and complement are combined in a test tube. 6) The mixture is allowed to incubate and if antigen–antibody complexes are present, complement will bind. 7) Sheep erythrocytes and antibody to sheep erythrocytes (8) are then added. 9) If antigen–antibody complexes were originally present in the serum, then the added complement activity is depleted, and no lysis of the erythrocytes will occur. If, however, lysis occurs, then antigen–antibody complexes were not present in the test serum.

Neutralizing antibodies

One of the functions of antibody is to bind to and inactivate a potential toxin or microbe before its interaction with a cell. **Neutralizing antibodies** prevent subsequent interaction of that toxin or microbe with a host cell by their binding to soluble molecules or cell-surface molecules on microbes. The neutralizing capacity of an antibody is determined functionally, most often in vitro (Fig. A-11). Virus particles incubated with cells in tissue culture normally kill the cells to cause zones of lysis or plaques (Fig. A-11.4). In the test, serum containing the antibodies is heated (56°C for 30 minutes) to inactivate complement and to prevent complement-mediated lysis. Virus particles are incubated with the serum once it returns to room temperature (Fig. A-11.6). The serum-treated virus particles are then incubated with the cells in culture (Fig. A-11.7). A decrease in the number of lytic plaques indicates an inhibition of viral infection caused by the presence of neutralizing antibodies in the test serum (Fig. A-11.8).

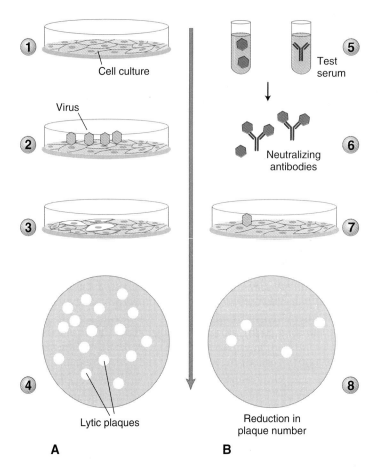

FIGURE A-11. Neutralizing antibodies. Antibodies can prevent entry of viruses or bacteria into cells. This can be assessed in the laboratory. **(A) Positive control**. 1) A cell line, permissive for viral growth, is grown in tissue culture until the cells reach confluence or a monolayer of adjacent cells. 2) Virus is added to the cell culture to infect the cells. 3) Infected cells undergo programmed cell death (apoptosis). 4) The cultured cells are stained with a dye and zone of viral-induced lysis are seen as nonstaining clear areas or lytic plaques. **(B) To test for neutralizing antibodies**, (5) viral particles are added to a test serum and allowed to incubate. 6) Antibodies will bind to the virus whether they are neutralizing. 7) Neutralizing antibodies will block viral (or bacterial) entry into the permissive cell lines. 8) With fewer cells infected with virus, the number of lytic plaques will be reduced, indicating the presence of neutralizing antibodies in the serum.

In vitro assessment of cellular function

Function of cells of the immune system can also be assessed in vitro.

Phagocytic function

Polymorphonuclear (PMN) cells, macrophages, and dendritic cells kill ingested microorganisms by a respiratory burst (release of superoxide). Phagocytes of individuals who lack or have defective NADPH oxidase activity, which prevents the production of reactive oxygen intermediates, can engulf microbes but fail to kill the ingested microorganisms. The nitroblue tetrazolium (NBT) dye reduction test is useful in identifying individuals with impaired respiratory burst activity, such as those with chronic granulomatous disease (CGD). In this test, PMNs are isolated from peripheral blood and are stimulated with phorbol myristate acetate (PMA) or yeast zymosan granules to produce superoxide. Phagocytes ingest yellow soluble NBT. Normal cells produce superoxide that reduces NBT to blue insoluble formazan crystals that are readily detected within the phagocyte microscopically. Phagocytes from individuals with impaired respiratory burst activity such as those with CGD are unable to produce superoxides and unable to reduce yellow NBT into blue crystals. The NBT test is also used to detect phagocytic defects in individuals with severe G6PD, myeloperoxidase, glutathione synthetase, or glutathione reductase deficiencies.

Proliferation responses

Naïve antigen-specific T lymphocytes are found in relatively low numbers in antigen-naïve individuals. An immunologic encounter with antigen causes a proliferative expansion in the number of antigen-specific T cells. Re-exposure to the antigen restimulates T cells and causes them to proliferate. Immunologists exploit this property to indicate whether an individual has had previous immunologic exposure to an antigen.

In this technique, mononuclear (lymphocytes, monocytes, and dendritic) cells are isolated from peripheral blood and placed in tissue culture with antigen for 48 to 72 hours. A radionuclide (such as ^{3}H-thymidine) is added for the final 18 to 24 hours of culture. Proliferation is measured by ^{3}H-thymidine incorporation into the DNA of dividing cells. Antigen-specific proliferation indicates that the individual has had previous exposure to the antigen.

T-cell proliferation can also be used to indicate MHC class II histocompatibility. For example, alloreactive cells from one individual (the stimulator), treated with mitomycin C or irradiated so that they cannot respond by DNA synthesis, are cultured with peripheral blood mononuclear cells from another individual (the responder). The cells are cultured for 3 to 7 days and ^{3}H-thymidine is added for the final 18 to 24 hours. Incorporation of ^{3}H-thymidine by the CD4$^+$ T cells of the responding individual indicates MHC class II differences between the two individuals.

Nonspecific simulators of proliferation, **mitogens**, can also be used to assess the potential ability of lymphocytes to respond to a stimulus. Phytohemagglutinin (PHA) and concanavalin A (con A) are lectins that bind to carbohydrate moieties found on T cells and act as mitogens. They are used to assess the ability of T cells to proliferate in response to a polyclonal stimulus. Likewise, a product of Gram-negative bacterial cell walls, lipopolysaccharide (LPS), acts as a mitogen to stimulate B cells to proliferate. Pokeweed mitogen (PWM) is used to assess the proliferative ability of both B and T cells.

Cell migration

Cell migration (homing) in response to a chemoattractant signal is important to innate and adaptive immune responses. Cell-migration assays can be used to assess the ability of cells to be attracted to a variety of molecules, as well as the ability of molecules to attract leukocytes. An assay device containing two chambers separated by a semi-permeable membrane is used. Cells are loaded into the upper chamber, and a diluted chemical attractant is used to fill the lower chamber. The semi-permeable membrane contains microscopic pores somewhat less than the diameter of a cell. Cells migrating in response to the increase gradient in chemoattractant will squeeze through the pores in the membrane and enter the lower chamber. Cells that cross the membrane are counted compared with the number of cells that cross the membrane in a replicate chamber without the chemical attractant. This system can assess the ability of cells to home to a chemical signal and, alternatively, assess the ability of a chemical signal to induce cell migration.

Cytotoxic T-lymphocyte assay

Activated CD8$^+$ T cells often recognize and kill cells that display a specific peptide–MHC class I complex on the cell surface. CD8$^+$ T-cell function may be readily assessed by the ability of these cells to kill radiolabeled target cells. Radioactive sodium chromate, $Na_2{}^{51}CrO_4$, readily crosses the cell membrane of live cells and binds to cytoplasmic proteins in the cell. The radiolabeled cells are washed to remove unbound sodium chromate, and the cells then are incubated with CD8$^+$ T cells in a test tube. Within 4 hours, CD8$^+$ T cells specifically destroy the cell membrane of specific peptide–MHC class I-bearing cells, causing the release of ^{51}Cr–protein complexes into the culture medium. Intact cells and cellular debris are separated from the medium by centrifugation and radioactivity detected in the cell-free medium is used as a measure of cytotoxicity.

In vivo assessment of immune function

Immune function can also be assessed in vivo.

Allergy skin tests

Hay fever, sensitivity to pet dander, and some cases of urticaria and gastrointestinal food reaction are common allergic disorders. Predisposition to allergen sensitivity is characterized by the development of specific IgE antibodies to the allergen (i.e., antigen). To test an individual's sensitivity to an allergen, a small amount of diluted antigen is introduced intradermally either by injection with a needle under the skin or by placing it on a scratch on the skin. Introduction of antigen-free diluent serves as a negative control and histamine may be used as a positive control. A **wheal-and-flare reaction** (swelling and redness) is evident in responding sites usually within 20 minutes after antigen application. Because an overt allergic reaction may occur in the skin test, antihistamine or epinephrine should be available during testing. Also, because the test depends on the degranulation of mast cells in the dermis, drugs that block the effect of histamine (anti-histamines, hydroxyzine) may interfere with the outcome of the test. An alternative test is called the **radioallergosorbent test** (**RAST**). Antigen bound to an insoluble matrix is incubated in vitro with a serum sample. IgE specific for the insoluble antigen binds to the matrix-bound antigen and unbound serum proteins are then washed away. Binding of a radiolabeled anti-IgE antibody to the IgE–antigen matrix complex allows quantization of specific IgE in the serum.

Contact dermatitis, delayed hypersensitivity, and Mantoux tests

Type IV hypersensitivity reactions may be determined by application of antigen to the surface of the skin (**contact dermatitis**) or by the introduction of antigen intradermally (**delayed hypersensitivity** and **Mantoux test**). All three tests evaluate whether a person has had previous exposure to and had a CD4$^+$ T-cell response to a specific antigen. In the contact dermatitis test, antigen is applied to the surface of the skin under a nonabsorbent dermal patch. A positive reaction is evident 48 to 72 hours after introduction of antigen by erythema and induration, similar to the wheal-and-flare reaction seen in a positive allergy skin test. In the delayed hypersensitivity test, antigen is injected intradermally. In a positive response, erythema and induration are evident after (but not before) 24 to 72 hours. The Mantoux test (also called the tuberculin skin test) is variation of the delayed hypersensitivity test. Killed *Mycobacterium tuberculosis* organisms are introduced into the dermis, often by pricking the skin. A positive reaction becomes apparent 24 to 72 hours after antigen introduction and indicates that the individual has had previous exposure to the tuberculosis bacterium.

Rebuck skin window

This test measures cell migration in vivo. The skin of the forearm is gently abraded with a scalpel and a sterile cover slip is placed on the abrasion. The sterile cover slip is replaced every 2 hours over an 8-hour period. The migration of leukocytes into the damaged skin can be monitored by the accumulation of white cells onto the cover slips.

CD Designation And Function

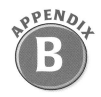

Antigen	Alternate names	Expressed by	Function
CD1a	R4; HTA1	Thy, T, DC	Non-peptide (glyco)lipid presentation
CD1b	R1	Thy, T, DC	Non-peptide (glyco)lipid presentation
CD1c	M241; R7	Thy, T, DC	Non-peptide (glyco)lipid presentation
CD1d	R3	Thy, T, DC	Non-peptide (glyco)lipid presentation
CD1e	R2	B, M	Non-peptide (glyco)lipid presentation
CD2	CD2R; T11; LFA-2	T	LFA-3 receptor, T cell activation
CD3δ	CD3d	T	TCR signal transduction
CD3ε	CD3e	T	TCR signal transduction
CD3γ	CD3g	T	TCR signal transduction
CD4	L3T4; W3/25	(T)	Co-receptor for MHC class II
CD5	Leu-1; Ly-1; T1; Tp67	T, (B)	Signal transduction
CD6	T12	Thy, T	Signal transduction
CD7	gp40	Thy, T	Signal transduction
CD8α	Leu2; Lyt2; T8	(T)	Co-receptor for MHC class I
CD8β	Leu2; CD8; Lyt3	(T)	Co-receptor for MHC class I
CD9	DRAP-27; MRP-1; p24	T*, (B), G, End, other	Cell adhesion
CD10	CALLA; enkephalinase; gp100; NEP	PB*, B*	Membrane metallo-endopeptidase, common acute lymphocytic leukemia antigen (CALLA)
CD11a	αL integrin chain; LFA-1α	all	Cell adhesion and co-stimulation
CD11b	CR3; Mac-1	(T, B), M, NK, G	Cell adhesion and co-stimulation
CD11c	CR4	M, NK, G, ~T, ~B	Cell adhesion and co-stimulation
CDw12	p90–120	M, G, NK	Unknown
CD13	APN; EC 3.4.11.2; gp150	pG, pM	Function unknown, receptor for coronaviruses
CD14	LPS-R	M	LPS-binding protein receptor
CD15u	Sulphated CD15		Carbohydrate structures
CD16a	FCRIIIA	M, NK	Low affinity IgG receptor
CD16b	FCRIIIB	G	Low affinity IgG receptor
CDw17	LacCer	M, G, P, (B, DC)	Binds bacteria, function unknown
CD18	CD11a β subunit; CD11b β subunit; CD11c β subunit; β-2 integrin chain	T, B, NK, M, G	Cell adhesion and signaling
CD19	B4	B, -PC	Signal transduction
CD20	B1; Bp35	B	Co-receptor with BCR
CD21	C3d receptor; CR2; EBV-R	B, -B*	Receptor for C3d and iC3b, receptor for EBV
CD22	BL-CAM; Lyb8	B	Cell adhesion and signaling
CD23	B6; BLAST-2; FcεRII; Leu-20;	B, M, (G, DC)	Low affinity IgE receptor
CD24	BA-1; HSA	pB, B, -PC	Unknown, may serve as co-stimulatory molecule
CD25	IL-2R α chain; IL-2R; Tac antigen	T*, B*, M*	IL-2 Receptor
CD26	EC 3.4.14.5; ADA-binding protein; DPP IV ectoenzyme	T*	T cell co-stimulatory molecule, exopeptidase
CD27	S152; T14	T	Tyrosine phosphorylation, co-stimulatory signal for T & B cell activation
CD28	T44; Tp44	T	Costimulation upon binding with CD80 or CD86

Antigen	Alternate names	Expressed by	Function
CD29	Platelet GPIIa; VLA-β chain; β-1 integrin chain	Leu~G	Leukocyte adhesion
CD30	Ber-H2 antigen; Ki-1 antigen	PMN, T*, M	Member of TNFR family, function unknown
CD31	GPiia'; endocam; PECAM-1	End, P, -M, -NK, (T)	Adhesion molecule, binds to CD31 on another cell
CD32	FCR II; FcγRII	M, G, End	Binds aggregated IgG, plays role on phagocytosis
CD33	gp67; p67	M, My	Binds to sugar chains containing sialic acid
CD34	gp105–120	SC	Binds to L-selectin, CD62L
CD35	C3bR; C4bR; CR1	G, M, EC, B, (DC)	Receptor for C3b and C4b and accelerates their decay
CD36	GPIIIb; GPIV; OKM5-antigen; PASIV	P	Scavenger receptor for oxidized low density lipoprotein
CD37	gp52–40	B, (T, T*, G, PMN. M)	Signal transduction
CD38	T10; cyclic ADP-ribose hydrolase	PC, pMy, also brain, muscle, kidney	Catalytic enzyme with multiple activities including NAD glycohydrolase, ADP-ribosyl cyclase, and cyclic ADP ribose hydrolase
CD39	ectonucleoside triphosphate diphosphohydrolase 1	T*, B*, NIC*	B cell adhesion, activation marker
CD40	Bp50	B, M, (DC), End, CD34$^+$ cells	TNFR family protein, involved in growth, differentiation, and isotype switching in B cells
CD41	GPIIb; α IIb integrin chain	P	Binds platelet fibrinogen receptor
CD42a	GPIX	P	Receptor for von Willebrand factor and thrombin
CD42b	GPIbα; Glycocalicin	P	Receptor for von Willebrand factor and thrombin
CD42c	GPIb-β	P	Receptor for von Willebrand factor and thrombin
CD42d	GPV	P	Receptor for von Willebrand factor and thrombin
CD43	gpL115; leukocyte sialoglycoprotein; leukosialin; sialophorin	All leukocytes except resting B	Anti-adhesive, barrier molecule, large number of sialic acid residues causes repulsion between leukocytes, may interact with CD54
CD44	ECMR III; H-CAM; HUTCH-1; Hermes; Lu, In-related; Pgp-1; gp85	Most cells	Leukocyte attachment and rolling on endothelial cells, T cell activation, leukocyte homing
CD44R	CD44v; CD44v9	Epi	Leukocyte attachment and rolling on epithelial cells
CD45	B220; CD45R; CD45RA; CD45RB; CD45RC; CD45RO; EC 3.1.3.4; LCA; T200; Ly5	T, T*, B, M, G, NK, DC	Tyrosine phosphatase, critical for TCR and BCR mediated activation
CD46	MCP	Leu, others	Cofactor for Factor I proteolytic cleavage of C4b and C4b
CD47R	Rh-associated protein; gp42; IAP; neurophilin; OA3; MEM-133	Leu, SC, Epi, End, brain, others	Adhesion molecule, thrombospondin receptor
CD48	BCM1; Blast-1; Hu Lym3; OX-45	Leu	Low affinity ligand for CD2
CD49a	α-1 integrin chain; VLA-1 α chain	T*, M	Leukocyte adhesion
CD49b	α-2 integrin chain; GPIa; VLA-2 α chain	P, T*, M, (B)	Leukocyte adhesion
CD49c	α-3 integrin chain; VLA-3 α chain	T, M, (B)	Leukocyte adhesion
CD49d	α-4 integrin chain; VLA-4 α chain	T, M, B	Leukocyte adhesion, binds to VCAM-α, MadCAM-1
CD49e	α-5 integrin chain; FNR α chain; VLA-5 α chain	T, M, (B)	Leukocyte adhesion
CD49f	α-6 integrin chain; Platelet gpI; VLA-6 α chain	P, T*, M	Leukocyte adhesion

Antigen	Alternate names	Expressed by	Function
CD50	ICAM-3	Leu, End, (DC)	Adhesion, regulates LFA-1/ICAM-1 and integrin-β1 dependent pathways
CD51	VNR-α chain; α V integrin chain; vitronectin receptor	End, (B), M, Mas	Forms a complex with CD61 to mediate cell adhesion
CD52	CAMPATH-1	Thy, L, M	Unknown
CD53	OX-44	Leu	Signal transduction
CD54	ICAM-1	End*, ~T*, ~B*, ~M	Adhesion, ligand CD11a/CD18 (LFA-1) and CD11b/CD18 (Mac-1), ligand for Rhinovirus
CD55	DAF	Many cell types	Binds C3b and C4b to inhibit formation of C3 convertases, receptor for echovirus and Coxsackie B virus
CD56	Leu-19; NKH1; N-CAM	(CD4$^+$ T), (CD8$^+$ T), brain	Adhesion, function unknown
CD57	HNK1; Leu-7	NK, (T), M	Unknown
CD58	LFA-3	Leu, E, End, Epi, others	Adhesion between killer and target cells, antigen presenting cells and T cells, and thymocytes with thymic epithelial cells, costimulatory signal, CD2 is the receptor for CD58
CD59	1F-5Ag; H19; HRF20; MACIF; MIRL; P-18; Protectin	Many cell types	Inhibits formation of the terminal steps of the MAC complex of complement
CD60a	GD3	(T), P, Thy	Carbohydrate structures, may provide costimulation
CD60b	9-O-acetyl-GD3	(T), P, Thy Epi, others	Carbohydrate structures, may provide costimulation
CD60c	7-O-acetyl-GD3	(T), P, Thy Epi, others	Carbohydrate structures, may provide costimulation
CD61	CD61A; GPIIb/IIIa; β 3 integrin chain	P, M, End, Leu	Adhesion
CD62E	E-selectin; ELAM-1; LECAM-2	End	Adhesion, mediates leukocyte rolling on endothelium at sites of inflammation
CD62L	L-selectin; LAM-1; LECAM-1; Leu-8; MEL-14; TQ-1	Leu	Adhesion, mediated T lymphocyte homing to high endothelial venules
CD62P	P-selectin; GMP-140; PADGEM	P, End	Adhesion, interacts with PSGL-1 to mediate tethering and rolling of leukocytes on activated endothelium
CD63	LIMP; MLA1; PTLGP40; gp55; granulophysin; LAMP-3; ME491; NGA	PMN, M, End, P*	Transmembrane adapter protein
CD64	FCγRI; FCR I	M, (DC), PMN*	Phagocytosis, receptor mediated endocytosis of antigen-IgG complexes, ADCC
CD65	Ceramide-dodecasaccharide; VIM-2	G	Unknown
CD65s	Sialylated-CD65; VIM2	G	Unknown
CD66a	NCA-160; BGP	G, Epi	Adhesion, E-selectin binding, receptor for *Neisseria gonorrhea* and *N. meningitidis*
CD66b	CD67; CGM6; NCA-95	G	Adhesion, function unknown
CD66c	NCA; NCA-50/90	G, Epi	Adhesion, E-selection binding
CD66d	CGM1	G	Unknown
CD66e	CEA	Epi	Adhesion, unknown
CD66f	Pregnancy specific b1 glycoprotein; SP-1; PSG	Placental syncytiotrophoblasts	Unknown, may protect fetus from maternal immune system
CD68	gp110; macrosialin	M, DC, G, T*, (B)	Unknown

Antigen	Alternate names	Expressed by	Function
CD69	AIM; EA 1; MLR3; gp34/28; VEA	Thy, T*, B*, NK*, PMN*, Eos*	Signal transduction, Ca^{2+} influx
CD70	CD27-ligand; Ki-24 antigen	T*,B*	Member TNF family, ligand from CD27
CD71	T9; transferrin receptor	Proliferating cells	Iron uptake
CD72	Ly-19.2; Ly-32.2; Lyb-2	B	Adhesion, ligand from CD5
CD73	Ecto-5'-nucleotidase	(T, B, DC)	Costimulatory signalling
CD74	Class II-specific chaperone; Ii; Invariant chain	B, T*, M, End*	Intracellular sorting of MHC class II molecules
CD75	Lactosamines	B, (T)	Carbohydrate structures
CD75s	α-2,6-sialylated lactosamines	B	Carbohydrate structures, cell adhesion, ligand for CD22
CD77	Pk blood group antigen; BLA; CTH; Gb3	(B)	Carbohydrate structures, induces apoptosis
CD79a	Ig α; MB1	B	B cell signal transduction
CD79b	B29; Ig β	B	B cell signal transduction
CD80	B7-1; BB1	DC, M, B*	Co-regulator of T cell activation
CD81	TAPA-1	Hematopoietic cells, -E, -PMN	Signal transduction
CD82	4F9; C33; IA4; KAI1; R2	Leukocytes, -E	Signal transduction
CD83	HB15	DC, (B)	Unknown
CD84		M, (T), B, P	Unknown
CD85	ILT/LIR family	DC	T cell activation
CD86	B7-2; B70	DC, M, B*	Co-regulator of T cell activation
CD87	uPAR	T, NK, M, PMN, others	Cellular receptor for uPA and pro-uPA
CD88	C5aR	G, M, DC, astrocytes, microglia	Receptor for C5a, when occupied stimulates GTPase activity of Gi2
CD89	Fcα-R; IgA Fc receptor; IgA receptor	Myeloid cells	IgA receptor; when occupied induces phagocytosis, degranulation, respiratory burst
CD90	Thy-1	SC, neurons, HEV	Role in T cell activation
CD91	α2M-R; LRP	M	Binds low density lipoproteins
CD92	CTL1	Myeloid cells	Unknown
CDw93		M, G, End	Unknown
CD94	Kp43	NK, (T)	Together with NKG2-A, inhibitory receptor for MHC class I molecules
CD95	APO-1; Fas; TNFRSF6; APT1	T*, B*, many others	Binds to Fas ligand, mediates apoptosis-inducing signaling
CD96	TACTILE	T	Unknown
CD97		B*, T*, M, DC, G	Unknown
CD98	4F2; FRP-1; RL-388	Many cell types	Regulation of cellular activation, perhaps an amino acid transporter
CD99	CD99R; E2; MIC2 gene product	Many cell types	Unknown
CD100	SEMA4D	Many cell types	Signaling
CD101	IGSF2; P126; V7	M, G, DC, T*	Inhibitory signaling
CD102	ICAM-2	End, (L), M, P, -PMN	Adhesion molecule, lymphocyte recirculation, costimulatory molecule
CD103	ITGAE; HML-1; integrin αE chain	IEL, (T)	Homing of intraepithelial T lymphoocytes
CD104	β4 integrin chain; TSP-1180; β4	Thy, Epi	Adhesion molecule
CD105	endoglin	End, M	Regulatory component of TGF-β complex
CD106	INCAM-110; VCAM-1	End, M, (DC)	Adhesion molecule
CD107a	LAMP-1	P, T*, End*	Lysosome-associated membrane protein expressed upon activation
CD107b	LAMP-2	P, T*, End*	Lysosome-associated membrane protein expressed upon activation

Antigen	Alternate names	Expressed by	Function
CD108	SEMA7A; JMH human blood group antigen	Non-lineage molecules	Unknown
CD109	8A3; E123; 7D1		Unknown
CD110	MPL; TPO-R; C-MPL	SC, P	Thrombopoietin receptor
CD111	PRR1; nectin-1	Many cell types	Poliovirus receptor-related, herpesvirus entry mediator
CD112	PRR2; nectin 2	Many cell types	Poliovirus receptor-related, herpesvirus entry mediator
CD113	Not yet assigned	Not yet assigned	Not yet assigned
CD114	CSF3R; HG-CSFR; G-CSFR	G	Granulocyte colony-stimulating factor receptor
CD115	c-fms; CSF-1R; M-CSFR	M	Receptor for macrophage colony stimulating factor (CSF-1)
CD116	GM-CSF receptor α chain	My, DC	Receptor for GM-CSF
CD117	c-KIT; SCFR	SC	Growth factor receptor
CD118	Not yet assigned	Not yet assigned	Not yet assigned
CDw119	IFNγR; IFNγRa	M, DC,B, T, End, Epi	Receptor for IFN-γ, mediates biologic effects of IFN-γ
CD120a	TNFRI; p55	Many cell types	Receptor for TNF-α, mediates biologic effects of IFN-γ
CD120b	TNFRII; p75; TNFR p80	Many cell types	Receptor for TNF-α, -β, mediates biologic effects of TNF
CD121a	IL-1R; type 1 IL-1R	Many cell types	Receptor for IL-1, mediates biologic effects of IL-1
CDw121b	IL-1R, type 2	Many cell types	Receptor for IL-1, mediates biologic effects of IL-1
CD122	IL-2Rβ	T, B, NK, M	Critical subunit of IL-2R and IL-15R
CD123	IL-3Rα	M	Receptor for IL-3, mediates biologic effects of IL-3
CD124	IL-4R	B*, T*	Receptor subunit for IL-4 and IL-13
CDw125	IL-5Rα	Eos, B*, Baso	Low affinity receptor for IL-5
CD126	IL-6R	B*, PC, T, M	Receptor for IL-6, mediates biologic effects of IL-6
CD127	IL-7R; IL-7R α; p90 Il7 R	pB, T	Receptor for IL-7, mediates biologic effects of IL-7
CDw128a	CXCR1; IL-8RA	PMN, Bas, (T)	Receptor for IL-8, mediates biologic activity of IL-8
CD129	Not yet assigned	Not yet assigned	Not yet assigned
CD130	gp130	Most cell types	Transduces biologic activities of IL-6, IL-11
CD131	common β subunit	My, early B	Component of high affinity IL-3, IL-5, and GM-CSF receptors
CD132	IL2RG; common cytokine receptor γ chain; common γ chain	T, B, M, NK, PMN	Common component of receptors of IL-2, IL-4, IL-7, IL-9 and IL-15
CD133	AC133	SC	Unknown
CD134	OX40	T*	Signal transduction, TNFR superfamily
CD135	flt3; Flk-2; STK-1	PMy, pB	Growth factor receptor for early hematopoietic progenitors
CDw136	msp receptor; ron; p158-ron	Epi and others	Role in cell migration
CDw137	4-1BB; ILA	T, B, M	Costimulatory molecule
CD138	heparan sulfate proteoglycan; syndecan-1	B	Cell surface proteoglycan, function unknown
CD139	None	B, M, G, ~E	Unknown
CD140a	PDGF-R; PDGFRα	Many cell types	Receptor for PDGF subunit, mediates biological
CD140b	PDGFRβ	Many cell types	Receptor for PDGF subunit, mediates biological
CD141	etomodulin; TM	End, P, PMN, others	Cofactor for thrombin-mediated activation of protein C

Antigen	Alternate names	Expressed by	Function
CD142	F3; coagulation Factor III; thromboplastin; TF	Epithelial keratinocytes, absent from cells in direct contact with plasma	Cofactor with factor VIIa to form enzymatic activity that initiates blood clotting
CD143	EC 3.4.15.1; ACE; kininase II; peptidyl dipeptidase A	End, Epi, M*, others	Angiotensin converting enzyme
CD144	cadherin-5; VE-Cadherin	End	Adhesion molecule
CDw145	None	Epi	Unknown
CD146	MCAM; A32; MUC18; Mel-CAM; S-endo	End, (T*), others	Adhesion molecule
CD147	5A11; Basigin; CE9; HT7; M6; Neurothelin; OX-47; EMMPRIN; gp42	Leu, E, P, End	Adhesion molecule
CD148	HPTP-ε; DEP-1; p260	B	Tyrosine phosphatase, function unknown
CD150	SLAM; IPO-3	B, DC	Signaling lymphocyte activation molecule, costimulatory molecule on B and DC
CD151	PETA-3; SFA-1	End, P, Epi	Adhesion, platelet aggregation
CD152	CTLA-4	T*	Negative regulator of T cell activation
CD153	CD30L	T*, B, G, Thy	Ligand for CD30, TNF superfamily member, inhibits Ig class switching, role in activation induced cell death
CD154	CD40L; T-BAM; TRAP; gp39	T	CD40 ligand, regulates B cell function
CD155	PVR	Many cell types	Poliovirus receptor, function unknown
CD156a	ADAM8	My	Leukocyte extravasation
CD156b	ADAM17; TACE; cSVP	Many cell types	Unknown
CD157	BP-3/IF-7; BST-1; Mo5	G, M, pB, others	Role in lymphocyte development
CD158	KIR Family	NK	Killer cell immunoglobulin (Ig)-like receptors, many members of this family
CD159a	NKG2A	NK	Killer cell lectin-like receptor subfamily C
CD160	BY55	NK, (T)	Unknown
CD161	KLRB1; NKR-P1A; killer cell lectin-like receptor subfamily B, member 1	NK	Role in NK activation, function unknown
CD162	PSGL-1, PSGL	T, M, G, (B)	Mediates leukocyte rolling on activated endothelium, selectin P ligand
CD162R	PEN5	NK, My	Post-translational modification of CD162, selectin P
CD163	GHI/61; M130; RM3/1	M	May mediate anti-inflammatory pathway accompanied by IL-10 release
CD164	MUC-24; MGC-24v	Epi, CD34+, B	Adhesion, signal transduction
CD165	AD2; gp37	L, Thy, M, P	Adhesion between thymocytes and thymic epithelium
CD166	BEN; DM-GRASP; KG-CAM; Neurolin; SC-1; ALCAM	T*, M*, Epi, neurons	Adhesion molecule that binds CD6
CD167a	Disoidin domain R (DDR1)	Epi, others	Adhesion molecule, a receptor tyrosine kinase
CD168	RHAMM	Thy	Adhesion molecule, hyalouronan (HA)-binding receptor
CD169	sialoadhesin	M	Adhesion molecule, recognizes sialyated ligands
CD170	Siglec-5	My	Adhesion molecule, binds sialic acid
CD171	L1	Neurons	Adhesion molecule, required for normal neurohistogenesis

Antigen	Alternate names	Expressed by	Function
CD172a	SIRP α	Mye and others	Adhesion structures, member of the signal regulatory protein (SIRP) family
CD173	Blood group H type 2	E	Carbohydrate structures
CD174	Lewis y	E	Carbohydrate structures, fucosyltransferase 3
CD175	Tn	E	Carbohydrate structures
CD175s	Sialyl-Tn	E	Carbohydrate structures
CD176	TF	E	Carbohydrate structures
CD177	NB1	MC	Unknown
CD178	Fas ligand	L	Fas ligand, member of the TNF family, induces trimerization of Fas on target cells that leads to apoptotic cell death
CD179a	VpreB	pB	Associates with CD179b to form surrogate light chain on pB
CD179b	lambda5	pB	Associates with CD179a to form surrogate light chain on pB
CD180	RP105	B	Regulates B cell recognition of lipopolysaccharide
CD183	CXCR3	T	CXC chemokine receptor for CXCL9, CXCL10, and CXCL11, induces chemotactic migration in inflammation-associated effector T cells
CD184	CXCR4	Many cell types	CXC chemokine receptor for CXCL12, function unknown
CD195	CCR5	T, M	CC chemokine receptor for CCL3, CCL5, important co-receptor for HIV
CDw197	CCR7	B, others	CC chemokine receptor for CCL19, CCL21, may be induced by Epstein-Barr virus (EBV)
CD200	OX2	Others	May regulate myeloid cell activity, delivers inhibitory signal to macrophage lineage cells
CD201	EPC R	End	Receptor for activated protein C
CD202b	tie2; tek	End	Receptor tyrosine kinase, important in remodeling and repair of blood vessels
CD203c	NPP3; PDNP3	Bas, Mas, others	Ectoenzyme involved in hydrolysis of extracellular nucleotides
CD204	macrophage scavenger R	M	Macrophage scavenger receptors, three types produced by alternative splicing that mediate endocytosis of low density lipoproteins (LDL), implicated in Alzheimer's disease, atherosclerosis, and host defense
CD205	DEC205	DC	Involved in dendritic cell activation/inflammation
CD206	MRC1; MMR	DC	Pattern recognition receptor also known as macrophage mannose receptor, involved in innate defense
CD207	Langerin	(DC)	C-type lectin with mannose binding specificity only expressed by Langerhans cells

Antigen	Alternate names	Expressed by	Function
CD208	DC-LAMP	DC	Lysosomal-associated membrane protein 3, function unknown
CD209	DC-SIGN	DC	Dendritic cell-specific ICAM3-grabbing nonintegrin, binding unknown
CDw210	IL-10 R	Many cell types	Receptor for IL-10, mediates biologic effect of IL-10
CD212	IL-12 R	Many cell types	Low affinity IL-12 receptor, co-expression with IL12RB2 forms high affinity IL-12 binding
CD213a1	IL-13 R α 1	Many cell types	Part of the IL-13 and IL-4 receptor complexes, necessary component for signal transduction by these cytokines
CD213a2	IL-13 R α 2	Many cell types	Binds IL-13 with high affinity, lacks cytoplasmic domain
CDw217	IL-17 R	Many cell types	IL-17 receptor, mediates biologic activity of IL-17
CD220	Insulin R	Many cell types	Insulin receptor
CD221	IGF1 R	Many cell types	High affinity insulin-like growth factor receptor, functions as anti-apoptotic agent
CD222	Mannose-6-phosphate/IGF2 R	Many cell types	Receptor for insulin-like growth factor II (IGF-II) and other mannose-6-phosphate containing proteins, internalizes ligands and directs them toward lysosomes
CD223	LAG-3	T*, NK	Associates with MHC class II expressed by macrophages and dendritic cells, binds MHC class II better than CD4, appears to be involved in cellular activation
CD224	GGT; EC2.3.2.2	Many cell types	Gamma-glutamyl transpeptidase (GGT) and ectoenzyme involved in the degradation and neo-synthesis of glutathione
CD225	Leu13	Many cell types	Unknown
CD226	DNAM-1; PTA1; TLiSA1	NK, P, M, (T)	Activation-induced surface glycoprotein, may be involved in the generation of CTL
CD227	MUC1	Many cell types	Large cell surface mucin glycoprotein, may be involved in modulation of cell adhesion
CD228	melanotransferrin	Many cell types	Iron binding molecule, function unknown
CD229	Ly9	T	Unknown
CD230	Prion protein	Many cell types	Major prion protein, membrane glycosylphosphatidylinositol-anchored glycoprotein, mutation in this gene associated with Creutzfeldt-Jacob disease, Huntington disease-like 1, and kuru
CD231	TALLA-1.A-15	Many cell types	Unknown
CD232	VESP R	Many cell types	Unknown
CD233	Diego blood group	EC	Erythrocyte membrane protein that functions as an anion exchanger

Antigen	Alternate names	Expressed by	Function
CD234	Duffy antigen	EC	Erythrocyte membrane acidic glycoprotein that carries determinants of the Duffy blood group, also a receptor for *Plasmodium vivax* the human malarial parasite
CD235a	Glycophorin A	EC	Erythrocyte membrane glycophorins A and B that carry determinants for the M or N and S or s blood groups
CD235b	Glycophorin B	EC	Erythrocyte membrane glycophorins A and B that carry determinants for the M or N and S or s blood groups, additional variants result from recombination
CD235ab	Glycophorin A/B crossreactive mabs	EC	Erythrocyte membrane glycophorins A and B that carry determinants for the M or N and S or s blood groups
CD236	Glycophorin C/D	EC	Unknown
CD236R	Glycophorin C	EC	Erythrocyte membrane glycophorin C that play an important role in regulating the mechanical stability of erythrocytes
CD238	Kell	EC	Kell blood group antigen, type II transmembrane glycoprotein
CD239	B-CAM	EC	Lutheran blood group antigen
CD240CE	Rh30CE	EC	Rh blood group C antigen, Rh blood group antigen Evans
CD240D	Rh30D	EC	Rh blood group D antigen, alternative splicing results in two isoforms
CD240DCE	Rh30D/CE crossreactive mabs	EC	
CD241	RhAg	EC	Rhesus blood group-associated glycoprotein
CD242	ICAM-4	EC	Intracellular adhesion molecule (ICAM)-4, binds to LFA-1 (CD11a)
CD243	MDR-1	SC	Member of ATP-binding cassette transporter family, protein is an ATP-dependent efflux pump for xenobiotic compounds, protein also functions as transporter in the blood-brain barrier
CD244	2B4; NAIL; p38	NK, (T, M, Bas)	Surface glycoprotein, engagement with its ligand CD48 enhances NK cytokine production and cytolytic function
CD245	p220/240	T	Unknown
CD246	Anaplastic lymphoma kinase	T	Anaplastic lymphoma kinase resulting from the 2;5 chromosomal translocation creating a fusion gene that is oncogenic
CD247	ζ chain	T	TCR signal transduction

T cell (T), B cell (B), dendritic cell (DC), basophils (Bas), leukocytes (Leu), lymphocytes (L), intraepithelial lymphocytes (IEL), eosinophils (Eos), macrophage/monocyte (M), mast cells (Mas), myeloid cells (My), epithelial cells (Epi), polymorphonuclear cell (PMN), granulocyte(s) (G), stem or progenitor cells (SC), NK cells (NK), erythroid cells (EC), endothelial cells (End), platelets (P), plasma cells (PC), and thymocytes (Thy). Parenthesis (cellular subset), activated cells (*), low density (tilde ~), precursor (p), expression absent on (-)

Source: prow@ncbi.nlm.nih.gov Revised 07/02/02 http://www.ncbi.nlm.nih.gov/prow/guide/45277084.htm

Chemokines, Cytokines and Their Receptors

Cytokine	Cellular source	Targets	Function [receptor]
IL-1α	M, B	T, B, M, End, other	Leukocyte activation, increase endothelium adhesion. Receptor [CD121a or CD121b]
IL-1β	M, B	T, B, M, End, other	Function is same as for IL-1α
IL-2	T	T, B, NK, M, oligo	T-cell proliferation, regulation [CD122/CD25]
IL-3	T*, Mas, Eos, NK, End	Ery, G	Proliferation and differentiation of hematopoietic precursors [CD123/CDw131]
IL-4	Mas, T, M	B, T, End	Differentiation of Th2 and B cells [CD124/CD132]
IL-5	Mas, T. Eos	Eos, B	Growth differentiation of B cells and eosinophils [CD125/CDw131]
IL-6	T, B, M, Astocytes, End	T, B, others	Hematopoiesis, differentiation, inflammation [CD126/CD130]
IL-7	Bone marrow and thymic stroma	pB, pT	Pre/pro-B cell proliferation, T cell, up-regulation of pro-inflammatory cytokines [CD127/CD132]
IL-8	M, L, others	PMN, Bas, L	Chemoattractant [CD128]
IL-9	Th2*	T, B	Potentiates production of IgM, IgG, IgE
IL-10	CD8+ T, Th2, (B) M	T, B, Mas, M	Inhibits IFN-γ, TNF-β, IL-2 by Th1 cells, DTH, stimulates Th2 [CD210]
IL-11		Bone marrow stroma	Osteoclast formation
IL-12	DC, B, T	T, NK	Potentiates IFN-γ and TNF-α production by T and NK, down-regulates IL-10 [CD212]
IL-13	Th2*, Mas, NK	Th2, B, M	Th2 modulator, down-regulated IL-1, IL-6, IL-8, IL-10, IL-12
IL-14	T	B*	Stimulates proliferation, inhibits Ig secretion
IL-15	M, Epi	T, B*	Proliferation
IL-16	Eos, CD8+ T	CD4+ T	CD4+ chemoattractant
IL-17	(T)	Epi, End, others	Osteoclastogenesis, angiogenesis
IL-18	M	Th1, NK	Induces IFN-γ production, enhances NK activity
IL-19	M	M, B	Produced in response to LPS, homologue of IL-10, down regulate antigen presentation
IL-20	Keratinocytes	Keratinocytes	Autocrine growth factor
IL-21	T, Mas	T, B, Mas, Eos	Acute phase reactant inducer after LPS
IL-22	T*	Th2, others	Inhibits IL-4 production
IL-23	M	(T)	Activates signal transduction on complexing with p40 subunit of IL-12
IL-24	Melanocytes, others	M, others	Suppresses growth of tumor cells, apoptotic
IL-25	Mas	Non T	Promotes Th2 polarization
IL-26	(T), NK	Unknown	Unknown
IL-27	M	CD4+ T	Drives proliferation
IL-28	M, others	Unknown	Protects against viral infection
IL-29	M, others	Unknown	Protects cells from viral infection like IFN-γ, does not appear to have anti-proliferative activity

IL-30	Unknown	Unknown	p30 Subunit of IL-27
TGF-β	Eos, others(?)	Many cell types	Anti-inflammatory; promotes wound healing
TNF-α	M*, PMN, T, B, NK	M, PMN, T, End, others	Mediator of inflammatory reactions [CD120a and CD120b]
TNF-β	L	Wide variety	Mediator of inflammatory reactions [CD120a and CD120b]
IFN-α	L, Epi, fibroblasts	Many cell types	Up regulates MHC class I; inhibits viral replication
IFN-β	Epi, fibroblasts	Many cell types	Up regulates MHC class I; inhibits viral replication
IFN-γ	CD8$^+$*, (CD4$^+$*), NK	T, B, M, NK, End	Anti-viral, anti-parasite, inhibits proliferation, enhances MHC class I and II expression [CD119]
M-CSF	L, M, G, End, Epi, others	M	Growth and differentiation of macrophages [CD115]
G-CSF	T*, M, End	G	Growth and differentiation of granulocytes
GM-CSF	T, M, End, Mas	PG, pMy	Stimulates growth and differentiation of granulocytes and myeloid lineage cells [CD116]
MIF	M	M	Anti-apoptotic activity for macrophages, promotes macrophage survival

Note: Several cytokines listed have been deduced by molecular techniques and cellular source, target, and/or function may not be known.

Chemokine family	Ligand	Alternate names	Chemokine receptors
CC Family	CCL1	I-309	CCR8
	CCL2	MCP-1, MCAF	CCR2
	CCL3	MIP-1α, LD78α	CCR1, CCR5
	CCL4	MIP-1β	CCR5
	CCL5	RANTES	CCR1, CCR3, CCR5
	CCL6	Unknown	Unknown
	CCL7	MCP-3	CCR1, CCR2, CCR3
	CCL8	MCP-2	CCR3
	CCL9	Unknown	Unknown
	CCL10	Unknown	Unknown
	CCL11	Exotoxin	CCR3
	CCL12	Unknown	CCR2
	CCL13	MCP-4	CCR2, CCR3
	CCL14	HCC-1	CCR1
	CCL15	HCC-2, Lkn-1, MIP-1δ	CCR1, CCR3
	CCL16	HCC-4, LEC	CCR1
	CCL17	TARC	CCR4
	CCL18	AMAC-1	Unknown
	CCL19	MIP-3β, ELC, exodus-3	CCR7
	CCL20	MIP-3α, LARC, exodus-1	CCR6
	CCL21	6Ckine, SLC, exodus-2	CCR7
	CCL22	MDC, STCP-1	CCR4
	CCL23	MPIF-1	CCR1
	CCL24	MPIF-2, Eotaxin	CCR3
	CCL25	TECK	CCR9
	CCL26	Eotaxin-3	CCR3
	CCL27	TACK, ILC	CCR10
CXC Family	CXCL1	GROα, MCSA-α	CXCR1, CXCR2
	CXCL2	GROβ, MGSA-β	CXCR2
	CXCL3	GROγ, MGSA-γ	CXCR2
	CXCL4	PF4	Unknown
	CXCL5	ENA-78	CXCR2

CXCL6	GCP-2	CXCR1, CXCR2	
CXCL7	NAP-2	CXCR2	
CXCL8	IL-8	CXCR1, CXCR2	
CXCL9	Mig	CXCR3	
CXCL10	IP-10	CXCR3	
CXCL11	I-TAC	CXCR3	
CXCL12	SDF-1α, SDF-1β	CXCR4	
CXCL13	BLC, BCA-1	CXCR5	
CXCL14	BRAK, bolekine	Unknown	

Chemokine family	Ligand	Alternate names	Chemokine receptors
CXC Family	CXCL15	Unknown	Unknown
C Family	XCL1	Lymphotactin, SCM-1α, ATAC	XCR1
	XCL2	SCM-1β	XCR1
CX₃X Family	CX3CL1	Fractalkine	CX3CR

http://www.nchi.nlm.nih.gov/

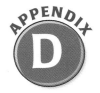
Answers to Review Questions

Chapter 1

1. The answer is C. The immune system is complex, involving the interactions of many different types of cells and molecules. It is concerned with protection of the body rather than the germline. It uses mechanisms that are also used by many other organisms, some of them quite simple. It must recognize both "self" and "non-self."

2. The answer is A. Humans use both innate and adaptive immune responses for defense. Adaptive responses are specific. Both types of defenses confront pathogens, and both types of defenses use cellular and soluble mechanisms.

3. The answer is B. He most probably has an immune deficiency disease. This condition may result from any of a variety of specific defects in the immune system. His immune system is not attacking his own cells and tissues. Because of the wide range and types of infections occurring, it is unlikely that the man's occupation or his reactions to specific antibiotics are involved without further significant evidence.

4. The answer is C. This woman's immune system has experienced a failure in one or more of the mechanisms used to prevent reactivity against self. Because the condition involves the production of antibodies, a shortage of B lymphocytes would not be suspected. Because the condition is not an infectious disease, there is no reason to suspect a defect in innate immunity. If the immune attack were directed against a "foreign" thyroid gland, it would be an attack against nonself rather than against self and thus not autoimmune.

5. The answer is B. Haptens are not capable, on their own, of generating immune responses against themselves. If coupled with an immunogen, however, they can generate responses that can specifically identify them. They are generally small or simple in structure and often are highly reactive in binding to other molecules.

6. The answer is D. PRR recognize structures that are most often associated with microbes not typically found on host cells. In a few cases, they may recognize molecules produced by host cells that are infected or stressed in some way.

7. The answer is B. Killer inhibitory receptors on NK cells are used to determine whether a target cell has the appropriate types and quantities of MHC I molecules. The presence of inappropriate MHC I molecules is an indicator that the cell bearing them is from a foreign source, and a subnormal quantity of MHC I molecules is an indicator that the cell is infected or otherwise abnormal.

8. The answer is D. The adaptive response generates receptors by rearrangement of DNA. Some will recognize and bind to self molecules, and some will recognize and bind nonself molecules.

9. The answer is A. Immunoglobulins and other receptors recognize epitopes and their binding can lead to immunological signals.

10. The answer is A. Immunogens are distinct from haptens that do not display immunogenicity as defined. Immunogens may occur in many forms, but in general the larger and more complex they are, the more potent they are in provoking responses.

11. The answer is C. Tolerogens are recognized by the immune system but cause diminished responses on re-exposure. They cause diminished responses only against themselves, but not against other immunogenic molecules.

Chapter 2

1. The answer is B. Basophils and mast cells, although morphologically distinct, are thought to be of the same embryonic origin. Cytoplasmic granules are rich in vasoactive amines and stain with basic dyes and are quite distinct from the granules of eosinophils and neutrophils. Lymphocytes do not normally contain granules.

2. The answer is B. The spleen is the largest lymphoid organ. The thymus increases in

size during fetal and neonatal life and progressively involutes after puberty. Lymph nodes and Peyer's patches are much smaller.

3. The answer is B. The B cells are the precursors of antibody-secreting plasma cells. Neither T cells, nor NK cells, nor their progeny are able to synthesize immunoglobulins.

4. The answer is A. Natural killer cells monitor the body's cells for the expression of MHC molecules; alteration in MHC surface density targets these cells for destruction. This process is independent of foreign antigen and CD4 or CD8 expression, and does not involve histamine.

5. The answer is C. T and B lymphocytes are similar in size and both have a nongranular cytoplasm and large unlobed nuclei. The only way to distinguish them is by testing for the presence of surface molecules such as immunoglobulin and CD3.

6. The answer is B. ADCC is performed by natural killer cells. T lymphocytes and neutrophils have other means of identifying and killing microbes or parasites. Mast cells have Fc receptors for unbound IgE.

7. The answer is B. Allergic rhinitis is a common disease. Allergic triggers include pollens (trees, grasses, and ragweed), molds, dust mites, and animal dander. This patient has symptoms consistent with allergic rhinitis caused by cat dander. The antigen (cat dander) associated with IgE and cytokines activate mast cells. The process of mast cell degranulation is responsible for the release of vasoactive amines that are responsible for the allergic symptoms.

Chapter 3

1. The answer is B. MBL binds to mannan. LPS, penicillin, and C3 are not recognized by MBL.

2. The answer is C. The most important products generated by the various pathways of complement activation are the generation of the C5 convertase that can then begin the construction of the membrane attack complex and a supply of C3b that acts as an opsonin, as well as helping to drive the alternative pathway. The membrane attack complex is not generated within the lectin-binding or alternative pathways, and neither are factors H and I. C4b fragments are not generated in the alternative pathway.

3. The answer is B. C3b is a highly effective opsonin. By itself, it cannot act as a C5 convertase, but it does contribute to the generation of C5 convertases that support rather than inhibit construction of the MAC. It is C3a rather than C3b that is an anaphylatoxin.

4. The answer is C. Formation of the MAC on the microbial membrane leads to lysis by forming open pores in the membrane. Cleavage of C3 is an earlier step that helps lead to MAC formation, but does not follow it. The MAC is not involved in opsonization or induction of fever.

5. The answer is C. NK cells can identify and directly kill virally infected cells; mast cells, basophils, and complement components do not.

6. The answer is C. α-Interferons and β-interferons induce neighboring cells to become more resistant to viral infection and stimulate increased activity on the part of NK cells. The other answers are incorrect because they fulfill neither function. In addition, production of α- and β-interferons is possible by almost all cells when so infected. Interferon-γ, IL-12, IL-2, IL-2R, and immunoglobulins are produced only by a narrow range of cells.

7. The answer is D. In humans, the killer activation receptor on NK cells is NKG2D, and it binds to MICA and MICB when they are expressed by infected or stressed cells. NK cells do not express T-cell receptors, IL-2, or CD40. KIRs have the opposite effect and inhibit killing by NK cells.

8. The answer is E. The KIR on NK cells are designed to bind to self MHC I molecules on the target cells. If the binding is sufficient, the NK cell does not proceed to kill the target cell. NK cells do not express T-cell receptors, IL-2, or CD40. KAR such as NKG2D have the opposite effect and activate NK cells to kill.

9. The answer is A. Binding of TLRs induces activation of phagocytes. It does not induce apoptosis. Phagocytes do not produce CD3, IL-2, IL-2 receptors, or MAC.

10. The answer is D. CRP can act as an efficient opsonin when it binds to phosphocholine on microbial cells. It does not act as an integrin, a receptor, a cytokine, or an addressin.

Chapter 4

1. The answer is E. Although IgM found in both monomeric and pentameric forms, it is the only immunoglobulin isotype found in the circulation as a pentamer. IgA forms

dimers, but with the attachment of secretory component by mucosal epithelial cells secretory IgA is transported to the mucosal surfaces. IgD, IgE, and IgG are found as monomers.

2. The answer is D. The classical complement pathway is initiated by the binding of C1q to antigen–antibody complexes, especially IgM and IgG isotypes. IgE does not activate any complement pathway C3b antigen, and factors B and P are part of the alternative complement pathway and MBL is part of the lectin-binding complement pathway.

3. The answer is A. The variable or antigen-binding region of antibody determines idiotype. The Fc, light chain constant, hinge, and heavy chain constant regions are distinct from the antigen-binding portion of the antibody molecule.

4. The answer is C. Only IgE is homocytophilic, binding to the FcεR on mast cells and basophils before antigen engagement. Other isotypes are bound by FcRs only *after* they bind antigen.

5. The answer is B. TNF is one of the acute phase proteins and functions to elevate body temperature. TNF is not directly responsible for isotype switching, nor does it induce IL-2 receptor expression. TNF, although it may cause cellular death, does not specifically target virus-infected cells. Cross-linking of cell-bound IgE results in degranulation of mast cells.

6. The answer is A. Adhesion molecules stabilize the interaction between leukocytes. Agglutination reactions and the quantitative precipitin reaction involve antigen–antibody reactions. The role for adhesion molecules in the immune response is significant; patients with adhesion molecule deficiency show increased susceptibility to infections. IgM monomers are joined by disulfide bonds.

Chapter 5

1. The answer is D. TAP or transporter of antigen presentation molecules are essential for the transport and loading of proteasome degraded peptides into newly synthesized MHC class I molecules in the endoplasmic reticulum. TAP molecules have no involvement in peptide loading into MHC class II, generation of B or T cell receptors, or the processing of particulate antigens.

2. The answer is E. B cells are negatively selected in the bone marrow. The thymus is the site for negative (and positive) selection of T cells. Negative selection of leukocytes

7. The answer is E. Although every cell does not display every CD molecule, every cell of the body expresses several different CD molecules. The exclusivity of CD molecules for T cells, B cells, erythrocytes, or leukocytes cannot be correct in light of the previous statement.

8. The answer is B. Chemokines are chemoattractant cytokines. No matter how powerful their attraction, they are not CD molecules dependent on steroids, nor are they adhesion molecules. Fragments of complement components such as C3a, C5a, and C4a have chemoattractant activity but are not considered chemokines. Cell-bound receptor molecules do not function as chemoattractants or chemokines.

9. The answer is A. IgA_1 antibodies are found primarily in the mucosal surfaces and secretions above the diaphragm. IgA_2 is found in the lower intestinal tract. Neither IgG nor IgE isotypes cross the epithelial barrier and they are not normally found in the oral cavity.

10. The answer is D. Antigen-bound IgM and IgG promote opsonization through FcR binding on phagocytic cells. IgD is bound to the surface of mature B cells and little is found in the circulation. Most IgA is secreted through the mucosa. IgE binds to FcεR found on mast cells and basophils *before* binding antigen. IgD, IgA, and IgE are not considered opsonizing antibodies.

11. The answer is A. The most common selective immune deficiency is selective IgA deficiency. Patients with IgA deficiency are at increased risk for a severe reaction from a blood transfusion. These patients may have IgE or IgG4 anti-IgA antibodies, which can cause anaphylaxis. Patients with IgA deficiency have the similar risk of adverse reactions to drugs as does the general population.

does not occur within the lymph nodes, blood vessels, or spleen.

3. The answer is C. Although both T and B cells undergo somatic mutation, only B cells fine-tune their fit with antigen by hypermutation; T cells cannot do this. Dendritic cells do not have antigen-specific receptors to somatically mutate.

4. The answer is B. IL-12 secretion by APC promotes Th1 differentiation. IL-4, IL-5, and IL-10 promote Th2 differentiation. TNF functions as an acute-phase protein.

5. The answer is E. Rag-1 and Rag-2 are en-

zymes for the DNA rearrangement essential for the generation of antigen-specific B-cell and T-cell receptors. They are not involved in antigen loading into MHC molecules or in the expression of IL-2 receptors.

6. The answer is B. Activated T cells secrete IL-2 and express IL-2 receptors forming an autocrine loop in which the cells are self-stimulatory. APC, NK, B, and follicular epithelial cells do not make IL-2.

7. The answer is B. Peptides loaded into MHC class I molecules derive from proteins degraded by the proteasome within the cell's own cytoplasm. Ingested antigens, opsonized microbes, and molecules bound by scavenger receptors enter the endocytic pathway and may be presented on MHC class II. Protease inhibitors have nothing to do with this process.

8. The answer is D. Macrophages are activated by IFN-γ. IL-4 and IL-2 are autocrine cytokines produced by Th2 and Th1, respectively, and neither activates macrophages. IL-12 is produced by macrophages.

9. The answer is A. Ingested antigens are degraded in the phagolysosome and peptides derived from them are loaded into MHC class II molecules. Cytoplasmic peptides are loaded into MHC class I molecules by TAP molecules. Neither ζ chain (CD247) nor protease inhibitors are involved.

10. The answer is A. Selectins expressed on the surfaces of lymphocytes bind to addressins on endothelial surfaces that overlie sites of inflammation. Vascular epithelium does not express CD40; IgG and C3b do not bind to vascular epithelium under nonpathogenic conditions. The ligand for LFA-3 is CD2, expressed by lymphocytes.

11. The answer is C. Antibody-dependent cell-mediated cytotoxicity (ADCC) involves NK cells using their FcR to bind surface-antigen bound by antibody on target cells, resulting in perforin and granzyme-induced lysis of the target cell. Activated macrophages and B cells, too, will kill antibody-coated cells, but they do this by phagocytosis and phagolysosomal killing. CTLs kill targets using perforin granules and granzymes but cannot recognize surface-bound antibody. Mast cells can only recognize IgE through their FcεR, but IgE does not induce ADCC, and mast cells do not have perforin or granzymes.

12. The answer is D. Only IgG immunoglobulins can cross the placental barrier to the fetus. All other isotypes are selectively excluded. This is particularly comforting to the fetus that IgE does not cross—the child will not be born with allergies! IgM in fetal circulation is of fetal origin and the vast majority of IgG is normally of maternal origin. The presence of fetal IgM antibodies against microbes is clinical indication of intrauterine fetal infection, a serious situation.

13. The correct answer is A. Patients with hyper IgM syndrome have low IgA and IgG levels and elevated IgM levels. Affected patients are infants within the first few months of life who have infections of the lungs, ears, sinus, and pharynx. In addition, these patients may have opportunistic infections. Most patients with IgA deficiency disorder are clinically healthy. Patients with bare lymphocyte syndrome have a decreased level of all immunoglobulins. Patients with X-linked agammaglobulinemia, most often boys, usually have clinical symptoms after the sixth month of life with an almost complete absence of immunoglobulins and small amounts of IgM.

Chapter 6

1. The answer is D. The cell-mediated inflammation of DTH is the effective agent for clearance of fungal infections. Antibodies are formed but are ineffective at clearance. Complement activation is also ineffective.

2. The answer is E. The inflammation generated by DTH and IgE inhibit attachment of the tapeworms to the intestinal wall. Eosinophilia is frequently seen in responses to roundworms, but not to flatworms. CTLs and NK cells are ineffective against tapeworms, as is lysis via the membrane attack complex of the complement system.

3. The answer is B. The absence of MHC class I and II molecules on erythrocytes prevents presentation of antigens derived from microbes within. Without surface MHC molecules, the erythrocytes are "invisible" to T-cell receptors. *Plasmodium* does not secrete IL-10 (as does Epstein-Barr virus), convert hemoglobin to a toxic form, or "cover" itself with host antigens (as does *Schistosoma*). The absence of B7 on erythrocytes is inconsequential, given the absence of MHC I and II molecules.

4. The answer is D. Live and attenuated vaccines are generally more effective. Killed vaccine often lack proteins synthesized during replication. Purified or recombinant vaccines often contain a limited number of epitopes. Synthetic peptides contain a limited number of epitopes.

5. The answer is B. Viral antigens are presented on MHC class I molecules. $CD8^+$ T cells effectively recognize and kill the infected cells. The antibodies generated by the infection are most effective at inhibiting reinfection. Although NK cells can kill virally infected cells as part of the innate immune response, activated macrophages are not responsible for preventing reinfection. Neutralizing antibodies are responsible for inhibiting reinfection, but not in clearance of infected cells. IgE and DTH responses do neither.

6. The answer is A. Activation of T cells occurs primarily in the lymph nodes. Once activated there, they can recirculate throughout the body to identify and kill infected cells. Activation does not occur in primary immune organs such as the thymus and bone marrow. T cells can be reactivated at inflammatory sites, but initial activation does not occur there. T cells of the lamina propria are usually initially activated in the mesenteric lymph nodes.

7. The answer is B. Apoptosis also causes the degradation of the nucleic acids of intracellular pathogens prevents them from escaping the dead host cell and infecting neighboring cells. Apoptosis is often induced by contact with cells such as CTLs that kill infected targets by multiple means. Complement is not involved. Speed of death between necrosis and apoptosis is not an important consideration here.

8. The answer is A. Schistosomes can, within hours of entering a host, cover themselves with host molecules (including MHC molecules) and evade the immune response by passing as "self." They do not use the other methods listed. Several viruses decrease MHC class I expression. HIV, influenza, *Neisseria gonorrhoeae*, and *Trypanosoma brucei* are examples of organisms that alter their antigens. HIV also kills $CD4^+$ T cells. *Plasmodium* evades the immune response by living within erythrocytes.

9. The answer is E. Reactivation of memory B cells induces proliferation and somatic hypermutation so that some cells have immunoglobulin binding sites that bind the antigen in question with greater or less affinity than previously. Cells bearing surface-bound immunoglobulin (antibody) molecules that bind more tightly to antigen proliferate more rapidly and come to dominate the response. The response does not spread from B cells to T cells, nor is aging involved.

10. The answer is B. Secretory IgA is the only isotype form that can be transported from the vasculature to the external environment. IgA and IgM cannot cross the placental barrier. Dimeric IgG does not exist.

11. The answer is A. Extracellular bacteria are accessible to serum complement and to antibody. Their roles in opsonization and lysis are often sufficient for clearance. T cell-mediated responses (CTLs and DTH) concentrate on intracellular microbes. The inflammatory mediators released by mast cell degranulation do not act on the bacteria.

12. The answer is C. *Mycobacterium* is an intracellular bacterium that lives in phagosomes/endosomes. Its antigenic fragments are therefore presented by the MHC class II pathway, which requires recognition and action by $CD4^+$ T cells. Antibodies are not effective in clearance. Although some role may develop for cytotoxic T cells, as microbial peptides get into the cytoplasm of the infected cells, DTH provides a far greater contribution.

13. The answer is E. Fungal infections are controlled and cleared primarily by DTH responses. Antibodies are formed, but are not effective at clearance. Extensive fungal infections suggest a defect in cellular immunity. If there are deficiencies in B cells or immunoglobulins, they do not impact the fungal growth. Hemophilia is not relevant.

14. The answer is D. It is an extract vaccine. Whole cells are not present, whether live, attenuated, or killed. No genetic engineering is involved.

Chapter 7

1. The answer is B. γc is critical to both cellular and humoral responses because the inability to respond to such a wide range of cytokines affects both T and B cells. Of particular importance is IL-7, a cytokine critical for early development in both T and B cells. Defects in *btk* and CD40L affect B cells, but not T cells. HLA and C3 defects are expressed in T cells.

2. The answer is C. Diminished T-cell function would be expected to result in increased risk of infection. The complement system should be unaffected, and answers C, D, and E would require elevated immune function, not diminished.

3. The answer is D. Immunoglobulins are effective in clearing infectious of free living extracellular bacteria. They are not effective in clearing intracellular bacteria or fungi. Decreased immunoglobulin levels should not increase complement activation and are not involved in DTH at all.

4. The answer is B. Decreased C3 should not el-

evate inflammation, whether resulting from autoimmune or other causes (including asthma). Anemia is unrelated.

5. The answer is D. The alternative pathway (and the lectin-binding pathway) would remain unaffected and functional. In these pathways, C3 convertases and cleavage of C3 can occur and the membrane attack complex can be formed.

6. The answer is B. Both T- and B-cell functions are usually deficient, although there are some cases in which the defect may have more severe consequences in one of the types of lymphocytes than in the other.

7. The answer is E. Administration of antibiotics, immunoglobulins, and thymic hormones must be frequently repeated to achieve permanent remission of immunodeficiency. Isolation is usually an additional precaution for patients already requiring passive therapy. The use of bone marrow transplantation to replace defective cells/tissues with normal ones provides an opportunity for a permanent repair that could last for life.

8. The answer is B. These conditions frequently accompany DiGeorge syndrome because they all involve defects in embryology of tissues derived from the third and fourth brachial arches. Distinctive facial and jaw features are also commonly present. None of the other listed immune deficiencies has such accompanying characteristics.

9. The answer is E. Hereditary angioedema is the condition associated with C1 inhibitor deficiency and is characterized by more frequent inflammatory episodes. T- and B-cell functions are normal. Wiskott-Aldrich and SCID are associated with T- and B-cell defects. C3 deficiency leads to decreased inflammation. Nutritionally based immune deficiency is usually reflected in generally diminished immune responsiveness.

10. The answer is D. CGD is characterized by the inability to destroy and degrade ingested microbes caused by defective lysosomal enzymes, oxygen metabolites, etc. The other listed components are normal in CGD.

Chapter 8

1. The answer is B. Histamine causes the junctions between the vascular endothelial cells to loosen and also promotes constriction of the smooth muscle of the arterioles. These effects increase the movement of fluid out of the vasculature and into the tissues.

2. The answer is C. The kidney glomeruli are one of the primary sites for accumulation of precipitated immune complexes. The bound antibody, IgG or IgM, activates complement via the classical pathway and triggers local inflammation. The inflammation is not triggered by IgE. The antigens triggering the response are fragments of nucleic acids or chromosomal proteins—soluble rather than membrane-bound antigens (as in type II hypersensitivity reactions). The damage is not inflicted by cellular responses such as DTH or CTLs.

3. The answer is D. Contact sensitivity (CS) is mediated by CD4$^+$ T cells. It is a type of DTH defined by the nature of the antigen. It is a type IV hypersensitivity that does not involve IgG, IgE, or immune complex deposition. CS is an adaptive immune response and does not involve natural killer cells.

4. The answer is C. The localization of the antigen determines the localization of the inflammation and, as a consequence, the nature of the symptoms. Type I hypersensitivity responses (triggered by IgE) do not involve activation of the complement system or activation of NK cells. Because almost all of the IgE secreted by plasma cells is bound to mast cell and basophil surfaces, IgE is rarely found in immune complexes. Immune complexes almost always involve IgG and IgM.

5. The answer is E. SLE is a condition in which high levels of soluble antigen can be present together with high levels of specific antibody (usually IgG). This combination can lead to immune complex disease. SLE is not caused by cell-mediated type IV hypersensitivity reactions (DTH and contact sensitivity), or by IgE (immediate hypersensitivity). SLE patients are not immunodeficient.

6. The answer is D. The most common sites for accumulation of precipitated immune complexes are the glomeruli of the kidney, synovial membranes, skin, and blood vessel walls. Other sites such as brain, liver, eyes, and bone are not.

7. The answer is A. Rheumatoid factor is the anti-IgM that is generated against exposed sites on antigen-bound IgG molecules in rheumatic diseases. Rheumatoid factor is not a cytokine or a complement component. It does not involve IgE or IgA.

8. The answer is A. Epinephrine provides a rapid counteraction of the effects of hista-

mine that induces smooth muscle contraction of the bronchioles. This situation can be life-threatening and requires immediate attention. Desensitization is a long-term procedure. Blockage of histamine receptors is inappropriate—the effects of the histamine are already evident. Treatment of the rash can be deferred until the emergency is dealt with.

9. The answer is A. Increased anti-immunoglobulin levels (rheumatoid factor) is a significant sign of rheumatoid arthritis. The other indicators are not useful in distinguishing rheumatoid arthritis from other inflammatory diseases.

Chapter 9

1. The answer is D. The presence of HLA-B27 is associated with several of the reactive arthritis groups, including ankylosing spondylitis.

2. The answer is B. Molecular mimicry (cross-reactivity of microbial antigens and self molecules) is thought to account for several diseases (e.g., rheumatic fever). IgE-mediated inflammation (allergy) is directed against foreign, but often benign, antigens. Total elimination of self-reactive T cells by negative selection would prevent any autoimmune disease in which T-cell activity is required. A similar effect might be expected from ablation of the thymus. Increased numbers of suppressor cells would be expected to reduce the incidence of autoimmunity.

3. The answer is C. SLE results in high levels of IgG antibodies specific for systemically distributed epitopes on fragments of chromatin (nucleic acids and proteins). The constant presence of the auto-antigens drives the production of additional autoantibodies. Simultaneous high levels of such antigens and antibodies are conditions inductive to the development of immune complex disease (type III hypersensitivity). Immediate hypersensitivity is IgE-mediated, whereas delayed hypersensitivity and contact sensitivity are entirely cell-mediated. Immunodeficiency generally lowers immune responsiveness.

4. The answer is D. Rheumatoid factors are antibodies (usually IgM) that can recognize and bind to sites on IgG molecules that become exposed when they undergo a conformational change as a result of binding to their antigen. C5a, IL-4, and IL-10 are not antibodies. IgE is not involved, and antibodies binding to epitopes not found on IgG are not rheumatoid factors.

5. The answer is E. Binding of the TCR of the naive T cells in the absence of the second signals normally provided by APCs renders the cell anergic. The anergized T cells do not die but are usually incapable of subsequent activation, proliferation, or effector function, even if they subsequently interact with APCs.

6. The answer is C. Binding of a reactive chemical to a self-molecule may induce a conformational change that makes the self-molecule appear to be foreign. The mere act of binding by an antibody does not create a neo-antigen, nor does normal processing and presentation or the appearance of normally sequestered antigens. By definition, a neoantigen is formed by an altered antigen, not by an altered receptor. In addition, recall that T-cell receptors do not undergo processes such as affinity maturation.

7. The answer is A. Approximately 2% to 5% of cases of male sterility are thought to result from autoimmune responses against sperm that result from their exposure to the immune system through injury or surgery. None of the other choices is associated with this type of autoimmunity.

8. The answer is B. Relative risk is a comparison of the frequency of a particular disease among individuals carrying a particular gene (or other risk factor) with the disease frequency among individuals who do not carry the gene (or other risk factor). It has no bearing on the blood relationship between individuals. It is not a measure of the frequency of the disease in the general population or within families.

10. The answer is D. The involvement of multiple sites and organs (particularly the combination of skin, kidney, and joints) fits best with a systemic immune complex disease (type III hypersensitivity reaction) such as systemic lupus erythematosus. These are all sites that are highly susceptible to deposition of immune complexes. The rash is consistent with an immediate hypersensitivity reaction, DTH, and contact sensitivity, but these do not typically also involve joints and kidneys. The anemia and rash are consistent with a drug-induced hemolytic anemia, but again the prominent involvement of joints and kidney are not typical.

Chapter 10

1. The answer is B. Cyclosporine and tacrolimus inhibit the proliferation and activation of T cells primarily by interfering with the production of IL-2 by lymphocytes. They do not inhibit CD40 expression or antigen processing/presentation by phagocytic cells. They do not target the bone marrow, nor are they responsible for thymic involution (shrinkage of the thymus), a change that occurs naturally with age.

2. The answer is D. Cyclosporine inhibits proliferation of T cells. The T cells that are proliferating most rapidly are those that are responding to the specific immunological stimulus in question. T cells specific for other antigens would not be proliferating rapidly and would largely remain unaffected by the treatment. All of the other agents listed act generally, damaging lymphocytes without regard to their antigen specificity.

3. The answer is E. Donor E is the best choice because he/she carries only one mismatched HLA gene (C6) that is not present in the donor. Donor A has four mismatches (A8, B7, B22, C4), donor B has two mismatches (B24, C12), donor C has six mismatches (A27, A44, B1, B8, C3, C6), and donor D has two mismatches (C2, C9).

4. The answer is B. Because bone marrow contains immunocompetent tissue, the primary threat from transplanted bone marrow is graft-versus-host disease (GVHD). Because the recipient is almost always immunocompromised (except in experimental situations), there is little danger of host-versus-graft responses. GVH responses are not allergic responses (type I hypersensitivities). Although type II hypersensitivity reactions are often autoimmune in nature, GVH responses are directed against host antigens that are "foreign" to the bone marrow and thus are not autoimmune responses.

5. The answer is D. HLA-matched grafts between unrelated individuals are almost certain to have numerous mismatches of minor histocompatibility genes. This situation usually results in chronic rejection occurring over months to years as opposed to hyperacute rejction (B) or acute rejection (C). Such grafts can sometimes (although rarely) survive permanently.

6. The answer is C. Of the possibilities listed, xenografts are highly susceptible to the action of natural antibodies that can cause hyperacute rejections. Graft-versus-host responses are not relevant except for bone marrow grafts, which are not likely to be used for nonhuman tissue. Orthotopic or heterotopic placement should not present any greater obstacles for xenografts than for allogeneic grafts. Cell-mediated responses, either by CD8$^+$ or CD4$^+$ T cells, do not play as large a role as hyperacute rejection caused by natural antibodies. Complement activation and NK cells usually destroy the xenografts before T-cell responses can be generated. In addition, it is questionable how well human CD8$^+$ T cells would be able to recognize and bind MHC I molecules on nonhuman cells.

7. The answer is D. The liver can be transplanted successfully despite considerable genetic mismatching of host and donor. Bone marrow, skin, kidney, and heart transplants require matching for a good chance of success.

8. The answer is A. The primary factor among those listed is the degree of genetic matching between host and donor. Graft size and placement (orthotopic or heterotopic) have little or no influence. Age and sex may have some influence on the recipient's physiology, but relative to genetic matching, play minor roles, if any.

9. The answer is A. Individual II-1 must be AO. She inherited A from I-1, but does not carry B, and so must have inherited an O allele from parent I-2. Individual II-2 must have inherited an O from parent I-4 (who must be OO) and a B from parent I-3, and therefore must have a BO phenotype. If II-1 is AO and II-2 is BO, they could produce offspring of four different genotypes: AO (phenotype A), AB (phenotype AB), BO (phenotype B), and OO (phenotype O).

10. The answer is C. Anti-Rh antibodies are produced by Rh$^-$ mothers in response to antigenic stimulation by Rh$^+$ fetal erythrocytes that may enter the maternal circulation during birth and sometimes during pregnancy as well. They are of the IgG isotype (not IgM or IgE). IgG is the only isotype capable of crossing the placenta. On entering the fetal circulation, they can bind to Rh$^+$ fetal erythrocytes, leading to hemolysis and possible additional severe problems.

Chapter 11

1. The answer is D. IL-12 is often produced by dendritic cells to help initiate a CD4$^+$ T-cell response. Neither IFN-α, IFN-γ, IL-2, nor IL-15 has been shown to augment vaccination.

2. The answer is A. Bacille Calmette-Guérin is a bovine strain of *Mycobacterium tuberculosis* and is used as an adjuvant in tumor immunotherapy. IFN-γ has no adjuvant activity and its polyethylene glycol-modified form of pegylated IFN-γ has a prolonged half-life in circulation. Rheumatoid factor is an auto-reactive antibody characteristic of rheumatoid arthritis. FK506 is an immunosuppressive drug. Nonsteroidal anti-inflammatory agents (NSAIDs) tend to minimize activation of the innate (inflammatory) immune processes.

3. The answer is C. Human immune globulin contains mainly IgG with only trace amounts of IgM and IgA antibodies. The half-life of IgG is 23 days. Neither IgM (half-life 1 day), IgD (half-life 2.8 days), IgA (half-life 5.8 days), nor IgE (half-life 2.5 days) would have sufficient duration in the serum to provide adequate protection. In addition, IgE antibodies would trigger atopy in the patient, IgM antibodies would be of low affinity, and it is unknown whether IgD antibodies would serve any useful therapeutic function.

4. The answer is C. Because the underlying mechanism of asthma is inflammation, an inhaled corticosteroid is recommended as first-line therapy. Antibiotics are not indicated because the subject does not have other symptoms such as fever or cough of productive sputum. NSAIDs are anti-inflammatory agents but do not treat inflammatory respiratory disorder. IgE antibody would exacerbate the patient's disorder. Additional medication is required because this patient has daily symptoms.

5. The answer is E. TNF-α inhibitors would be the next best option. Clinical trials using TNF-α inhibitors in RA patients have demonstrated clinical benefits in decreasing both the signs and symptoms of RA, and the progression of joint damage and their onset of action is faster than DMARDs. Other DMARDs can slow the disease but it may take many weeks to up to 6 to 8 months to demonstrate a response to treatment. IL-1 would only exacerbate her condition.

6. The answer is B. Aspirin inhibits platelet aggregation and has been shown to reduce the incidence of unstable angina. Corticosteroid is used to treat many diseases and autoimmune disorders and other conditions, but not myocardial ischemia. NSAID is not used to treat myocardial ischemia. Epinephrine is an α-adrenergic, β1-adrenergic, and β2-adrenergic receptor. It is the initial drug of choice for treating bronchoconstriction and hypotension resulting from anaphylaxis, as well as all forms of cardiac arrest. Cyclosporine is frequently used to inhibit unwanted T-cell proliferation and/or activation in graft rejection.

Glossary

ABO blood groups: Complex carbohydrate molecules most often found on the surfaces of erythrocytes. The ABO locus has three alleles: A, B, and O. The A and B alleles produce glycosyl transferases for *N*-acetylgalactosamine and galactose, respectively, whereas the O allele fails to produce a functional enzyme.

Absorption: Removal of an antibody or antigen from a solution using antigen or antibody, respectively.

Acquired immune deficiency syndrome (AIDS): A severe, often fatal human disease caused by a retrovirus (formerly called HTLV-III; currently termed HIV). It preferentially infects CD4⁺ human T lymphocytes and macrophages. First identified in the United States as infecting primarily homosexuals, AIDS has now reached epidemic proportions worldwide in both heterosexual and homosexual populations. The long latency period (often >5 years) for disease onset contributes epidemiologically.

Activated lymphocytes: White blood cells of the lymphoid series stimulated by specific antigen or nonspecific mitogen. Activated lymphocytes often increase in size, a phenomenon known as BLAST TRANSFORMATION; these proliferating cells are detected by an increase in tritiated thymidine incorporation.

Activated macrophages or phagocytes: Macrophages displaying increased phagocytic activity and size. Macrophage activation is often caused by a LYMPHOKINE signal from sensitized T lymphocytes or from binding of PRR.

Activation: For lymphoid and phagocytic cells, the transformation from a resting state to a functionally active state. For molecules, the transformation of inactive molecules into an enzymatically active state.

Active immunity: Immunity of an individual caused by sensitization of and response by his/her own immune system, as distinguished from PASSIVE IMMUNITY.

Acute phase proteins: Proteins that induce a loosening of the junction between endothelial cells lining the vasculature to permit freer entry of blood-borne cells and molecules of into the infected tissues.

Adaptive immunity: The ability of the immune system to acquire specific protection as the result of intentional immunization or infection.

Adherent cells: Cells, usually macrophages, from lymphoid tissues or inflammatory exudates that adhere strongly to glass or plastic surfaces.

Adhesion molecules: Provide stable cell-to-cell contact.

Adjuvant: Any of many foreign materials injected along with an antigen to enhance its immunogenicity. These include killed bacteria (*Bordetella pertussis*, mycobacteria) or bacterial products (such as endotoxin) or emulsions (Freund's complete adjuvant, alum).

Afferent lymphatic vessel: Part of the lymphatic circulatory system. Conveys lymph that contains fluid, leukocytes and debris to a lymphoid organ.

Affinity: The thermodynamic quantification of the noncovalent interaction between two molecules, usually that of an antibody with its corresponding antigenic determinant, *see also* AVIDITY.

Agammaglobulinemia: Severe deficiency or absence of one or more immunoglobulin isotypes.

Agglutination: Clumping of bacteria, cells, or other particulate antigens caused by cross-linking by antibody. As a technique, agglutination provides a simple and rapid means of determining blood groups such as ABO.

Allelic exclusion: Phenomenon whereby a B lymphocyte will produce immunoglobulin of only one allelic form (i.e., ALLOTYPE) of the light chain and the heavy chain. In cells containing two different alleles for those genetic loci, only a single allele is expressed. In heterozygotes, a mixture of two cell populations, each expressing one of the alleles, is seen.

Allergen: ANTIGEN and often an IMMUNOGEN that provokes ALLERGY.

Allergy: A type I HYPERSENSITIVITY response to an agent (i.e., ALLERGEN) that is nonantigenic for most individuals in a population. Most often, an antibody response of the IgE class is seen.

Allo-: *Prefix*, meaning between genetically different members of the same species.

Alloantigen: An antigen obtained from another individual or inbred line of the same species. Such antigens are the result of genetic polymorphism. Histocompatibility molecules are common examples.

Allograft: Tissue transplanted between genetically nonidentical individuals of the same species, also called HOMOGRAFT.

Allotype: A structural site on the heavy chain of a particular immunoglobulin class or on the light chain that differs among individuals or inbred lines of the same species. It can be used as a marker for genetic studies.

Alternative complement pathway: Complement activation that involves the binding of components C3 and B by certain PAMP on microbes.

Anamnestic response: *Same as* SECONDARY IMMUNE RESPONSE.

Anaphylactoid reaction: Nonimmunological local or systemic reaction often resulting from a physical stimulus such as trauma, heat, cold, etc.

Anaphylaxis: Systemic immediate hypersensitivity reaction resulting in respiratory distress or vascular collapse.

Anaphylatoxin: Small fragment of C3 (C3a) or of C5 (C5a) that causes degranulation of mast cells and liberating vasoactive amines.

Anergy: Immune nonresponsiveness (see SUPPRESSION and TOLERANCE).

Antibody: Immunoglobulin molecule capable of combining specifically with a known substance (antigen) (see IMMUNOGLOBULIN). The term antibody implies that the specificity is known.

Antibody-dependent cell-mediated cytotoxicity (ADCC): The ability of nonsensitized cells (i.e., cells from an unimmunized animal) to lyse other cells that have been coated by specific antibody.

Antigen: Molecule or part of a molecule recognized by the immune system. A specific target of the immune response. An antigen may be composed of many determinants or EPITOPES, *see also* DETERMINANT, EPITOPE, IMMUNOGEN.

Antigen binding site: That portion of an antibody molecule that binds with the corresponding epitope, located in the Fab portion of the molecule.

Antigen presentation: Display of antigenic peptide bound to MHC CLASS I or MHC CLASS II molecules on the cell surface. T LYMPHOCYTES recognize antigen only when presented in this manner.

Antigen processing: Intracellular enzymatic degradation of an antigen occurring before ANTIGEN PRESENTATION. It is usually attributed to macrophages and dendritic cells.

Antigen suicide: Method to specifically destroy cells carrying receptors for a particular antigen by exposing the cells to antigen of very high specific radioactivity. The localized irradiation leads to death of the cells. Alternatively, any toxic molecule attached to an antigen (e.g., ricin) that would lead to the destruction of a cell bearing a specific receptor for that antigen.

Antigenic determinant: Minimum recognition unit of the immune response also known as an EPITOPE. It is generally believed to be as small as 4 to 6 amino acids.

Antigenic drift: Error-prone genetic accumulation of errors during replication.

Antigenic shift: A process in which recombination creates major changes in the dominant antigen expressed by the virus.

Antigenic universe: Epitopes that may be recognized by the immune system, including immunogens, haptens, and tolerogens.

Antigenicity: Property of a substance permitting it to react with antibody or an antigen-specific T-CELL RECEPTOR, but an antigen does not necessarily induce an immune response, *see also* IMMUNOGEN.

Antihistamine: Pharmacological substance (not an antibody) that blocks the effect of histamine.

Antiserum: The fluid, acellular portion of the blood (serum) containing antibody molecules of known specificity. Antisera often are prepared by IMMUNIZATION with ANTIGENS.

Antitoxin: Protective antibodies that inactivate soluble toxic proteins of bacteria.

Apoptosis: Programmed cell death that follows a sequence of events including DNA degradation, nuclear condensation, and plasma membrane blebbing leading to the phagocytosis of the apoptotic cell. Importantly, this type of cell death does not lead to an inflammatory response.

Arthus reaction: Local immune (hypersensitivity) reaction mediated by antigen–antibody complexes and resulting in vascular injury, thrombosis, hemorrhage, and acute inflammation.

Association: A statistical correlation between two events.

Association constant: Or K_a value, the mathematical expression of affinity of binding between antigen and antibody.

Ataxia-telangectasia: A complex syndrome with neurological and immunological abnormalities. *Ataxia*—imbalance of muscular control. *Telangectasia*—dilated capillary blood vessels.

Atopy: A genetically determined abnormal state of hypersensitivity, as distinguished from hypersensitivity responses in normal individuals.

Auto-: *Prefix*, meaning within the same individual.

Autoantibody: An antibody produced by an individual directed against that individual's own epitopes.

Autoimmune: Immune response(s) directed against an individual's own tissues, cells, or fluids.

Autoimmune disease: Tissue injury and inflammation resulting from an autoreactive immune response, which gives rise to clinically manifested anomalies and demonstrable pathological changes.

Autologous: Originating from the same individual.

Autoreactivity: Immunologic activity, either humoral or cell-mediated, directed against host native or "self" antigenic component(s).

Autosomes: Chromosomes other than the X and Y sex chromosomes.

Avidity: Measure of binding strength of antibody and antigen molecules—usually involving multiple different molecular interactions, *see* AFFINITY.

B: Symbol for a component of the ALTERNATIVE PATHWAY of complement activation, also known as C3 proactivator.

B cell: One of the two major classes of lymphocytes. B cells derive from the BURSA OF FABRICIUS in birds or the BONE MARROW of mammals, and respond to an immunogenic signal by differentiating into antibody-producing cells (i.e., PLASMA CELLS).

B-cell receptor: Immunoglobulin produced by and expressed on the surface of B lymphocytes that function as antigen-specific receptors.

B1 cell: A self-renewing class of B lymphocytes most often found in the peritoneal and plural cavities.

B$_2$ cell: Conventional B lymphocytes.

Basophil A white blood cell of the granulocytic series (see MAST cell) that has receptors for the Fc portion of homocytotropic or heterocytotropic antibodies. Important in the allergic response.

β$_2$-Microglobulin: A 12,000-dalton polypeptide, whose amino acid sequence shows homology with an immunoglobulin heavy chain domain, found in association with histocompatibility antigens on the surface of cells.

Binding site: That portion of a receptor (e.g., T-CELL RECEPTOR or IMMUNOGLOBULIN molecule) that displays a significant AFFINITY for a ligand.

Blood: The circulating tissue of the body, it is composed of a pale yellow fluid called plasma, erythrocytes (red cells), leukocytes (white blood cells), and cellular fragments (platelets).

Blood groups: Surface molecules on red blood cells that may vary between individuals of the same species. The most important blood groups in humans are the ABO and Rh blood groups.

Bone marrow: Hemopoietic tissue, precursors (stem cells) of most of the cellular elements of the blood are located here. Lymphocytes differentiating at this site are referred to as B CELLS, and cells of this lineage give rise to immunoglobulins.

Booster: Secondary challenge with antigen.

Bruton's agammaglobulinemia: Sex-linked genetic inability to form B cells and, hence, immunoglobulins.

Bursa of Fabricius: Hindgut lymphoid organ in birds that influences B-CELL development. BONE MARROW is the mammalian equivalent.

Bystander: A cell or tissue not actively involved at the site of an immune reaction, but close proximity to that reaction makes it subject to damage as a consequence of an immune reaction.

C3 Receptor (C3R): A site on the surface of B cells and phagocytes able to bind activated C3 or fragments of C3.

Calnexin: Chaperone protein found within the endoplasmic reticulum.

Calreticulin: Chaperone protein found within the endoplasmic reticulum.

Candidiasis: Oral candidiasis is a fungal infection of the oropharynx characterized by white plagues lesions.

Capping: The coordinated surface movement of membrane molecules to one region of the cell surface after binding by a multivalent ligand such as an antibody or an antigen.

Caspases: Intracellular cysteine proteases involved in apoptotic death pathways.

CD: Cluster of differentiation.

Cell-mediated immunity (CMI): Immune responses mediated by cells. Includes CYTOTOXIC T-LYMPHOCYTE REACTIVITY, DELAYED HYPERSENSITIVITY, ANTIBODY-DEPENDENT CELL-MEDIATED CYTOTOXICITY, and, in general, any cell-mediated immunological effector function.

Cellular immunity: *See* CELL-MEDIATED IMMUNITY.

Central lymphoid organs: Lymphoid tissues that serve as the differentiation sites for lymphocytes. In mammals, these are THYMUS (T CELLS) and BONE MARROW (B CELLS). Birds have a defined organ for B-cell differentiation called the BURSA OF FABRICIUS.

C_H region: Segment of the heavy chain of immunoglobulin with a relatively constant amino acid sequence. There are several of these regions of homology or DOMAINS on the heavy chain that are sequentially labeled C_{H1}, C_{H2}, C_{H3} (sometimes C_{H4}).

Chaperone: A molecule controlling the three-dimensional folding and transport of another molecule.

Chediak-Higashi syndrome: Disease based on faulty phagocytic destruction of ingested microbes and related to lysosomal membrane abnormalities.

Chemokine: A member of a large family of low-molecular-weight cytokines that stimulates lymphocyte movement and migration from the circulation into the tissues.

Chemotactic factor for macrophages: Produced by TH1 CELLS, provokes migration of macrophages to the site of cell-mediated immune reactions.

Chemotaxis: A process whereby phagocytic cells are attracted to the vicinity of invading pathogens.

Chronic granulomatous disease (CGD): An inherited disorder of phagocytes. Occurs in neutrophils and macrophages that are unable to make superoxide anion and thus unable to kill an ingested organism.

Cis: Two linked genes on the same chromosome (as opposed to *trans*).

C_L region: The region of the light chain of immunoglobulins with a relatively constant amino acid sequence in different antibodies.

Class (antibody): The major molecular types of immunoglobulin, IgM, IgG, IgA, IgE, IgD, *see also* ISOTYPE.

Class I molecules: The classical transplantation antigens or MHC MOLECULES. Glycoproteins of approximately 45,000 daltons. Products of HLA-A, HLA-B, HLA-C loci.

Class II molecules: Products of HLA-D/DR regions. These are noncovalently associated heterodimers consisting of α (approximately 33,000 daltons) and β (approximately 28,000 daltons) chains, *see also* Ia ANTIGENS.

Class III molecules: Complement proteins (C2, C4, factor B) encoded by genes within the major histocompatibility complex.

Classical complement pathway: The mechanism of complement activation by antigen–antibody complexes involving the binding of C1, C4, and C2 to activate C3.

Clonal anergy: A theory stating that the interaction of B cells with antigen may lead to the selective inactivation of specific B cells resulting in tolerance during ontogeny.

Clonal deletion: Concept that tolerance results from the elimination (i.e., deletion) of self-reactive clones.

Clonal restriction: The ability of a lineage of cells only to react only on stimulation with a ligand in the context of a particular MHC MOLECULE.

Clonal selection theory: Hypothesis explaining the specific nature of the immune response in which the diversity among various cells for the recognition of specific antigens exists before their exposure to the antigen. Subsequent exposure to a particular antigen causes the proliferation of the appropriate antigen-specific cells.

Clone: A group of genotypically *and* phenotypically identical cells, all of which are the descendants of a single cell.

Cluster of differentiation (CD): Term used to serologically identify lymphoid cell surface molecules as detected by different monoclonal or polyclonal antibodies.

Colony-stimulating factor: Molecules that stimulate the growth of cells.

Colostrum: First milk secreted by mother after birth.

Complement: A set of serum proteins activated in sequence by antibody–antigen complexes or by bacterial products (ALTERNATIVE PATHWAY) and responsible for many biological defense mechanisms such as lysis, opsonization, leukocyte chemotaxis, inflammation, etc.

Complement fixation: The binding of COMPLEMENT to an antigen–antibody complex.

Complementation test: A genetic test for determining whether two variants involve the same locus or chromosomal segment.

Congenital: Existing at birth, may be hereditary trait or caused by some other influence arising during gestation.

Constant region: That region of an immunoglobulin chain with a close sequence homology to other chains of that class or subclass.

Contact dermatitis: Delayed or cell-mediated hypersensitivity response to cutaneously applied immunogens.

Contact sensitivity: Form of DELAYED HYPERSENSITIVITY in which sensitivity to topically applied simple chemical compounds is manifested by a skin reaction.

Cortex: The peripheral region of the lymph node or thymus.

Cortical thymocytes: T-cell precursors that populate the outer layer of the thymus.

Costimulation: A second stimulatory signal provided to a T cell.

Creutzfeld-Jacob disease (CJD): Prion-related disease in humans.

Cross-link: The joining of two similar or dissimilar molecules or cells by a chemical by covalent or noncovalent means.

Cystic fibrosis: A fatal genetic disorder caused by a defective gene product that interferes with normal chloride ion permeability resulting in thickend, viscous secretions of the respiratory tract.

-cyte: *Suffix*, meaning cell, e.g., splenocyte or spleen cell.

Cytokines: Protein molecules that act as messengers between cells affecting their behavior.

Cytotoxic T lymphocytes: Lymphocytes (T CELLS) that have been sensitized and are able, by direct contact, to specifically lyse target cells to which they bind, *see* CML.

D: Symbol for a component of the ALTERNATIVE PATHWAY.

Death domain: Portions of protein molecules involved in the apoptotic death pathway. Their definition has now been expanded to include other protein–protein interactions.

Defensins: Small proteins that kill microbes by disrupting their membranes.

Degranulation: A process whereby cytoplasmic granules of phagocytic cells fuse with phagosomes and discharge their contents into the phagolysosome thus formed.

Delayed (-type) hypersensitivity: Specific inflammatory immune reactions elicited by antigen in the skin of immune individuals. Takes 24 to 48 hours to develop and is mediated by T cells and macrophages, but not by antibodies.

Deletion: Loss of a section of genetic material from a chromosome.

Dendritic cell: Specialized antigen-presenting cells, the most potent stimulator of T-cell responses.

Desensitization: The reduction of abolition of allergic reactivity. This term is really a misnomer, because, in fact, the patient is actively immunized with the allergen in hopes of producing an IgG response that will supplant IgE.

Determinant: That part of the structure of an antigen or immunogen that binds to the antibody combining site of an immunoglobulin or that part of an antigen or immunogen specifically recognized by the T cell receptor, *see* EPITOPE, HAPTEN.

Dextran: High-molecular-weight glucose polymers. Often *these are T-independent antigens*.

Diapedesis: The outward passage of cells through the intact vessel walls.

Differentiation antigen: A serologically detectable cell-surface antigen expressed at a particular stage of differentiation.

DiGeorge syndrome: Birth defects in embryonic development of the thymus resulting in loss of immune competence requiring T lymphocytes.

Direct sensing: Engagement of PRRs expressed by dendritic cells that recognize PAMPs on viruses, bacteria, or fungi.

Discriminate: To tell the difference between two antigens and especially between "self" and "non-self" (foreign) antigens, a fundamental property of the immune system.

Diversity: The large number of antigen-specific receptors produced by the immune system.

Domain: A single homology region of an immunoglobulin, encompassing approximately 110 amino acids, and held together by a disulfide bridge spanning the central approximately 60 residues.

Dominant: An allele whose phenotypic effect is evident whether in the homozygous or heterozygous state.

Edema: Accumulation of fluid in a tissue.

Effector cell: A leukocyte that responds to a stimulus and performs an immune function without the necessity of further proliferation or differentiation.

Efferent lymphatic vessel: Part of the lymphatic circulatory system. Convenes fluid and leukocytes away from a lymphoid organ.

Endocytosis: Internalization extracellular molecules or particles by pinocytosis or phagocytosis.

Endogenous: Having origin within the organism.

Endotoxin: A lipopolysaccharide derived from cell walls of Gram-negative—has multiple biological effects—stimulates the immune response nonspecifically, stimulates mouse B lymphocytes, and activates the alternative complement pathway.

Enzyme-linked immunosorbent assay (ELISA): An immunoassay employing an enzyme covalently bound to either antibody or antigen as a marker. A chromogenic substrate is used to detect the presence of enzyme and hence antibody or antigen.

Eosinophil: A leukocyte with a bilobed nucleus and red-staining cytoplasmic granules, often found at sites of parasitic infections.

Epistasis: A form of gene interaction in which expression of one gene is dependent on the expression or activity of another nonallelic gene(s).

Epitope: A single antigenic determinant—the portion of a molecule that will combine with a particular antibody combining site. Multiple epitopes usually found on the same antigen, *see* HAPTEN, IDIOTOPE, ANTIGENIC DETERMINANT.

Equivalence: A ratio of antigen–antibody concentration in which maximal precipitation occurs.

Erythroblastosis fetalis: Medical term for Rh incompatibility disease of the newborn.

Extracellular bacteria: Bacteria that live freely and can reproduce in body fluids or extracellular spaces.

Extravasation: Movement of the fluids and/or cells from the blood vessels into the surrounding tissue.

Exudation: Discharge of plasma into a tissue.

Fab fragment: A product of papain digestion of immunoglobulins; contains one intact light chain and part of one heavy chain. Fab fragments have one combining site for antigen.

F(ab ′)₂ fragment: A product of pepsin digestion of immunoglobulins, containing two intact light chains and parts of two heavy chains. It has two combining sites for antigen, but lacks the Fc region.

Fas (CD95): Member of the TNF receptor family expressed on the cell surface. Engagement of Fas triggers apoptosis of the Fas-bearing cell.

Fc fragment: A product of papain digestion of immunoglobulin with parts of two heavy chains and no combining sites for antigen. This fragment has sites for activation of complement. It contains no antigen-binding capacity, but determines important biological characteristics of the intact molecule.

FcR: *See* Fc receptor.

Fc receptor: A receptor for the Fc fragment of immunoglobulins; present on various subclasses of lymphocytes.

Fd fragment: N-terminus, papain cleavage fragment of the heavy chain of an immunoglobulin molecule. This fragment linked by disulfide bond to a light chain forms a Fab fragment.

Fluorescein (FITC): An organic molecule that absorbs light at 485 nm and emits light at 535 nm. This property is exploited immunologically in that the isothiocyanate form of this molecule (FITC) is used to react with α and ε amines as a convenient label for both antibodies and antigens.

Fluorescence: The emission of light of one color while a substance is irradiated with a different wavelength.

Follicle: A circumscribed region in lymphoid tissue, usually in the superficial cortex of lymph nodes, containing mostly B cells.

Foreign: A chemical, organism, or substance not naturally found in your body, something that triggers the immune system to make a protective response.

Gamma (γ) globulin: γ globulins with slow electrophoretic mobility in the γ region, including most immunoglobulin molecules. This term is sometimes used to refer to all immunoglobulins of various classes or isotypes.

Gammopathy: Protein disorder involving abnormalities of immunoglobulins.

Gastrointestinal associated lymphoid tissue (GALT): Those accumulations of lymphoid tissue (e.g., tonsils, appendix, Peyer's patches, and in lamina propria) that are responsible for monitoring and protection of the gastrointestinal tract.

Gene: A distinctive hereditary unit located on a chromosome at a specific site or locus which codes for a functional product, e.g., tRNA, rRNA, or a polypeptide chain.

Generation of diversity: The generation of a vast diversity of antibodies (and T-cell receptors to recognize approximately 10^6 to 10^7 different antigens.

Germinal centers: A collection of metabolically active lymphoblasts, macrophages, and plasma cells that appear within the primary follicle of lymphoid tissues after antigenic stimulation.

Germ-line: The genetic lineage of an individual or cell.

Germline theory: The explanation proposed for receptor diversity in which all of the genes responsible for all the possible receptors are fully formed and transmissible within the genome.

Graft rejection: An immune reaction elicited by the grafting of genetically dissimilar tissue onto a recipient. The reaction leads to destruction and ultimate rejection of the transplanted tissue.

Graft-versus-host reaction (GVH): The pathological reactions caused by transplantation of immunocompetent T lymphocytes into an incompetent host. The host is unable to reject the T lymphocytes and becomes the target of their attack.

Granuloma: A local accumulation of densely packed macrophages, often fusing to form giant cells, and sometimes including lymphocytes and plasma cells. Seen in chronic infections such as tuberculosis and syphilis.

Granzyme: A collective term for several enzymes (serine proteases) contained within the granules of cytotoxic T lymphocytes (CTL) and natural killer (NK) cells. Granzymes are released upon perforin exocytosis, become activated in the extracellular fluid, and enter target cells through perforin-induced target cell lesions, where they proteolytically cleave caspases and initiate apoptosis.

Graves' disease: Autoimmune disease in which antibodies are produced against thyroid-stimulating hormone receptor, stimulating thyroid hormone secretion and hyperthyroidism.

Growth factors: Soluble molecules that promote the growth or proliferation of a particular cell or tissue.

H2 or H-2: The major histocompatibility complex (MHC) of the mouse.

H2K, H2D, H2L: MHC class I loci of the mouse. They are the equivalent of the HLA-A, B, and C loci in the human MHC.

Hay fever: A seasonal allergic disease causing inflammation of the eyes and nasal passages.

Heavy chain: The higher molecular weight polypeptide chain of an immunoglobulin molecule—the one determining the CLASS or ISOTYPE of the immunoglobulin.

Helper T cells: A class of specific CD4$^+$ T lymphocytes that are necessary to "help" B lymphocytes produce antibody to thymic-dependent immunogens and effector T cells to perform their respective functions.

Hemagglutination: *See* AGGLUTINATION.

Hemagglutination inhibition: A technique for detecting small amounts of antigen in which homologous antigen inhibits the agglutination of red cells or other particles coated with antigen by specific antibody.

Heterologous: From a different individual, inbred strain, or species. Sometimes applied to a different carrier molecule.

Heterophil antigen: An antigen found on seemingly unrelated organisms, cells, or molecules.

High endothelial postcapillary venules (HEV): Specialized vessels that allow the passage of circulating lymphoid cells into the parenchyma.

Hinge region: That portion of the immunoglobulin molecule lying between the Fc and Fab portions; so named because of the "flexibility" of this region of the molecule, most likely caused by proline residues in this region.

Histamine: An amine found in all plant and animal tissues, it causes vasodialation and hence lowers blood pressure.

Histiocytes: Fixed or immobile macrophages.

Histocompatible: The ability to transplant tissues between individuals without rejection.

HLA-A, HLA-B, HLA-C: Three distinct genetic loci in the human MHC encoding class I major histocompatibility antigens. Equivalent of the H2K, H2D, and H2L loci in the mouse H2 complex.

HLA-D/DR: A region of the human HLA comples encoding class II major histocompatibility complex antigens expressed primarily on B cells and macrophages and that stimulate the specific proliferation of allogeneic T cells in culture. Equivalent to the I-region in the mouse H2 complex.

Hole in the repertoire: The concept that during the random generation of T-cell and B-cell receptors that receptors toward some epitopes are not generated.

Homocytotropic antibody: Antibody that attaches to mast cells of the species producing it; IgE is an example.

Human immunodeficiency virus (HIV): Retroviruses that cause human acquired immunodeficiency syndrome AIDS.

Human leukocyte antigen (HLA) complex: The major histocompatibility complex of humans.

Humor or Humoral: Pertaining to the fluids or humors of the body. In immunology, this term refers antibodies and/or complement. According to the ancient Greeks, the body is governed by the four humors: PHLEGM, BLOOD, CHOLER (or yellow bile), and BLACK BILE.

Humoral immunity: Immune response involving soluble effector molecules such as antibody or complement.

Hybridoma: A hybrid cell derived in the laboratory from the somatic cell fusion of a normal B or T cell with a tumor cell line of either B-cell (myeloma) or T-cell (thymoma) origin, respectively. Such hybrid cells have the ability to produce antibody (B cell) or T-cell products (T cell) of the normal "parent" and are immortalized by the tumor cell 'parent'.

Hyper-IgM syndrome: An X-linked disease in which affected individual have elevated levels of IgM but low levels of IgG and IgA. Caused by a defect in the CD40 ligand (CD154).

Hyperplasia: Physical increase in size of an organ or tissue caused by an increase in cell number.

Hypersensitivity: A term usually applied to those immune phenomena that are in some way damaging to the host animal.

Hypervariable region: Defined portions of the variable region of either heavy or light immunoglobulin chains having extreme variability in amino acid sequence in different molecules. The antibody combining site includes the hypervariable regions.

Idiopathic: Primary disease or pathological state arising from uncertain causes.

Idiotype: An antigenic determinant on a specific antibody, characteristic of that antibody and different from others even of the same ISOTYPE and ALLOTYPE—idiotypes are usually located in or near the antigen binding site, see EPITOPE.

Immediate hypersensitivity: A specific immune reaction taking place within minutes to hours after the administration of antigen and is mediated by antibodies, see ARTHUS REACTION, ANAPHYLAXIS.

Immune adherence: Adhesive nature of antigen–antibody complexes to inert surfaces when complement is bound into the complex.

Immune complexes: Antigen–antibody complexes.

Immune deficiency: A defect in immune responsiveness due to environmental insult or genetic factors.

Immune memory: The primary tenet of the immune system, allowing a rapid response to subsequent exposure to the same or related immunological stimulus.

Immunity: An active process performed by leukocytes and their products in the repulsion of a foreign organism or substance.

Immunization: The process of inducing a state of immunity. This can result from the conscious introduction of immunogen (antigen) into the body as in VACCINATION or can result from the introduction of a foreign organism such as a microorganism to the immune system.

Immunoabsorption: Removal of particulate or soluble substance from solution by antibodies specific to these substances. Often the antibodies are bound to a solid matrix such as beaded agarose or are precipitated from solution by chemical means.

Immunodeficiency: Genetic absence of a cell type or tissue or the acquired inability of the immune system to respond to a particular stimulus or stimuli.

Immunoelectrophoresis: A technique combining an initial electrophoretic separation of proteins with an immunodiffusion resulting in precipitation arcs.

Immunofluorescence: A histochemical or cytochemical technique for the detection and localization of antigens in which specific antibody is conjugated with fluorescent compounds, resulting in a sensitive tracer that can be detected by fluorometric measurements.

Immunogen: A substance that, when introduced into an animal, stimulates an immune response.

Immunoglobulin: The various classes of gamma globulin molecules having antibody activity.

Immunological unresponsiveness or **tolerance:** Inhibition, by any one of several mechanisms, of activation and proliferation of an immunocompetent clone of lymphoid cells.

Immunoreceptor tyrosine-based activation motifs (ITAMs): A structural motif of two tyrosines separated by approximately 13 amino acid residues that are part of invariant molecules in association with the T-cell receptor complex. ITAMs are phosphorylated by protein tyrosine kinase and adapter protein.

Indirect sensing: Engagement of toll-like receptors (TLRs), cytokine receptors, TNF family receptors, etc., in response to PAMPs.

Inflammation: Redness, swelling, and pain in a tissue resulting from the infiltration of the tissue by infectious agents and/or lymphoid cells.

Inflammatory cells: T lymphocytes (Th1 and CTL) and monocytes or macrophages that mediate an inflammatory response.

Innate immunity: The mechanical (e.g., skin), chemical (e.g., pH), and biological (e.g., symbiotic flora of the gut) components that provide natural barriers to infectious agents.

Inoculation: Introduction of a substance into the body or into a culture.

Intercellular adhesion molecules (ICAMs): Ligands for leukocyte integrins crucial for the binding of leukocytes to other cells, e.g., antigen-presenting cells and endothelial cells.

Interferon-α, β, or γ: A CYTOKINE showing nonspecific activity in providing protection against viral infection and tumor growth. Three varieties, IFN-γ produced by lymphocytes and NK CELLS.

Interleukin: A term applied to any of a group of peptides signals that are produced by activated lymphocytes or monocytes.

Intracellular bacteria: Bacteria that enter and reproduce within cells.

Intravenous immunoglobulin: A therapeutic method for augmenting insufficient immunoglobulin levels by intravenous injection.

Invariant (Ii) chain: Associates with MHC class II molecules within the endoplasmic reticulum.

Isotype: The class or subclass of an immunoglobulin.

Isotype switching: The ability of B cells to alter the class or isotype of antibody produced without significantly altering antibody specificity.

J chain: A small polypeptide found in IgM and IgA polymers—responsible for maintaining the polymeric form of the immunoglobulin.

Janus kinases (JAK): Intracellular cytokine signaling molecules.

Junctional diversity: Diversity created by the process of joining V, D, and J gene segments.

Kappa (κ) chain: Immunoglobulin light chain, one of two types known to exist, *see* LAMBDA CHAIN. Classification is based on the amino acid sequence of the constant portion of the light chain.

Killer cell or **K cell:** A class of null lymphocytes able to mediate ADCC. Most likely these are NK CELLS.

Killer activation receptors (KARs): Recognition receptor, also called NKG2D, that provides a "kill" signal that induces a NK cell to kill a target cell.

Killer inhibition receptors (KIRs): Receptors expressed by NK cells for MHC class I molecules. This recognition signals NK cells from destroying the cell expressing MHC class I.

Kuru: Prion-related disease in humans.

Lambda (λ) chain: An immunoglobulin light chain, one of two types known to exist (see KAPPA CHAIN). Classification is based on the amino acid sequence of the constant portion of the light chain.

Langerhans cell: Epidermal dendritic cells.

Late-phase reaction Antihistamine resistant type I hypersensitivity reaction.

Lectin: Any of a number of plant products that bind to cells, usually by means of a combining site for specific sugars.

Leprosy: Infectious disease caused by *Mycobacterium leprae* that may lead to either a tuberculoid (Th1-mediated) form or a lepromatous (antibody-mediated) form.

Leukocytes: Circulating white blood cells. There are approximately 9,000/mm^3 in human blood, divided into granulocytes (polymorphs 68%–70%, eosinophils 3%, and basophils 0.5%) and mononuclear cells (monocytes 4% and lymphocytes 23%–25%).

Ligand: Any molecule that forms a complex with another molecule.

Light chain: The lower-molecular-weight polypeptide chain present in all immunoglobulin molecules, *see also* LAMBDA CHAIN, KAPPA CHAIN.

Lipopolysaccharide (LPS): Active component of endotoxin, derived from bacterial cell walls, a B-cell mitogen in the mouse.

Locus: A position on a chromosome at which the genes for a particular trait are be found.

Lupus erythematosis: Fatal autoimmune disease characterized by the production of antinuclear antibodies, *see also* SLE.

Lymph fluid: The acellular serous exudate from capillaries picked up by the lymphatic drainage vessels, and thus circulated throughout the lymphatic network.

Lymphatics: Vessels of the immune system that drain interstitial tissues of fluids, debris, and leukocytes.

Lymphocyte: A white blood cell of the lymphoid series, the "workhorse" cell of the immune system. It is capable of recognizing and responding to antigens in a specific manner.

Lymphoid organs: Accumulations of lymphoid cells into regular anatomical structure, e.g., spleen, thymus, lymph nodes, appendix, etc.

Lymphokines: A group of substances produced by lymphocytes having diverse effects on other cells.

Lymphokine-activated killer cell (LAK): A cytotoxic leukocyte requiring a lymphokine as one of its inductive signals.

Lymphoma: A cancer of the lymphoid organs.

Lymphotoxin: A lymphokine (tumor necrosis factor-β, TNF-β) that directly causes cytolysis. It is released from stimulated lymphocytes.

Lysosome: Cytoplasmic organelle present in many cells, bounded by a lipoprotein membrane, which contains various enzymes. Plays an important role in intracellular digestion.

Lysozyme: An enzyme present in the granules of polymorphs, in macrophages, in tears, mucus, and saliva. It lyses certain bacteria, especially Gram-positive *cocci*, by splitting the muramic acid- & (1-4)-N-acetylglucosamine linkage in the bacteria cell wall. It potentiates the action of complement on these bacteria.

Macrophage: An ubiquitous phagocytic cell found in tissues and blood. When found in blood it is called a monocyte. It is sometimes referred to as a histiocyte.

Major histocompatibility complex (MHC): A region of genetic material containing genes coding for certain predominant histocompatibility antigens, immune response and suppression loci, some lymphocyte and macrophage antigens, and complement components. Three classes of MHC molecules are recognized. Class I molecules are single-chain, 245,000-dalton molecules that associate with b2-microglobulin. Class II molecules are heterodimers termed α (alpha) and β (beta) chains (229,000 and 233,000 daltons, respectively) that are not covalently linked. Class III MHC molecules are complement proteins whose genetic loci lie within the MHC. In humans the MHC is called HLA, in mouse H2, in rat Rt-1.

Mannin-binding lectin (MBL): An acute-phase protein that binds to mannin residues and can activate the complement system and is important in innate immunity.

Mannin-binding lectin pathway: A complement system pathway activated by mannin residues.

Mast cell: A leukocyte of the granulocytic series which mediates anaphylactic reactions. Mast cells have been shown to bear Fc receptors for anaphylactic antibody (IgE). Interaction of IgE antibodies on the surface of mast cells with antigen results in the degranulation of the cell and the release of vasoactive amines (i.e., histamine, heparin, etc.).

Medulla: The central region of a lymph node or the thymus, consisting of lymphatic sinuses and medullary cords.

Megakaryocyte: Multinuclear giant cell of the bone marrow, portions of which break off to form the platelets.

Membrane attack complex (MAC): Those components of the terminal pathway of complement ($C\overline{5b678}$) that forms a stable macromolecular complex serving as the building block for the final and lytic component of complement (C9).

Memory: The ability of the immune system to mount a specific secondary response to an immunogen that was previously introduced.

Memory cell: A lymphocyte, either B or T, that has undergone the first stages of differentiation as a consequence of have been specifically stimulated by immunogen.

MHC class II transactivator (CIITA): A protein that activates the transcription of MHC class II genes.

Microglia: Phagocytic cells of the nervous system, some investigators report the expression of MHC class II molecules by these cells.

Microorganism: Microscopic organisms that include bacteria, fungi and protozoans.

Migration inhibition factor (MIF): A protein produced by lymphocytes upon interaction with antigens. It inhibits mobility of macrophages in culture.

Mistaken identity: The concept that sometimes self molecules or cells are erroneously recognized as nonself.

Mitogen: A substance which stimulates lymphocytes to proliferate independently of any specific immunogen.

Mitogen-activated protein (MAP) kinases: Proteins that are phosphorylated and activated on cellular stimulation by a variety of ligands.

Mixed lymphocyte reaction (MLR) or culture (MLC): The in vitro proliferation of T lymphocytes as the result of "recognition" of foreign antigen on another lymphocyte or monocyte.

Modulation: Temporal variation in the expression of a particular alloantigen on the surface of a cell or population of cells.

Molecular mimicry: Induction of an immune response to a infectious organism, the consequence of which is a cross-reactive immune response to self antigens that may have close structural similarities to molecules of the infectious agent.

Monoclonal: Derived from a single clone of cells. Recently this has come into use to describe antibodies made from a HYBRIDOMA.

Monoclonal antibody: Antibody originating from cells having a single cell precursor as its origin. Often this is applied to HYBRIDOMA-derived antibodies, but is also applicable to paraprotein antibodies derived from myeloma (B cell tumor) cells.

Monocyte: A phagocytic blood leukocyte, precursor of most tissue macrophages. Monocytes originate from cells in the bone marrow.

Monokine: Soluble factors released by activated macrophages/monocytes.

Monomer: A single polypeptide chain.

Mononuclear cells: Leukocytes with a single, non-lobed nucleus, included in this group are monocytes and lymphocytes.

Mononucleosis: A disease characterized by the increased number of atypical lymphocytes, including CD8$^+$ lymphocytes and NK cells, in the circulation and enlarged spleen and lymph nodes caused by Epstein-Barr virus (EBV) infection.

Mucosal cell adhesion molecule-1 (MadCAM-1): The ligand for lymphocyte surface proteins L-selectin and VLA-4 that allows the specific homing of lymphocytes to mucosal tissues.

Multiple myeloma: A disorder typically consisting of the presence of serum paraprotein, anemia, and lytic bone lesions.

Multiple sclerosis: A presumed autoimmune neurological disease that results from the demyelination of proteins.

Myasthenia gravis: An autoimmune disease involving the production of antibodies against acetylcholine receptor on skeletal muscle leading to progressive weakness and death.

Myeloblast, myelocyte: An immature cell derived from the bone marrow that gives rise to cells of the polymorphonuclear series.

Myeloma: A plasmacytoma—a tumor of the immunoglobulin secreting cells.

Naïve lymphocytes: Cells that have never encountered specific antigen.

Natural immunity: Immunity conferred without known sensitization.

Natural killer cell: Type of NULL CELL involved in destruction of tumor cells thought to be one of the cells responsible for IMMUNE SURVEILLANCE.

Necrosis: Death of cell or tissue caused by chemical or physical injury, as opposed to APOPTOSIS.

Negative selection: Deletion of thymocytes that recognize self during intrathymic development.

Neoantigens: Spontaneously arising nonself antigens found on cell membranes, usually associated with neoplasia.

Neutralization: The process by which antibody and complement neutralizes the activity of microorganisms, particularly viruses or soluble substances such as toxins.

Neutralizing antibodies: Specific immunoglobulins that inhibit the infectivity of a virus or the toxicity of a molecule.

Neutrophil: The most prominent leukocyte in the circulation, accounting for more than 90% of the circulating granulocytes or 60% to 70% of the circulating leukocytes. A pinocytotic cell involved in complement-mediated and DTH reactions. An increase in the number of circulating neutrophils indicates chronic infection.

Nonself: Molecules, cells, tissues, and organs that originate from an individual other than the one the immune system calls its own. Because of extensive genetic heterogeneity, the majority of individuals are seen as nonself by an individual's immune system.

Nuclear factor of activated T cells (NFAT): A transcription factor that on activation (serine/threonine dephosphorylation and dissoci-

ation from the Fos/Jun dimer, AP-1) moves from the cytoplasm to the nucleus.

Neutropenia: A neutrophil count of less than 1000 cells per milliliter, indicating that the individual is at increased risk of infection.

Null cell: A class of lymphocytes without markers for either T cells or B cells.

Oncogene: A gene involved in regulating cell growth, defect structure, or function of these genes leads to the continuous growth of cell forming a tumor.

Ontogeny: The developmental history of an individual organism within a group of animals.

Opportunistic infection: Infection caused by a microorganism in individuals with a compromised immune system.

Opsonin: Any substance that enhances phagocytosis of a cell or particle. Antibodies appear to be the only opsonin occurring normally in the body.

Opsonization: Enhancement of phagocytosis of a particle or a cell (especially bacteria) by virtue of its being coated by antibody.

Parasite: An organism that obtains sustenance from a live host.

Paratope: The antigen binding site of an antibody molecule.

Passive immunity: Immunity transferred to an individual with serum or immune cells as distinguished from ACTIVE IMMUNITY.

Patching: Aggregation of membrane molecules into many small regions on the cell surface after cross-linking by a multivalent ligand such as antibody.

Pathogen-associated molecular patterns (PAMPs): Genetically conserved molecules expressed by molecules that are recognized by PATTERN RECOGNITION RECEPTORS (PRRs).

Pathology: Study of disease mechanisms.

Pattern-recognition receptors: Genetically encoded receptors expressed by a variety of leukocytes that recognize and bind to molecules found on a wide variety of microbial cells and on damaged or infected host cells.

Perforin: Produced by NK and cytotoxic cells that polymerizes to form pores in a membrane, important in cell-mediated killing.

Peripheral lymphoid tissues: Spleen, lymph nodes, tonsils, Peyer's patches, etc. These are lymphoid accumulations in which an antigen-driven immune response can occur, *see* CENTRAL LYMPHOID ORGAN.

Peripheral tolerance: Induction of post-thymic antigen unresponsiveness.

Peyer's patches: Collections of lymphoid tissue in the submucosa of the small intestine that contain lymphocytes, plasma cells, germinal centers, and T-dependent areas.

Phagocytes: Cells that can ingest particulate matter.

Phagocytosis: The engulfment of microorganisms or other particulate matter by phagocytic cells.

Pharyngeal pouch: Ectodermal embryological structure occurring as blind sacs in the cervical region of the embryo, give rise to the epithelial tissues of the thymus, parathyroids, etc.

Phenotype: Characteristic of an individual or cells of that individual that reflect the genes expressed by that individual or cell.

Pinocytosis: The ingestion of soluble materials by cells.

Plasma: The fluid phase of whole blood, containing water, salts, proteins, and clotting factors.

Plasma cell: A fully differentiated cell of the B lymphocyte lineage, actively secreting large amounts of immunoglobulin.

Platelet or thrombocyte: A cell fragment deriving from a prothrombocyte, responsible for the activation of the clotting mechanism.

Platelet-activating factors (PAF): Substances released immunologically and able to aggregate and degranulate platelets.

Pluripotent cell: A stem cell that has the capacity to produce cells of several lineages.

Poison ivy: A plant that elicits contact sensitivity to the pentadecacatechol present in its leaves.

Pokeweed mitogen (PWM): A lectin derived from pokeweed which stimulates both B and T lymphocytes in humans.

Polyclonal: Immunologically, arising from cells of differing antigenic specificities.

Positive selection: Double-positive, $CD4^+CD8^+$, thymocytes that escape apoptosis within the thymus because they recognize MHC class I or II molecules.

Post-capillary venules: Small vessels found downstream of the capillary bed through whose walls lymphoid cells are often found to migrate.

pre-B cells: Immature cells developmentally destined to become B CELLS, in contrast to B cells pre-B cells express immunoglobulin only in their cytoplasm.

Precipitin: The insoluble aggregate formed from the interaction of soluble antigen with soluble antibody, *see also* PRECIPITATION.

Precipitation: A reaction between a soluble antigen and soluble antibody in which a complex lattice of interlocking aggregates forms and falls out of solution.

Prednisone: Anti-inflammatory synthetic steroid.

Presentation: The display of small peptide fragments by specialized proteins on the surface of antigen-presenting cells or virus-infected cells.

Primary follicles: Tightly packed accumulations of lymphoid cells (primarily B cells) in spleen and thymus, destined to become germinal centers.

Primary immune response: Response occurring upon first exposure to an immunogen.

Primed: Refers to an animal or cell population that has been previously exposed to an immunogen and that is capable of making a secondary response.

Privileged sites: Anatomical site thought to be exempt from normal immune monitoring.

Processing: Uptake and breakdown of antigen by host accessory cells leading to the presentation of antigen in an immunogenic form. Macrophages may process antigens and present them to lymphocytes in association with self Ia molecules.

Professional antigen presenting cells: Cells that initiate response of naïve T cells, e.g., dendritic cells, macrophages, and B cells.

Progenitors: Cells that give rise to distinct subsets of mature blood cells.

Programmed cell death: Apoptosis, cell death triggered from within the cell.

Properidin: A component of the ALTERNATIVE COMPLEMENT PATHWAY.

Properidin pathway: *See* ALTERNATIVE COMPLEMENT PATHWAY.

Prostaglandins: Liphatic acids with a wide variety of biological activities including vasodilatation and smooth muscle contraction.

Proteasome: A large protease that degrades cytosolic proteins.

Protective immunity: Resistance from specific infection caused by previous infection or immunization.

Protein A: A protein derived from the *Cowan* strain of *Staphylococcus aureus* that has binding affinity for the Fc portion of several different IMMUNOGLOBULIN ISOTYPES.

Prothymocyte: A precursor to the thymus cells, the embryological origin is the bone marrow in mammals and the yolk sac in birds.

Protozoa: Single-celled, nonphotosynthetic eukaryotic organisms.

Pus: A fluid product of inflammation containing leukocytes.

Pyrogens: Substances often derived from bacteria (e.g., endotoxins) that cause a characteristic rise in body temperature of an individual.

Radioallergosorbent test (RAST): A radioimmunoassay that measures the amount of serum IgE antibody bound to a specific allergen or immunogen.

Radioimmunoassay (RIA): A test that measures radiolabeled ligand (or antibody) binding to an antibody (or ligand).

Receptor: Immunologically a chemical structure on the surface of any immunocompetent cell.

Receptor-associated tyrosine kinases: Bind to receptor tails via Src family SH2 domains.

Recessive: An allele whose phenotypic effect is evident only when present in the homozygous state.

Recombination activating gene (RAG): Encode proteins RAG-1 and RAG-2 that are critical to receptor gene rearrangement.

Red pulp: Erythrocyte-rich portion of the spleen.

Rejection: Unsuccessful transplant because of an immune reaction (both cellular and humoral) against the transplanted tissue.

Repertoire: The entirety of antigens that are recognized by an individual's immune system.

Respiratory burst: The metabolic change in neutrophils and macrophages that occurs after phagocytosis of opsonized particles.

Reticuloendothelial system: A system of cells that take up particles and certain dyes injected into the body. Composed of Kupffer cells of the liver, tissue histiocytes, monocytes, and the lymph node, splenic, alveolar, peritoneal, and pleural macrophages.

Reticulum: Framework or structural elements of a tissue or organ.

Rhesus (Rh) system: A system of human red cell protein antigens under complex genetic control. Rh-negative mothers who bear Rh-positive offspring may develop Rh antibodies, which can cross the placenta and produce hemolytic disease in newborn babies.

Rheumatoid factor (RF): An anti-immunoglobulin antibody directed against denatured IgG present in the serum of patients with rheumatoid arthritis and other rheumatoid diseases.

S value: Sedimentation constant of 1×10^{-13}, usually used as a measure of relative protein size and determined by centrifugation.

Secondary follicle: A GERMINAL CENTER.

Secondary immune response: The response occurring on the second and subsequent exposures to an immunogen (memory). The secondary immune response is usually characterized by a much more rapid immune response than is seen in a primary reaction.

Second set rejection: Rapid graft rejection caused by previous sensitization of the graft recipient.

Secretory component: A 70-kDa molecule produced in epithelial cells and associated with secretory immunoglobulins, e.g., IgA, *also called* TRANSPORT PIECE.

Secretory IgA: A dimer of IgA molecules with a sedimentation coefficient of 11S, linked by the J chain and secretory component.

Selectins: Leukocyte cell-surface adhesion molecules that bind to specific glycoproteins and mucin-like molecules.

Self: Molecules, cells, tissues, and organs that belong to the body that the immune system recognizes as its own. Because of extensive genetic heterogeneity, each individual is unique and each individual's immune system has a different perception of "self."

Self education: The process occurring in the thymus in which thymocytes "learn" to distinguish MHC molecules and self peptides.

Self tolerance: Failure to respond to antigen expressed by self tissues.

Sensitization: Exposure to an individual or cell to an immunogenic form of antigen.

Sensitized cell: A cell that has been exposed to a specific stimulatory signal, e.g., exposed to immunogen.

Sepsis: Bloodstream infection.

Seroconversion: First appearance of antibodies in the blood against a particular infectious agent.

Serologically defined (SD) determinant: A determinant defined by serological methodology. Sometimes used to refer to class I alloantigens of the MHC, although they can also be defined by cellular methods.

Serology: The study of serum.

Serum: The liquid portion of the blood remaining after cells and fibrin have been removed.

Serum sickness: Systemic syndrome resulting from the deposition of circulating immune complexes, leading to complement-mediated inflammation in blood vessels and glomeruli of the kidney.

Severe combined immunodeficiency (SCID): A recessive genetically determined stem cell deficiency affecting both T and B lymphocytes; may be caused by autosomal or X-linked genes.

Sib: Sibling, one or more offspring of the same parents.

Signal transduction: The series of molecular steps that begin with the ligand binding by a receptor, activation of a sequential series of enzymes leading to the activation of their substrate molecules, resulting in altered metabolism, cell movement, and protein expression.

Specificity: The ability of antibodies and T lymphocytes to distinguish between different determinants (epitopes). Also used to refer to a specific determinant.

Spleen: The ductless vascular lymphoid organ located in the upper left quadrant of the abdomen divisible into white pulp (lymphoid cell rich) and red pulp (erythrocyte rich) regions.

Splenomegaly: Increase in spleen size. Often used as an assay for graft-versus-host reactions.

Src family tyrosine kinases: Receptor-associated protein tyrosine kinases; have domains termed Src-homology domains-1, -2, -3, or SH1, SH2, SH3.

Stem cell: A multipotent precursor cell that may give rise to cells of different morphological and functional specificities.

Subclass: Immunoglobulins of the same class (e.g., IgG), but differing in electrophoretic mobility or in an antigenic determinant detectable in the C_H region (e.g., IgG_1, IgG_2, IgG_3, IgG_4).

Superantigen: Molecule that stimulates T-cell subsets by binding to parts of the T cell receptor other than the antigen binding groove.

Suppressor T cells: A class of T lymphocytes able to suppress the immune response to an antigen. There are specific and nonspecific suppressor T cells.

Systemic lupus erythematosis (SLE): An autoimmune disease characterized by the production of autoantibodies to different autoantigens and especially to DNA.

T cell: A class of lymphocytes derived from the thymus and able to respond to thymic dependent antigens and major histocompatibility complex gene products. T cells do not produce antibodies. They mediate cellular reactions, "help" B cells and regulate responses.

T-cell receptor: A heterodimer molecule consisting of α–β or γ–δ chains.

T cell-replacing factor (TRF) A molecule, produced by CD4+ T cells, that induces B-cell differentiation.

T regulatory (Treg) cells: A subpopulation of CD4+CD25+ T cells that inhibit effector CD4+ T cells either by contact-dependant suppression or by the production of immunosuppressive cytokines.

TAP-associate protein: Tapasin, a key molecule in the assembly of MHC class I molecules.

Tapasin: A chaperone protein associated with TAP molecules within the endoplasmic reticulum.

Target cells: Are used to measure the function of effector cells.

Tat: Protein product of the *tat* gene of HIV, binds to a transcriptional enhancer of the long terminal repeat of the provirus, thus increasing transcription.

Template theory: Proposed that lymphocytes use antigen as a mold for the construction of a receptor. Theory discarded when each lymphocyte was found to be inherently antigen specific.

Th1 cells: A subset of CD4 T cells characterized by the cytokine they produce. Often involved in cell-mediated immune responses.

Th2 cells: A subset of CD4 cells characterized by the cytokines they produce. Often involved in stimulating B cells to produce antibody, *see also* HELPER T CELLS.

Thymocyte: A lymphocyte resident in the thymus; generally considered to be maturing functionally, once the cell leaves the thymus it is called a T CELL.

Thymus: A central lymphoid organ, the site of T-cell development.

Thymus-dependent area: Region within peripheral lymphoid tissue containing mostly B cells, which does not atrophy after thymectomy (*e.g.*, the follicle of lymph nodes and spleen found in the superficial cortex).

Titer: A term used to connote the relative strength of an antiserum. An antiserum is progressively diluted until some measurable property of the antiserum (agglutination, facilitation of complement mediated lysis, etc.) is reduced by some predetermined amount. That dilution (e.g., 1:256) is then defined as the titer for that particular antiserum.

Tolerance: Failure of the immune system, as the result of previous contact with antigen, to respond to the same antigen on subsequent occasions, although able to respond to others. Tolerance is best-established by neonatal injection of antigen.

Tolerogen: A substance that preferentially induces tolerance.

Toll-like receptors: A set of PATTERN–RECOGNITION RECEPTORS (PRRs) that recognize a diverse range of viral, bacterial, and fungal components.

Tonsils: Any collection of lymphoid tissue, in particular those lymphoid accumulations surrounding the pharynx (pharyngeal and palatine tonsils).

Toxic shock syndrome: A systemic toxic reaction to *Staphylococcus aureus* resulting in the massive production of cytokines by CD4+ T cells.

Toxin: A poisonous substance that is either the intracellular or the extracellular part of the cell or tissue.

Toxoid: A toxin treated in a manner that inactivates or removes its toxic activity.

Trans: Linked, nonallelic genes located on different members of the homologous chromosome pair (as opposed to *cis*).

Transduction: The transfer of a genetic fragment from one cell to another, especially the transfer of bacterial genes from one bacterium to another by a bacteriophage.

Transfection: Insertion of segments of DNA into cells. A stable transfection results when the DNA fragment integrates into host DNA; if not, it is called a transient transfection.

Transplantation antigen: A histocompatibility antigen.

Transport piece: A polypeptide found in association with secreted IgA, but not with serum IgA; also called SECRETORY COMPONENT.

Transporters associated with antigen processing (TAP-1, TAP-2): ATP-binding cassette proteins involved in the transport of short peptides from the cytosol to the lumen of the endoplasmic reticulum for loading into MHC class I molecules.

Tuberculin test: A clinical test in which purified protein derivative (PPD) is injected subcutaneously to elicit a delayed hypersensitivity reaction, a positive reaction indicates that the individual has been infected by or has been immunized against *Mycobacterium tuberculosis*.

Tuberculosis: An infection caused by *Mycobacterium tuberculosis*.

Tumor necrosis factor – α (TNF-α): A cytokine produced by macrophages and T cells with multiple functions.

Tumor specific transplantation antigens (TSTA or TSA): Antigens found on the membranes of tumor cells, but not on normal cells from the same or identical individuals, against which immunological reactions are directed.

Uticaria: Or hives, red welts usually caused by an allergic reaction.

Vaccination: Inoculation of a nonvirulent or inactivated virus or bacterium as a means of inducing specific immunity. The term derives from *vaccinia* or the cowpox virus, used by Edward Jenner to induce a specific immunity to smallpox.

Vaccinia: Or cowpox virus, causes limited infection in humans, but leads to immunity to smallpox virus.

Valence: Term applied to antibody molecules indicates the number of epitopes to which an antibody molecule can bind. Serum IgG, IgE, IgD, and IgA have a valency of two, secretory IgA has a valency of four, and serum IgM has a valence of 10.

Variable region: That portion of an immunoglobulin molecule, T-cell receptor, etc.

that conveys antigen specificity to the molecule. By its very name, the amino acid sequence of one molecule varies as compared to another molecule of differing specificity.

Vasoconstriction: Narrowing of the blood vessels, often caused by the contraction of smooth muscle fibers.

Vasodilation: Temporary enlargement of the lumen of the blood vessel.

Vasculitis: Dilation of a lymphatic or blood vessel.

V_H region: The variable amino acid sequence region of the heavy chain.

V_L region: The variable amino acid sequence region of the light chain.

Wheal: An acute swelling of a circumscribed area of the skin as the result of edema of the skin.

Wheal-and-flare reaction: Raised area of the skin, the result of an allergic reaction to dermally injected allergen.

White blood cell: A LEUKOCYTE.

White pulp: The leukocyte-rich area of the spleen.

Wild type: The allelic form of a gene most frequently found in nature, which is arbitrarily designated as "normal."

Wiskott-Aldrich syndrome: Sex-linked genetic disease with combined losses of B and T lymphocytes, especially affecting IgM production.

Xeno-: *Prefix*, between species.

Xenogeneic: Originating from a different species, *see* ISOGENEIC and ALLOGENEIC.

Xenograft: Exchange of tissue between members of different species.

Zymosan: A preparation of yeast cell walls that activates the alternative pathway of complement.

Index